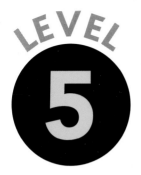

LEVEL
5

DIPLOMA IN LEADERSHIP FOR HEALTH & SOCIAL CARE

SECOND EDITION

Tina Tilmouth
Jan Quallington

HODDER
EDUCATION
AN HACHETTE UK COMPANY

Although every effort has been made to ensure that website addresses are correct at time of going to press, Hodder Education cannot be held responsible for the content of any website mentioned in this book. It is sometimes possible to find a relocated web page by yping in the address of the home page for a website in the URL window of your browser.

Hachette UK's policy is to use papers that are natural, renewable and recyclable products and made from wood grown in sustainable forests. The logging and manufacturing processes are expected to conform to the environmental regulations of the country of origin.

Orders: please contact Bookpoint Ltd, 130 Milton Park, Abingdon, Oxon OX14 4SB. Telephone: (44) 01235 827720. Fax: (44) 01235 400454. Email education@bookpoint.co.uk Lines are open from 9 a.m. to 5 p.m., Monday to Saturday, with a 24-hour message answering service. You can also order through our website: www. hoddereducation.co.uk

ISBN: 978 14718 6792 7

© Tina Tilmouth and Jan Quallington 2016

First published in 2016 by

Hodder Education
An Hachette UK Company
Carmelite House
50 Victoria Embankment
London EC4Y 0DZ

www.hoddereducation.co.uk

Impression number 10 9 8 7 6 5 4 3 2 1

Year 2020 2019 2018 2017 2016

Cover photo © FotografiaBasica/istockphoto.com

Illustrations by Integra

Typeset by Integra Software Services Pvt. Ltd., Pondicherry, India

Printed in Slovenia

A catalogue record for this title is available from the British Library.

Contents

Acknowledgements

Every effort has been made to acknowledge ownership of copyright. The publishers will be glad to acknowledge any copyright holders whom it has not been possible to contact.

The HSE text on pages 74, 75, 82, 85-86, 242 (adapted case study), contains public sector information published by the Health and Safety Executive and licensed under the Open Government Licence.

Photo credits: **p.1** © Alexander Raths – Fotolia; **p.12** *t* © Stratol – iStock via Thinkstock/Getty Images; **p.12** *b* © CandyBox Images – Fotolia; **p.28** © Lisa F. Young/Fotolia; **p.50** © Katarzyna Biasiewicz – 123R; **p.73** © David Fernandez – 123RF; **p.81** © David J. Green/Alamy Stock Photo; **p.83** © nirat makjantuk – 123RF; **p.87** © belchonock – 123RF; **p.93** © Hero Images Inc./Alamy Stock Photo; **p.116** © CaiaImage – Getty Images; **p.134** © Agencja Fotograficzna Caro/Alamy Stock Photo; **p.135** © JPC-PROD – Fotolia; **p.158** © ginasanders – 123RF; **p.168** © kzenon – 123RF; **p.178** © Kacso Sandor – 123RF; **p.187** © ponsulak kunsub – 123RF; **p.190** © Barry Diomede/Alamy Stock Photo; **p.198** © Juice Images/Alamy Stock Photo; **p.200** © Alamy Stock Photo; **p.203** *t* © SFM Archivio Storico/Alamy Stock Photo; **p.203** *b* © gwimages – Fotolia; **p.204** © Alexander Raths – 123RF; **p.217** © Jules Selmes; **p.228** © Alexander Raths – 123RF; **p.229** BSIP SA/Alamy Stock Photo; **p.230** © Stockbyte via Thinkstock/Getty Images BSIP SA; **p.234** © monkeybusinessimages – iStock via Thinkstock/Getty Images; **p.245** © Alexander Raths – 123RF; **p.257** © katiemartynova – 123RF; **p.267** © Monkey Business – Fotolia; **p.270** © Rafał Olechowski – 123RF; **p.284** © Monkey Business – Fotolia; **p.292** © Ocskay Bence – Fotolia; **p.301** © goodluz – Fotolia; **p.312** © Adam Gregor – Fotolia.

The photos on **p.100**, **p.108**, **p.217** and **p.279** are taken by Jules Selmes.

How to use this book

This book will provide you with the knowledge and information required to complete your Level 5 Diploma in Leadership for Health and Social Care and covers all 14 mandatory units of the Adults' Social Care pathways as well as three popular optional units.

Key features of the book

LO2 Be able to support a positive culture within the team

Understand all the requirements of the qualification with clearly stated learning outcomes and assessment criteria fully matched to the specification.

AC 2.1 Identify the components of a positive culture within own team

Learning outcomes

By the end of this unit you will:

1 Be able to address the range of communication requirements in own role.

Prepare for what you are going to cover in the unit.

Key term

Team culture is the behaviour, values, thoughts and norms of an organisation – the unspoken rules.

Understand important terms.

Reflect on it

3.4 Effects of change

Write a reflective account of a recent change you made, looking specifically at the response

Learn to reflect on your own skills, experiences, and see how concepts are applied in settings.

Reflective exemplar

You may wish to use this to write your own reflective account and use it as an example of how to evidence this assessment criterion.

Explore examples of reflective accounts tailored to the content of the unit and understand how you can write your own accounts.

In practice

2.1 Induction into a team

a Conduct some primary research. Interview a new member of staff and find out how they

Test your understanding of the assessment criteria, apply your knowledge in the work setting and generate evidence.

Case study

1.3, 1.4 Barriers

A member of staff has recently undergone a traumatic separation from her husband. She has

See how concepts are applied in settings with real life scenarios.

Research it

1.1 Assessment tools

Research a couple of the assessment tools discussed and identify their use in your

Enhance your understanding of topics with research-led activities encouraging you to explore an area in more detail.

Legislation

● The Health and Social Care Act 2012 brings together the White Papers which led to its

Legislation sections summarise the legislation relevant to the study of the unit.

LO	Assessment criteria and accompanying activities	Assessment methods *To evidence these assessment criteria you could:*
LO1	1.1 1.2 Reflect on it (p. 108)	Write a journal piece to use as part of the evidence you require for assessment criteria. You may wish to use Tuckman's Stages of Development.

Assessment methods tables compile all of the activities covered in the unit and summarise suggestions for how you can use the activities to provide evidence for the assessment criteria. These are suggestions and your tutor will be able to offer more guidance on this.

Further reading and useful resources

Alton Barbour, A. and Koneya, M. (1976) *Louder Than Words: Non-verbal communication.* Columbus, Ohio: Merrill.

Includes references to books, websites and other various sources for further reading and research.

Unit SHC 51

Use and develop systems that promote communication

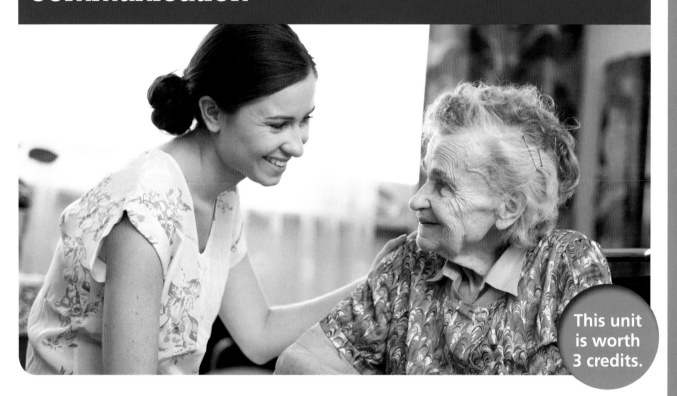

This unit is worth 3 credits.

Effective interpersonal or social skill demands that we know ourselves well, are aware of what we bring to the relationship, and how we might impact on those we communicate with.

The purpose of this unit is to revisit the systems of communication we use in care work and in particular in managing a care setting. In any relationship, be it personal or working, effective interpersonal skills play an essential part and being able to communicate well is one of the most important aspects of your role as a leader and manager. Misunderstanding and misinterpretation of the message can lead to team conflict and disruption to the smooth running of the organisation. It can, moreover, lead to ineffective delivery of services and unproductive teamwork. Being an effective communicator then, holds the key to successful working.

We'll explore the range of communication, challenges and barriers to communication and the importance of effective management of information will be addressed, as will types of communication and the means of working in partnership with others.

Learning outcomes

By the end of this unit you will:

1 Be able to address the range of communication requirements in own role.
2 Be able to improve communication systems and practices that support positive outcomes for individuals.
3 Be able to improve communication systems to support partnership working.
4 Be able to use systems for effective information management.

LO1 Be able to address the range of communication requirements in own role

AC 1.1 Review the range of groups and individuals whose communication needs must be addressed in own job role

Defining communication

To be skilled in communication requires us to be able to use a variety of interpersonal techniques. As a manager your particular skills lie in listening actively to staff and others you meet in your work in order to make decisions and to negotiate issues that may arise. Your role requires that you deliver information and also provide feedback. You will use several methods to do this, including attendance at meetings, training staff, assessing service users and writing reports. See ACs 1.3 and 1.5 for information on different types of communication.

Crawford *et al.* (2006) suggest that:

'Communication is something we do in our internal world of thoughts and in our external world by speaking, writing, gestures, drawing, making images and symbols or receiving messages from others.'

So effective communication is the means by which we deliver and receive a message and both need to be congruent in order for the communication to work.

Communication is the basis of interaction, so skills in speaking, writing and, in particular, listening are essential in health and social care. As a manager, you will be interacting and communicating with a range of people within health and social care settings, including service users (who may be vulnerable) and their families as well as staff, visitors and other professionals. You may sometimes communicate with people who are going through personal crisis or are feeling upset, for example, and this therefore requires skill in making sure they feel supported and valued.

The effectiveness of your communication skills as a manager and leader within the care setting will undoubtedly lead to the success of the organisation and the team with which you work.

Groups and individuals

Who will you be communicating with in your setting? Look at the 'Reflect on it' activity and figure 1.1 on page 3 and think about the groups and individuals you communicate with in your setting.

Addressing communication needs

You may have more than the ones shown in Figure 1.1, but the point is that with such a diverse group of people interacting with you each day, there is a need for the use of a variety of communication skills, all highly dependent on the position of the person and the context in which the communication takes place. Recognising this is paramount since many barriers to communication arise as a result of inappropriate language and terminology being used, which effectively means the message is lost. For example, the delivery of factual information can be quite impersonal and may be totally inappropriate when dealing with a vulnerable child or adult who requires an empathetic response to a problem. However, a member of the medical staff may require just such a response. Therefore, in order for the message to be received and understood you must match appropriate communication with the individual to whom you are speaking and the circumstances in which the interaction takes place.

Research in this area has been well documented. Davis and Fallowfield (1991) reported on the general failure of communication and lack of empathy, and Graham (1991) described breakdown in respectful relationships leading to poor communication. Hewison, in 1995, highlighted the power relationships and barriers to communications. It would also be useful to research further and explore more recent texts dealing with communication and interpersonal skills by Burnard (1996) and Donnelly and Neville (2008), or the TED talks available on the internet. TED talks are usually 20-minute instructive talks from leaders in their field and cover communication, among other topics.

AC 1.2 Explain how to support effective communication within own job role

What is 'effective communication'?
Three-skill management approach
Robert Katz's skills approach to management and leadership has had a far-reaching effect in

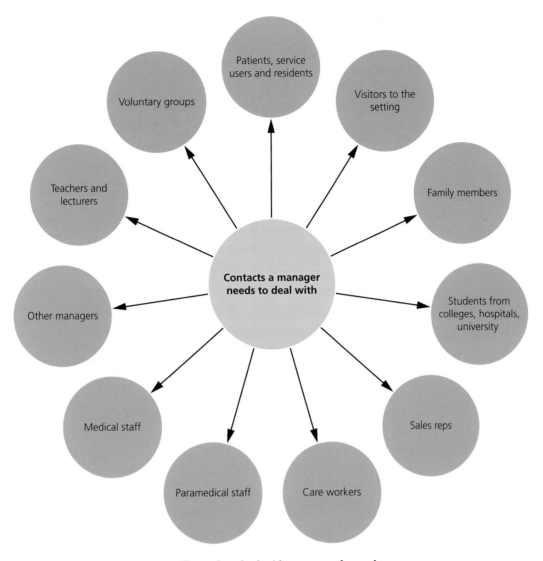

Figure 1.1 As a manager, you will need to deal with a range of people

Reflect on it

1.1 Contacts

Think about and make a list of all the relationships and contacts you may have within the course of your managerial role.

You may come up with the contacts shown in Figure 1.1.

shaping our thinking about what constitutes the skills required by a good and effective leader. Katz (1955) suggested in his Three-Skill Approach that three basic personal skills – technical, human and conceptual – were competencies that all leaders and managers could acquire, quite separately from the traits or qualities that many researchers had focused on. These three skills were not innate, as some leadership skills are often thought to be, but were achievable through learning.

In Katz's model, human skills refer to how we work with people effectively, creating an atmosphere of trust and cooperation, and being sensitive to the needs of others, involving them in the planning and decision making of the organisation where possible. The way in which we interact with each other in this respect will go a long way to achieving this. When we look at the skills identified for leaders and managers we are made aware of the importance of communication.

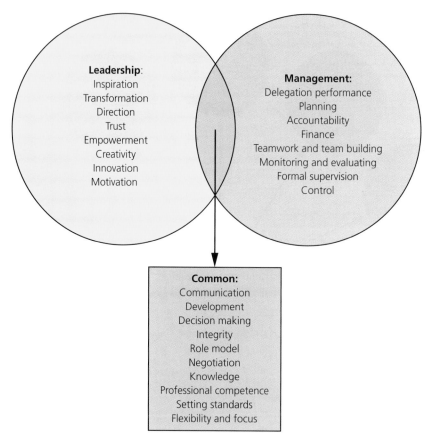

Leadership:
Inspiration
Transformation
Direction
Trust
Empowerment
Creativity
Innovation
Motivation

Management:
Delegation performance
Planning
Accountability
Finance
Teamwork and team building
Monitoring and evaluating
Formal supervision
Control

Common:
Communication
Development
Decision making
Integrity
Role model
Negotiation
Knowledge
Professional competence
Setting standards
Flexibility and focus

Figure 1.2 The importance of communication

Skills for Care (2006) published the diagram shown in Figure 1.2 to emphasise this.

Of all the skills involved in leading and managing, communication crosses both divides. Being effective is crucial. When we communicate effectively, we invariably use a variety of skills, but more importantly, it is how we develop our relationships with others in the setting that is paramount to getting the message across and being effective.

In management roles we communicate with people who may be in a subordinate position to ourselves, those in more senior roles, peers and others such as visitors or other service providers, and they may have different communication needs. The direction of the communication will have a bearing on how you address these groups. For example, have a look at Figure 1.3.

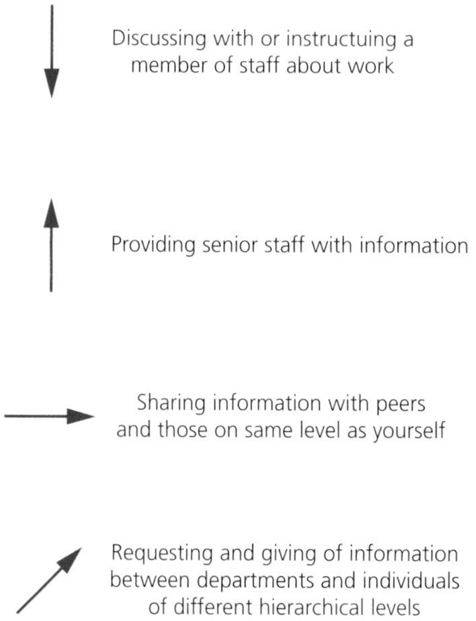

Discussing with or instructuing a member of staff about work

Providing senior staff with information

Sharing information with peers and those on same level as yourself

Requesting and giving of information between departments and individuals of different hierarchical levels

Figure 1.3 Direction of communication

Source: Gopee and Galloway, 2009, p. 20

4

Communicating as a manager

There are a number of reasons for communicating as a manager and leader, including:

- delegation of work
- conducting meetings
- presentations
- supervision and appraisal
- report writing
- building the team
- negotiation
- interviewing.

All of these tasks in themselves are detailed and can be further broken down to reveal more complex levels. An example might be helpful to explain what we mean here.

Let's look at supervision. Before undertaking such roles we need to be aware of what they entail. Our list might look like this:

- function of supervision
- who requires it?
- mechanics of how it is carried out
- record-keeping policies
- conduct of the interview
- evaluating the process.

Meeting communication needs

Whatever the communication need or type, a good working relationship is essential, and one which demands that there is trust and the ability to be able to talk openly and honestly. The other person may need to feed back to you, report complaints of abuse, for example, and as a manager you should ensure you equip them with the skills to do so. In all communication that occurs in the course of your daily work you will undertake a variety of roles and will therefore need to adjust your communication to each circumstance. It is thus important to know what role you are fulfilling in any interaction in health and social care settings. As mentioned above, the different people to which you will have access will require different types of communication and throughout a span of duty you may find yourself advising, instructing, welcoming, assessing, observing, informing, counselling.

Effective communicators make appropriate choices when it comes to deciding how they intend to interact and when they are clear about the purpose of the interaction.

In practice

1.1, 1.2 A 'communication diary'

Keep a communication diary for one span of duty. Use the questions below to show how you have undertaken the different types of communicating:

- advising
- instructing
- welcoming
- assessing
- observing
- informing
- counselling.

1 Who were the groups or individuals whose communication needs were addressed in the diary?
2 In what context did the communication take place?
3 What purpose did it have?
4 How successful was it?
5 How did you ensure the communication was effective? What did you do?

How can you support effective communication?

By now you will have realised that effective communicators are those people who adapt their communication style to the situation and respond in sensitive and empathetic ways to the needs of those to whom they are communicating. In supporting others to become effective communicators, it is necessary for you as a leader to be an effective role model and, where you are able to, reflect effectively on how you are communicating your messages.

Effective communicators are just as much aware of the skills and types of communication as they are of the need to affirm the self-worth of the person with whom they are interacting. What do we mean by this?

Be empathetic

Key term

Empathy is being able to understand and share the feelings of another or having the ability to experience another person's condition from their perspective.

Rogers (1980) referred to the term '**empathy**', which is the ability to 'put yourself in the shoes of others' or to understand the client's frame of reference, and active listening skills are the best way to show this. This is different from showing sympathy, which might make a person feel pitied.

Take a non-judgemental approach and listen

If we support all our communication by accepting and valuing the people with whom we interact in the expression of warmth and a non-judgemental attitude, we will improve our communication skills no end.

Have you ever been dealt with in a manner in which you felt judged or where you felt the other person was not listening to you? In this sort of situation it is very difficult to be open and honest about our feelings and needs. If we judge the people with whom we are interacting, whether they are staff or service users, they may feel they are unable to open up to us, which might be detrimental to the organisation's aims and objectives. In other words, your failure to communicate effectively or ingrain this principle in your staff will lead to lack of success.

Help staff to support communication with service users

Therefore, as a manager and leader you can support effective communication by ensuring that your staff are all aware of the need to be flexible in the way in which they communicate within varied contexts and to engage in communication that is empathetic and values the people with whom they interact. It is also useful if staff understand the communication plans which may be developed in partnership with speech and language therapists to enable continuity of care. Users will have different communication needs and it is important that staff can address these needs by having a firm understanding of different communication methods such as sign language. They may need to have specialist training in these.

AC 1.3 Analyse the barriers and challenges to communication within own job role

Having looked at what makes for effective communication we can identify areas where barriers hinder communication. Sometimes when we feel

Reflect on it

1.3 Barriers to communication

List two reasons (one internal and one external factor) that may have been the reasons for the blocks or barriers in communication. For example, an external barrier may be a poor environment for the communication which lacks privacy, leading to an internal barrier in that you are unsafe talking about a matter.

that we are not communicating well we need to reflect on the reasons for the problem. A common complaint in large organisations is one of poor communication which often leads to conflict. It can be a major issue in whether or not the job gets done.

You may have come up with some of the following:

- Difference in culture, values and language.
- Dealing with different viewpoints and values/ negative feelings about the person you are speaking to or getting upset about what they are saying, leading to conflict.
- Body language and non-verbal communication (NVC), as well as general personality issues where some people will be more confident communicators than others.
- Conflict and resistance to change causing upset.
- Personal issues which may make it difficult to concentrate and communicate effectively.
- Power dynamics, i.e. where some people are perceived to be in higher/lower levels of powers, affecting their ability to communicate/ or how they are expected to communicate.
- Self-esteem may affect confidence and thus someone's ability to communicate.
- Tiredness, personal issues or other health issues or disabilities, including sensory loss. Health issues may include people who suffer from depression and anxiety, for example, which may affect their ability to communicate.
- Environmental issues, including noise and/or poor lighting.
- Feeling unsafe, due to the person's demeanour or behaviour.
- Not listening effectively.

Differences in culture, values and language

We talk at length about 'fostering equality and diversity' and the importance of respecting the differences we may come across in people. We are not talking only about cultural differences or language differences where people may come to us with English as a second language but also about the differences in values that people hold. This can have a huge impact on our ability to communicate, not only because words can have different meanings across different **cultures** but also our understanding of other cultures can impact on this.

Living in a multi-cultural society it is important to be culturally aware in our interpersonal interactions. Miller (2006) says that defining the term culture is complex. When we talk about race, we often confuse the term with ethnicity and culture. Ethnicity, gender and social class, while all being relevant, should additionally include religious beliefs, sexuality, rationality, skin colour and experience of oppression (Miller, 2006). Miller suggests that by developing a respectful curiosity about the beliefs and practices within all service users' lives, we are able to communicate in more meaningful ways.

Dealing with different viewpoints/negative feelings about the person you are speaking to or getting upset about what they are saying

We occasionally meet with people who, for whatever reason, we just don't 'click' or get on with.

In settings where there is a diverse group of people, we come into contact with all types of characters, all of whom have their own feelings, values and attitudes. Sometimes these may clash with how we see the world. We may not share their views or particularly like the stance the person takes, but as the manager and leader in a setting we have to show tolerance of these views (providing they are not contravening any anti-discrimination policy) and, in this instance, we need to be fully aware of how we come across to those we are communicating with. It is possible that we may communicate our dislike of somebody through our body language or the way we speak to them; this will have a negative effect on the interaction and may lead to conflict in the workplace.

Body language and non-verbal communication (NVC)

One of the things that we often do not pay enough attention to is our body language.

Argyle (1978) pointed out that non-verbal communication can have as much as five times the impact on a person's understanding compared with the words spoken, so if we are displaying negative non-verbal signals this can prove problematic. Communication can be broken down as follows:

● 7 per cent is what you say in words.
● 38 per cent is contributed to how you say it (volume, pitch, tone, rhythm, etc.).
● 55 per cent reflects your body language (facial expressions, gestures, posture, etc.).

It is also useful to remember that service users in a health and social care setting may have communication difficulties and may not pick up the non-verbal cues communicated (Crawford *et al.*, 2006).

The way in which we present ourselves can have as much if not more impact on whether our message is listened to and understood.

When communicating:

> *'Our attention is focused on words rather than body language. But our judgement includes both. An audience is simultaneously processing both verbal and non-verbal cues. Body movements are not usually positive or negative in and of themselves; rather, the situation and the message will determine the appraisal.'*

(Givens, 2000, p. 4)

It is vital to ensure that our behaviour and bodily actions match our speech. Awareness of the way in which we conduct our non-verbal communication is just as important as what we say in some cases.

Conflict and resistance to change causing upset

When we come across a situation that is causing some **conflict**, this again may cause us to have negative feelings about a person, which in turn may become a barrier to communication.

Key terms

Culture is the customs, attitudes and beliefs that distinguish one group of people from another.

Conflict is a disagreement or argument.

Case study

1.3 Jim

Jim is the union representative for Unison and is trying to encourage the union members into action over the spending cuts in the setting which have been enforced by the recent recession and the potential redundancy situation that has arisen. There have been government cutbacks on staffing and this has meant that you, as a manager, have had to look closely at the workforce and make decisions that are not palatable with respect to reducing the number of staff. Five people are now at risk of losing their jobs.

Jim has sent an email to all Unison members and is seeking the following commitment from union members:

- one-day strike action and protest outside the workplace.
- non-cooperation at meetings, with all the Unison members turning their chairs to face the back of the room, staging a protest while being present.

Think about the following:

1 Comment *honestly* on how this makes you feel about Jim and his potentially disruptive influence.
2 What is your initial response to the actions as a manager?
3 Now reflect on the above and say why you reacted this way and how you will respond to the situation.

It is possible that your thoughts about Jim in the case study are negative and it would be difficult to have any sort of dialogue with him that could be positive at the present time. Perhaps you feel his actions are unjust and unfair; the cuts are not your fault, after all, but a result of a government drive to reduce costs in the NHS. You may even take this stance personally.

Your reactions are perfectly reasonable in such a situation, but as a manager you have to now detach yourself from the subjective emotions of the situation, i.e. your personal feelings about Jim, and deal in a more objective way with the task at hand, that of reducing the impact of these actions and raising staff morale. A tall order!

Conflict is often viewed as a negative issue and becomes a problem when it affects our work, causes inappropriate behaviour and lowers morale, impacting on the workforce and the service users.

John Adair, in his book *Effective Teambuilding* (2000), came up with the following five strategies for dealing with conflict:

1 **Competing** – forcing your own ideas through because you believe your way is right.
2 **Confronting/collaborating** – by bringing all the issues into the open and exploring all feasible options you are showing an openness to change.
3 **Compromise** – negotiating halfway.

4 **Avoid** – opt out altogether and avoid taking up any position.
5 **Accommodate** – allowing the change to happen in order to not hurt feelings.

In the incident regarding Jim, the conflict is about the budget cuts impacting on your workforce. It is unavoidable and therefore you are unable to change it. But the way in which you approach the inevitable redundancies and unrest will go a long way to securing a happier outcome in the long run. The strategy that appears to be the most useful will be that of collaboration and confronting the issue and employing the views of all the workforce in exploring all the options.

What is happening here is a huge change to the way in which the people in this organisation are operating and any change is a difficult area to deal with.

The people in the organisation face a loss in a small way. If you are faced with the same or similar situation, your understanding of their emotions will help you in dealing with how to address the changes in an effective way. See Unit LM1c on leading and managing a team for more information.

With effective communication that encourages the person/team within the institution to accept and understand the reason for the change, you can move to a new way of working that is embraced by everyone (Cole, 2011).

Reflect on it

1.3 Listening

Think of a time when you know that you were not being listened to and heard.

- What was going on at that time?
- How did it affect the interaction?
- What do you think was going on for the person you were trying to communicate with at that time?

Key term

Active listening is listening clearly and ensuring that you understand what the sender intends to communicate and the content of the message.

Not listening effectively

If we are to understand our staff and service users and be able to communicate, we need to listen to what they are saying, a very difficult skill to do well.

Active listening shows that our staff and service users have been heard and the way in which we do this is with the following skills:

- acknowledging and reflecting feelings
- body language
- restating
- paraphrasing
- summarising
- questioning.

Acknowledging and reflecting feelings

When we undertake this activity, all we are doing is repeating back to the person a word, phrase or sentence that they have spoken. They become aware that we are paying attention to what they are saying and are inviting them to continue with the conversation.

Body language

We mentioned the importance of this briefly above and we now turn to the work of Egan, who gave us the acronym **SOLER** in order to help us remember how to create a good relationship with reference to our non-verbal communication (see Table 1.1).

Restating

This means:

- Repeating back to the person words or short phrases that they have used shows that they have been heard and understood.
- It encourages the person to continue with the conversation and explore what they are saying more deeply.

Paraphrasing

In order to show a person that you understand their concerns from their point of view:

- Rephrase what you understood to be the core message of their communication.
- Check your understanding of what the person has said.

Table 1.1 Explanation of Egan's 'SOLER' model

Source: Tilmouth *et al.*, 2011

S	Sit squarely	Sit slightly opposite the other person so that you are either side of an imaginary corner. This allows you to see all aspects of non-verbal communication, which you might not see if you were sitting side by side, and is less threatening than sitting face on.
O	Open position	Sit with uncrossed arms and legs; this conveys to the client that you are open and not defensive.
L	Lean slightly towards the client	Leaning slightly towards the client shows that you are interested and want to understand their problem.
E	Eye contact	It is important to get the balance right. The client will feel uncomfortable if you stare and will think that you are not interested if you do not look at them at all.
R	Relax	If you are relaxed, you can concentrate on listening rather than worrying about how to respond to the service users.

- By using such phrases as 'It sounds like...' or 'It seems that...' or 'I'm wondering if you mean' and 'I have got it right that…', you are testing your accuracy and perception of what is being said.

Summarising

This means:

- to gather together the person's statements to identify their thoughts and feelings – this helps us to get a grasp on the main problem
- clarifying content and feelings
- reviewing what has been said and bringing the communication to an end.

A summary is simply a longer paraphrase that enables you to bring together the important aspects of what the person is saying.

Questioning

This is an essential skill, but too many questions can make the person feel as though they are being interrogated. You will be aware of the types of questions, but here is a reminder:

- **Open questions** – these are the 'what', 'where', 'how' and 'who' questions. 'Why' might also be included, but it can be a difficult one for somebody to answer and puts pressure on them to justify their position. Think about the last time you were asked why you felt that or did that. Open questions can be useful as they involve the person more and encourage exploration and thoughtfulness.
- **Closed questions** – these non-exploratory-type questions elicit only 'yes' or 'no' answers and may shut down the communication.

The way in which we ask the question is also important. We can be:

- direct
- concise – i.e. specific and brief
- clear – saying precisely what we mean.

Silence

- There are different kinds of silences: thoughtful silences, which give us space to process our thoughts, or angry, tense silences, which can sometimes be uncomfortable and difficult to bear.
- Be aware of what kind of silence it is.

- Allow the person space to process their thoughts before stepping in to help by breaking the silence.
- By being aware of eye contact or body language, we can ascertain if the silence is uncomfortable.

Listening is an art, and active listening leaves people feeling appreciated and heard.

Personal issues making it difficult to manage or lead

In all management and leadership situations you will be dealing with your own issues, as well as those of others, and sometimes this can affect the way in which you are perceived, understood or viewed. You may well have come across situations that touch you because they reflect a problem you may have yourself. Or you may simply be dealing with a person you find particularly difficult, perhaps even aggressive. As a manager, you have a responsibility to ensure that your communication is positive where it can be and this requires a certain amount of self-awareness. Being aware of who you are will have an impact on others. This means you need to attend to your personal growth and development.

Emotional intelligence

Daniel Goleman (1995) stated that emotional intelligence is:

> *'the capacity for recognising our own feelings and those of others for motivating ourselves, for managing emotions well in ourselves as well as others.'*

(Goleman, 1995, p. 137)

For Goleman, self-awareness is about knowing our own emotions and recognising those feelings as they happen. So, we may feel angry at something somebody has said, but as a manager and leader, showing that anger inappropriately will have a negative effect on relationships.

Social awareness refers to the empathy and concern we have for others' feelings; the acknowledgement that people under threat in an organisation may show aggression and anger. Decisions affecting people's jobs may have to be made, and the manager who sees only the task in hand is failing to acknowledge the effect this is having on those at risk and

Case study

1.3, 1.4 Barriers

A member of staff has recently undergone a traumatic separation from her husband. She has three small children and is struggling to make ends meet. She finds it difficult to get to work on time and has been late a number of times recently. You know she does not have family to help her get the children to school.

When you ask to see her to try to resolve some of her issues, she is aggressive and quite rude. This may make you feel angry, particularly when you are trying to come up with a solution. However, fighting anger with anger does not work and you need to consider how you might approach this problem in a different manner.

How might you deal with this situation?

Perhaps you will have empathised with the staff member's plight and asked her how she might see a way forward. It is likely, she has been unable to take time out to note the decline in her work or her lateness. You might suggest a change in hours to help her to get to work on time, or a reduction in her hours of work until she can settle her children into a more favourable routine. Perhaps she might work the same number of hours but at times when the children are at school.

The way you deal with the situation will have an effect on the whole workforce.

---

those who have to continue to work in such a climate of change.

Relationship management is the ability to handle relationships competently in order to best deal with conflict, and to develop collaboration in the workforce.

Finally, Goleman refers to motivation, particularly of ourselves, to enable the workforce to meet goals.

In a management situation our awareness of the impact of our actions and responses can go a long way towards defusing situations that might be potentially threatening. We may not be feeling very happy or friendly ourselves, but being in a position of authority demands that we have some awareness of the feelings of others. A good manager is one who has a level of emotional intelligence.

Inappropriate environment

Another area where communication is apt to break down is being in an inappropriate environment. You will be aware of the need for privacy when carrying out sensitive types of communication, breaking bad news or reprimanding someone. But have you thought about the impact your own setting will have on others?

The initial impact of a room or building can have a huge effect on how people feel when they enter the building and can influence the success of an interaction.

Reflect on it

1.3, 1.4 Overcoming barriers

'I remember attending an informal interview where I was asked to sit in an easy chair. The interviewer sat in an upright chair next to me and towered over me. The effect this had on me, as I sank down into the soft cushions, was of being vulnerable. I am sure the interviewer had not intended for me to feel that way but it certainly changed the way in which I responded to his questions.'

Have a look around the room in which you are sitting. How does it make you feel? Think about it for a moment. Is it welcoming, untidy, too busy, crammed, too large, are the chairs too far apart?

It is as well to take a good look at where and when you conduct important communications with staff. Noisy environments may mean your message is not heard, impacting on the outcomes you may have expected.

Have you thought about where you conduct your staff meetings? Again, even the position of the chairs can affect the interactions. For example, look at the two photographs of different types of classroom set-ups in Figure 1.4.

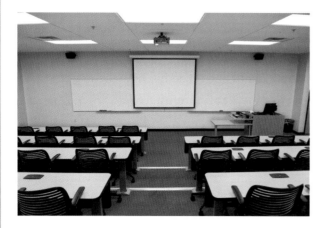

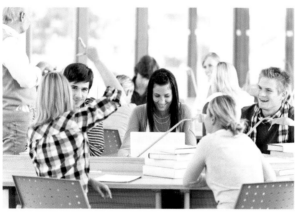

Figure 1.4 Different types of classroom set-ups

Which classroom set-up do you prefer? Does the set-up in the first image bring up memories of school? Perhaps those memories are less than happy? The way that our environment communicates with us is extremely important.

In practice

1.3 Analysing barriers and challenges to communication

Analyse the communication barriers present in your working environment and write a short piece to show your understanding of the effects these have.

AC 1.4 Implement a strategy to overcome communication barriers

Dealing with communication barriers

Much of the last section highlighted the types of communication barriers and these fall into two groups, internal and external.

Overcoming external barriers

External barriers refer to environmental and cultural barriers and these can be dealt with by making changes to the actual fabric of the environment and improving the general layout of the place in which communication is to occur. As a manager, you should critically examine the environment where you and staff engage with visitors and other staff, when you communicate bad news for example, or where supervision and team meetings are held. If you feel uncomfortable and unsettled in this setting, then the chances are that your staff and visitors will too.

With respect to cultural barriers, we are aware that this is about recognising that everybody is different and you may have identified in your own settings areas where there is a shortfall in this aspect. For example, you may have noticed that some of the care workers fail to respond to some of the service users in appropriate ways simply because they lack an understanding of the condition or culture of the client. For example, a deaf client may be excluded from certain social activities or a client who wishes to practise his religion is not given the opportunity.

In ensuring that your staff respond to the differences of their service users, you need to ensure they are aware of the responsibilities they have to *all* individuals in the setting. Have you checked your anti-discrimination policy? You may need to revise and update the policy to ensure that all staff are aware of how they can implement it in their practice and how they address the issues of cultural sensitivity and diversity.

There may be a need for more training to raise awareness of cultural and religious differences in your workforce. The key here is to determine how well your own setting delivers 'holistic and person-centred care' or care that is user focused, promoting independence. Only you can say what you need to do in your own workplace.

Overcoming internal barriers

The internal factors pertaining to communication barriers require you to be aware of your own emotions and feelings about how you are dealing with the problems you come across. Our awareness of the way in which we portray ourselves to others can only come about with a true reflection of ourselves, and this can sometimes reveal uncomfortable traits. We sometimes need to move out of our comfort zone and identify areas for our own self-development in terms of how we communicate. Donnelly and Neville (2008) comment that being aware of oneself enables you to review your personal values against the professional standards that you are now expected to work within. According to Geldard and Geldard (2003), through the development of your self-awareness you can resolve past and current issues, and by doing so you can improve on your skills in the role of manager.

In an effort to improve our management and leadership skills, we also need to be aware of the way in which we communicate.

AC 1.5 Use different means of communication to meet different needs

The means of communication you use to meet different needs will include:

- verbal
- non-verbal
- sign
- pictoral
- written
- electronic
- assisted

The information may be:

- personal
- organisational
- formal
- informal
- public (information/promotional)

In the study of communication we might come across the following three terms:

- **Interpersonal communication**, which involves non-verbal, paralinguistic and verbal communication.
- **Environmental communication**, which involves the way in which our environment affects our interactions.
- **Intra-personal communication**, which takes place within ourselves, or 'self-talk'.

Verbal communication

Verbal communication can be complex since the meaning of words changes between cultures and generations. On its own it can be an ineffective form of communication. For example, words such as 'wicked' and 'bad' mean something very different to the youth of today than they may have done to older generations. There are many more examples of how words change. The words we use alter depending on the situation and the people involved and because of this, we can never be sure that a word has the same meaning for two people (Porritt, 1990). This is particularly important when communicating feelings, as the strength of the word may differ between people.

Choice of words

Our choice of words is important and we need to be careful not to use jargon and abbreviations or language that is too complex, that our service users or staff may not understand. Keep in mind the person you are speaking to and tailor your language to them. We need to be aware of cultural differences in language and conscious of the diverse nature of our service users. Similarly, we should avoid the use of euphemisms, which we might refer to as 'double speak', such as saying someone has 'passed away' instead of died. One example is of a student nurse who, for weeks, lacked understanding about the term 'she has gone to Rose Cottage' and thought the patients she had nursed had all been taken to a care home of that name! In fact, they had died. Just another use of a euphemism.

Avoid clichés and alienating language

One of the things that might alienate your staff can be the use of cliché and 'management-type' speak. Terms such as 'thinking outside the box', 'blue-sky thinking', 'scoping' and other such clichés can sound over – used and inauthentic and may also be misunderstood.

Be culturally sensitive and speak clearly

Speaking clearly and ensuring that you are not covering your mouth or turning away from a person when speaking will help those who need to lip read or listen carefully due to hearing problems. It is also important to consider cultural sensitivities around communication.

Paralinguistic communication

When we moderate our speech, for example changing the pitch, volume, rhythm, tone of voice and timing, occasionally lapsing into the odd grunt, 'ums' and 'ahs', we are using paralinguistic communication. The words we use are very important, but the way we say something is of equal importance and can affect how our message is perceived. Yawning, sighing, coughing, tutting, laughing and groaning can also be mentioned here as forms of paralinguistic communication. How do we communicate these aspects of language in written communication though? In such cases we may change the colour or size of the font, or use capital letters and exclamation marks.

Paralinguistic communication can offer us a clue to how a person is feeling and this can help in our dealings with them.

Table 1.2 shows the types of non-verbal communication we use.

Non-verbal communication

Table 1.2 Non-verbal communication

Source: Tilmouth, *et al.*, 2011

Facial expression	Our facial expression communicates emotions unless we train ourselves to mask our feelings. If you say you are angry while smiling, it gives a confusing message.
Eye contact and gaze	The way you look into another person's eyes during conversation is what is known as eye contact. If somebody can hold eye contact through a conversation, it can communicate a level of confidence and willingness to communicate fully. Some of the people you communicate with will have a very low level of eye contact, which might communicate a lack of ease with the conversation or a lack of confidence. It is a good idea to reduce the level of your eye contact to reflect theirs, otherwise it can feel threatening. The appropriateness of maintaining eye contact differs according to culture.
Gestures	Gestures are movements of your arms and hands that accompany speech. Gestures can help communication – for example, pointing in the direction in which a person needs to go can add emphasis to the communication. However, too much gesturing can be distracting.
Body position, posture and movement	The body position of a client can tell you a lot about how they are feeling – if they are hunched over, with arms and legs crossed, they are probably feeling quite anxious. Rogers (2002) recommends that we relax and it is important not to appear too formal and distant. However, if we are too laid back in our posture, we could appear uninterested. Sitting with our arms and legs crossed can appear closed off and defensive. However, in some circumstances, it may be a good idea to mirror the body posture of the person we are with.
Personal space and proximity	Two to three feet in distance between the chairs is about right for me; however, you may notice that some service users push their chairs back as soon as they sit down in the prearranged chairs. This may be because the space does not feel comfortable to them. People seem to have their own invisible boundaries, which change according to who they are interacting with and how comfortable they feel. Porritt (1990) calls it a bubble that surrounds us.
Clothes	The clothes you choose to wear say a lot about you. Dressing too informally or too formally may alienate you from service users.
Therapeutic touch	Touch can be a contentious subject. On the one hand, there is evidence of touch having therapeutic benefits; on the other, it can be misinterpreted and seen as an invasion of a person's personal space. Bonham (2004) suggests it may be appropriate and supportive for staff to touch when service users are distressed as it may validate the degree of their suffering. He suggests that appropriate places to touch in this situation are hands, forearms, upper arms and shoulders.

Sign language, Braille and Makaton

Additionally, sign language, Braille, Makaton, assisted technology and other non-verbal methods of communication are useful aids for those service users who cannot communicate verbally, and as a manager you will need to ensure that staff are equipped to support service users who may need to use such methods.

Assisted communication

Assisted communication refers to use of aids such as picture and symbol communication boards and electronic devices, which help individuals who have difficulty with speech or language problems to express themselves.

Written communication

Written reports, notes, email and other forms of electronic communication are all important, and being able to maintain clear and accurate records is a legal requirement.

As Donnelly and Neville (2008) point out, written communications should be accurate, in detail, up to date, non-judgemental and legible so that others are able to read them. We also need to comply with confidentiality guidelines and as such, all forms of written communication must be kept safely.

As a manager you will undoubtedly favour one form over another, but you do need to be aware of the advantages and disadvantages of written communication.

Electronic communication

Email is a quick and convenient method of communication with the added bonus that people can respond immediately or when it is suitable for them. As a written record of a communication, it can be accessed afterwards for evidence in a way that a telephone communication cannot. We can also add attachments and links to relevant internet sites into the mail, allowing the respondent to go straight to the information. There is no postage to pay and it can save on journey time to and from meetings.

There are disadvantages with emails, however, due to their impersonal nature and the inability to pick up paralinguistic and non-verbal signals. Short and to-the-point emails can sometimes appear rude and there is also the tendency for people to not reply to emails they do not understand, so you could be waiting for an answer for a while.

Confidentiality is another important consideration, with the potential for confidential information going to the wrong person by mistake or accidentally forwarded on by the respondent to someone who would not be included by the first writer.

The importance of good communication

Miscommunication must be avoided and we need to ensure that messages are clear and understood. Good communication is vital as it enables us to make decisions and promote rights, and give choice to service users. This means we promote a person-centred service. Good communication ensures that staff and service users are empowered and can support each other well in their work.

Personal, organisational, formal, informal or public information

The type of communication we use in our personal communication with members of staff and friends will be different to that we might use in an organisational context. For example, our language may be more formal when we speak to service users or other members of the multidisciplinary team and less formal in our everyday lives. When we impart information to members of the public or if we are engaged with promotional work, again the type of language we use would be very different from our usual way of speaking.

In practice

1.5 Using different means of communication

Which different means of communication do you use in the course of a span of duty? Write a short piece to show the types of communication you use and make a comment upon the effectiveness of each. You might address verbal, non-verbal, sign, pictoral, written, electronic and assisted methods. The means of communication may be personal, organisational, formal, informal or public (information/promotional).

LO2 Be able to improve communication systems and practices that support positive outcomes for individuals

AC 2.1 Monitor the effectiveness of communication systems and practices

In monitoring something, we look at whether there are any deficiencies we need to address and whether changes need to be made to address new initiatives (McGrath, 1985).

We can do this in two ways:

1 Search for information to support the current level of function with respect to communication.
2 Analyse and interpret that information to decide on a plan of action.

Our communication systems need to be monitored as to their effectiveness. The policy on record keeping, for example may state how staff should record complaints but this needs to be monitored as to how the process is being used and whether in fact it is efficient and maintains confidentiality. You may have a system of checks in place to determine how well staff are managing to record the complaints in line with the policy.

In determining the effectiveness of a system or practice it is essential to monitor its use and review it regularly.

In practice

2.1 Monitoring effectiveness of communication systems and practices

Design a questionnaire to obtain feedback from the following groups of people about your communication systems in place at this time:

● service users
● staff
● visitors
● other professionals you deal with.

You may have collected information from personal files and care plans, minutes of meetings, diaries, staff communication systems and emails.

You may also have gained the views of staff and visitors on how the systems work.

AC 2.2 Evaluate the effectiveness of existing communication systems and practices

Having collected the information, you now need to analyse and evaluate it. To do this you should examine all the data you have and then determine the positive and the negative aspects of what you have.

One way this can be carried out is on an informal basis where you obtain casual feedback from individuals as to how well your systems work. However, it is far better to collect information that may be used in auditing your service and can provide evidence to external bodies of your continual progress and quality assurance in the organisation.

There are a number of useful ways in which you can formally ask for feedback. For example, you may use service-user forums (groups of service users who meet to discuss the quality of the service) and meetings when the quality of these services can be discussed and minuted. This provides valuable information as to how the service users feel about the organisation. Other ways may be through a complaint and compliment system, questionnaires, appraisal and focus groups.

The care you give and the way you deliver the care has a significant impact, not only on the users of the service but also on staff morale, and as such, any feedback is essential in measuring the quality of the care you provide.

In practice

2.2 Evaluating effectiveness of existing communication systems and practices

Choose one of the systems in place (maybe you could look at the complaints procedure, for example) and compile a report evaluating the quality of the organisation's performance of the particular communication system.

How do you evaluate the effectiveness, quality and performance of communication systems in your setting? What standards do you use?

AC 2.3 Propose improvements to communication systems and practices to address any shortcomings

Improving communication problems can be done through staff and service-user meetings and reports. For example, a member of staff may suggest a change to current practice and it is important that the idea is considered and discussed at a team meeting. The change may be useful but may require some further refinement before full implementation.

AC 2.4 Lead the implementation of revised communication systems and practices

Any proposed change will require you as the manager to ensure that all staff are aware of what needs to be done and that a plan of action is in place. Any revised working practice must be discussed and fully understood by staff and others involved in the setting. New responsibilities may arise that may require training and time. By communicating all the information to staff and having guidelines in place, the changes can be presented in a clear and efficient way to ensure success.

Reflect on it

2.4 Revised communication systems and practice

Reflect on the way in which you led the implementation of a revised practice of your communication systems in your setting.

Research it

2.1, 2.2, 2.3, 2.4 Improving communication systems

Serious case reviews often comment upon poor communication as requiring attention to improve care. Under take a small scale study monitor the communication practice within your own setting and comment upon and evaluate how effective it is. Identify any improvements to the practices and make recommendations for revised systems.

In practice

2.3, 2.4 Proposing improvements and leading the implementation

Using the information from the questionnaire in AC 2.1, complete the following and compile a report for evidence of:

1 Which aspects of the communication system in your organisation need to be changed?
2 How did you come to this decision and what methods did you use to collect the information?
3 How did you determine which practices should stay, and why?
4 Who was involved in the decision?
5 What will you do to change the systems and lead the implementation?

LO3 Be able to improve communication systems to support partnership working

AC 3.1 Use communication systems to promote partnership working

Partnership working is an important means of making improvements in health care for people and this depends on effective partnerships between the different professions and organisations involved in commissioning and delivering services and interventions. It requires shared communication systems, including shared databases, records and files to ensure that consistency in care is maintained and decision-making processes are clear. In 2014, the Care Act brought about national changes to care and support in England.

The Care Act 2014 simplified and improved the existing legislation in care and the changes mean that more people are now able to access the care and support, from local councils or other organisations in the community. They also have more choice

Key term

Partnership working is the use of inclusive and mutually beneficial relationships in care work that improve the quality and experience of care. This refers to the relationships between individuals with long-term care conditions, their carers, and service providers and care professionals.

about the type of support and care they need. In addition, different ways to pay for care and support are now available. This meant that communication between partners had to be firmly established to ensure that all parties were talking to each other and had the service user at the heart of the care.

This new duty to promote people's well-being will now apply not just to users of services but also to carers. The Children and Families Act 2014, which was introduced at the same time as the Care Act, also applied a duty of care for parent carers of disabled under-18s.

Under this legislation service users receiving care and support from any regulated provider will now be covered by the Human Rights Act and local councils are responsible for helping the service user to access independent financial advice to help them with care funding.

New national changes put the individual requiring care firmly at the centre of that care, allowing them more control, with their carers' needs also being met.

Communication and working collaboratively

All partnership working depends on effective communication and good working relationships. As part of a care team that goes beyond the boundaries of your own organisation, you need to be aware of the need to build team links with external bodies.

Effective health and social care is that which is provided in collaboration and partnership with others, either in the same team or across a range of agencies and disciplines within the care sector.

Reflect on it

3.1 Communication systems

Think about the communication systems discussed and reflect on how they might be misused or fail.

Research it

3.1 The Care Act 2014

Go to www.skillsforcare.org.uk/Document-library/ Standards/Care-Act/learning-and-development/ introduction-and-overview/care-act-overview-fact-sheet.pdf and research the Care Act 2014.

In practice

3.1 Using communication systems to promote partnership working

Which partnerships currently exist for your organisation? Show how you fit into these. What communication systems are in place to promote partnership working?

Communication systems

The types of communication systems the partnerships are likely to rely upon include:

● written records, such as email and letters
● electronic databases
● service users' personal notes
● daily records of care and nursing/medical notes.

Your policy for partnership working and sharing information

The way we work with others demands that we are open about what we do and effective in sharing information. As an integral way of working, local strategic partnerships have been able to share information and sometimes services to enable service users to be cared for in a more effective way. You need to ensure that as a manager you are aware of the policy in place for partnership working. This policy will detail how information is to be shared and stored to protect the confidentiality of the client as well as detailing referral processes and recording procedures.

We want to ensure that the service we offer improves the experience and outcomes of the people who use that service. This can only be done by minimising the barriers between different services and ensuring that the lines of communication are not blurred.

AC 3.2, 3.3 Compare the effectiveness of different communications systems for partnership working and propose improvements to communication systems for partnership working

Different communication systems are likely to be used for partnership working. However, in different settings within a partnership, it is likely that record keeping for example may be carried out in a variety of ways. This can lead to communication issues

In practice

3.2, 3.3 Comparing effectiveness of communication systems and proposing improvements

Compile a questionnaire or set up an action research group to compare and determine the effectiveness of your current working across partnerships with respect to communication. The following questions may be helpful:

- Where does communication break down?
- What is good about our communication?
- What needs to be changed?
- Is there anything that we are missing?

When you feel you have the information you need, set down some proposals to improve the communication systems for partnership working.

particularly if staff do not clearly understand how records are being stored and shared. Confidentiality may be compromised when there is confusion about how the records are sent between several partners. For example, some settings may favour sending records via email attachments but this can be problematic if confidential information is sent to a central email system in another setting and not to the right person. See AC 2.2, which discusses how we can evaluate the effectiveness of communication systems.

For effective partnership, communication systems must be robust, confidential and standardised so that all staff who need to access records understand how they can do this without compromising confidentiality. If improvements to the ways in which this is done are to be made then all partners need to be involved in the change. Clear protocols as to who is responsible for updating information and who is allowed access to data need to be in place to ensure effective use. See AC 2.3 for information on proposing improvements.

LO4 Be able to use systems for effective information management

AC 4.1 Explain legal and ethical tensions between maintaining confidentiality and sharing information

Beauchamp and Childress (1994) define confidentiality as 'keeping secret' information given to a person by another. Infringement occurs when that information is disclosed to someone else without the giver's consent.

Health and social care staff are required to fulfil their duty of care and maintain confidences obtained via their work and you as a manager need to meet this requirement with respect to the staff you deal with. However, if there is a public interest issue at stake, then confidence may be broken. For example:

- if a crime has been committed or you believe it is about to be
- if malpractice has occurred
- if abuse is suspected
- in order to prevent harm to self or to others
- if professional misconduct has occurred.

If a breach of confidentiality occurs within your workplace, then you as the manager are obliged to take disciplinary action and/or legal action.

From a legal point of view, you are obliged to follow the laws associated with maintaining confidentiality:

- Data Protection Act (1998)
- Human Rights Act (1998)
- The Freedom of Information Act (2000)
- The Equality Act (2010)
- Public Interest Disclosure Act (1999) (often referred to as the 'Whistle Blowing Act').

Other guidelines are:

- clinical governance requirements
- essential standards for quality and safety (CQC)
- Caldicott recommendations
- Skills for Care guidelines
- Disability Discrimination Act (1995).

From an ethical point of view, in maintaining confidentiality, health professionals explicitly or implicitly make a promise to their service users to keep confidential the information they provide them with, thus respecting the

In practice

4.1 Legal and ethical tensions

Explain the legal and ethical tensions between maintaining confidentiality and sharing information in your own workplace and write a short piece about them.

autonomy of the client. But problems arise when decisions need to be made as to the sharing of certain personal information. For example, Article 10 of the Convention on Human Rights and Biomedicine states: 'Everyone has the right to respect for private life in relation to information about his/her health care' (European Parliament & Council of the European Union, 1995).

Another of the tensions with respect to confidentiality lies with the use of information and its safekeeping.

> 'The Health and Social Care Information Centre (HSCIC), formed in April 2013, was set up to improve health and social care in England by putting technology, data and information to work. One of the promises within the document is the assurance that every citizen's data will be protected by ensuring that the quality, safety and security of data and information flow across the health and social care sector so that citizens will willingly share their data in the knowledge that it will be kept confidential and secure.'

Health and Social Care (2015) Information and technology for better care. Information Centre Strategy 2015–2020

AC 4.2 Analyse the essential features of information-sharing agreements within and between organisations

The DOH (2003) Confidentiality NHS Code of Practice identifies the best practice for information sharing and the guidance outlines the NHS commitment 'to the delivery of a first class confidential service ensuring that all:

- patient information is processed fairly, lawfully and as transparently as possible so that the public:
  - understand the reasons for processing personal information;
  - give their consent for the disclosure and use of their personal information;
  - gain trust in the way the NHS handles information and;
  - understand their rights to access information held about them.

The recommendations within the Caldicott Report should also be taken into account here.

In 1997 the government appointed a committee to recommend how the information collected for

patient records should be processed. The principles produced by the committee became part of the Data Protection Act in 1998 and recommended the appointment of a person in every organisation to be responsible for the maintenance of confidentiality. In care homes this would be a senior staff member (or manager) who would be legally required to ensure that a policy was in place to protect the individual in the home.

The most important of the principles outlined were:

- The purpose of the information and the transfer of such should be clearly justified.
- Client-identifiable information should be limited if possible.
- Accessibility – staff should be permitted to access information on a need-to-know basis only.
- Staff should be made aware of their responsibilities with respect to confidentiality.
- All information kept on the client must conform to law such as the Data Protection Act (1998) and the Freedom of Information Act (2000).

Source: Tilmouth *et al.*, 2011

Any patient information you keep may be passed on for a particular purpose with the patient's consent or on a need-to-know basis. You also need to ensure that the patient is fully informed about how the information about them may be used.

The guidance stresses the importance of anonymising personal information wherever possible in order to minimise the risk of security breaches into your systems. Threats to security can be accidental and due to human error or failure, or naturally occurring events such as fire, or from deliberate breaches from external hackers.

The responsibility for maintaining confidentiality lies with the manager and you need to be convinced that your policies and procedures are appropriate and operational within your area.

Reflect on it

4.2 Essential features of information sharing agreements

What are the essential features of information sharing agreements within the organisation and between those you deal with in your workplace?

AC 4.3 Demonstrate use of information management systems that meet legal and ethical requirements

Storage of confidential information needs to be secure and policies put into place to show how your setting intends to meet legal and ethical requirements. As a manager, one of your responsibilities is to ensure that information is accessible to the relevant people only and that staff understand how the information is to be used. The service user must be aware of how the information about them is used and how such use conforms to legal and ethical principles.

One of the main legal requirements in any information system deals with the quality of the reports collected and the way in which the system is implemented. As a manager there are four key areas which you need to monitor and evaluate:

1 **Purpose** – clarity about why you need to collect data.
2 **Collection** – the processes by which data is collected.
3 **Storage** – the processes and systems used to store and maintain patient information and notes.
4 **Analysis** – the process of translating data into information that can be used to improve the organisation and its care-giving.

Taking this a step further, the actual information that is collected must also comply with legal requirements of accuracy.

Go to Unit M1 on health and safety for information on Dimond, who highlighted major areas of concern in care reports. Accurately documenting what happened provides an account of what actually was done at the time and what took place.

In practice

4.2, 4.3 Essential features of information sharing agreements and use of systems that meet legal and ethical requirements

In your own setting, prepare an analysis of the essential features of information-sharing agreements within and between organisations and show how the information management systems meet legal and ethical requirements.

We rely on these records, and if years later the case becomes part of a legal process, we need to be able to return to the records to remind us of what actually was done at the time.

Records then:

- provide an account of the care given (although they do not show what the quality of that care was)
- give a record of continuous care (in the case of nursing and medical records)
- provide a source of reference for care
- provide an audit and quality assurance trail
- are a legal requirement.

Legislation

- **The Care Act (2014)** simplified and improved the existing legislation in care, changing the way in which access and financing care were carried out. People requiring care are now able to access the care and support from local councils or other organisations in the community and have more choice about the type of support and care they need.
  Under this new legislation service users receiving care and support from any regulated provider will now be covered by the Human Rights Act and local councils are responsible for helping the service user to access independent financial advice to help them with care funding.
- **Human Rights Act (1998)** protects the human rights of individuals to privacy, among other rights.
- **Data Protection Act (1998)** deals with the processing and protection of data on individuals.
- **The Freedom of Information Act (2000)** allows individuals to see all the information of a personal nature held about them.
- **The Equality Act (2010)** is an umbrella act bringing together legislation that deals with race, disability and gender. It highlighted protected characteristics of age, gender reassignment, pregnancy, religion, marriage and civil partnerships, and sexual orientation in an attempt to end discrimination.
- **Public Interest Disclosure Act (1999)** safeguards individuals by providing them with the means to speak out about issues of negligence, miscarriages of justice, crime and dangers to health. It is commonly referred to as the 'Whistle Blowing Act'.

Research it

4.3 Legal and ethical requirements

The following are adapted from the National Occupational Standards for Managers Unit B8: Ensure compliance with legal, regulatory, ethical and social requirements.

Evaluate your own performance against these standards and then ask a colleague or your manager to verify your judgement. Keep the completed work in your portfolio as evidence.

Management standard	How do I do this and what evidence do I have to show completion?	Verification by manager or colleague	Further action needed
What are the national and international legal, regulatory, ethical and social requirements of my area and how do I monitor them? What effect do they have on my area of responsibility, and what will happen if I don't meet them?			
What are the policies and procedures which make sure my organisation meets all the necessary requirements?			
How do I make sure relevant people have a clear understanding of the policies and procedures and the importance of putting them into practice?			
How do I ensure that policies and procedures are put into practice and provide support?			
How do I encourage a climate of openness about meeting and not meeting the requirements?			
What failures to meet the requirements have I identified and corrected?			
What reasons have I identified for not meeting requirements and how have I adjusted the policies and procedures to reduce the likelihood of failures in the future?			
Have I provided full reports about any failures to meet the requirements to the relevant stakeholders?			

Assessment methods

LO	Assessment criteria and accompanying activities	Assessment methods *To evidence coverage of the ACs you could:*
LO1	1.1 Reflect on it (p. 3)	Think about and make a list of all the relationships and contacts you may have within the course of your managerial role. Discuss this with your assessor. You may come up with the contacts shown in Figure 1.1.
	1.1, 1.2 In practice (p. 5)	Keep a communication diary for one span of duty. Use the questions below to show how you have undertaken the different types of communicating listed in the activity (i.e. advising, instructing, welcoming, assessing, observing, informing and counselling. You might construct a table to evidence this. You could also write a short piece to answer the questions in the activity and place a copy in your portfolio. I.e. 1 Who were the groups or individuals whose communication needs were addressed in the diary? 2 In what context did the communication take place? 3 What purpose did it have? 4 How successful was it? 5 How did you ensure the communication was effective? What did you do?
	1.3 Reflect on it (p. 6)	Discuss with your assessor reasons (one internal and one external factor) for the blocks or barriers in communication. For example, an external barrier may be a poor environment for communication which lacks privacy, leading to an internal barrier in that you are unsafe talking about a matter.
	Case study (p. 8)	Read the case study for 1.3 and then answer the questions. 1 Comment honestly on how this makes you feel about Jim and his potentially disruptive influence. 2 What is your initial response to the actions as a manager? 3 Now reflect on the above and say why you reacted this way and how you will respond to the situation. Alternatively, provide your own case to show how you would respond to a similar issue.
	1.3 Reflect on it (p. 9)	Write a reflective piece which shows: A time when you know that you were not being listened to and heard, then write your responses to the following or discuss them with your assessor: ● What was going on at that time? ● How did it affect the interaction? ● What do you think was going on for the person you were trying to communicate with at that time?

→

LO	Assessment criteria and accompanying activities	Assessment methods *To evidence coverage of the ACs you could:*
	1.3, 1.4 Case study (p. 11)	Read the case study and explain how you would respond. How might you deal with this situation? See the case study for some of the ways in which the situation may have been dealt with.
	1.3 1.4 Reflect on it (p. 11)	Undertake an observation of the care setting with your assessor and discuss with them the barriers you see with respect to the environment. Alternatively read the account in the activity and answer the questions: Have a look around the room in which you are sitting. How does it make you feel? Think about it for a moment. Is it welcoming, untidy, too busy, crammed, too large, are the chairs too far apart?
	1.3 In practice (p. 12)	Provide a written analysis showing the communication barriers present in your working environment. This should show your understanding of the effects these have.
	1.4 In practice (p. 13)	Consider the next communication you have with each a client and a member of staff. Write a brief description of the circumstances in which the interaction took place. Comment on the following: ● your body language with respect to SOLER ● your listening skills ● your ability to show unconditional positive regard and empathy. Reflect on your strengths and areas for improvement and develop a strategy to show how you intend to undertake these improvements.
	1.5 In practice (p. 15)	Write a short piece to show the types of communication you use and make a comment upon the effectiveness of different means of communication that you use in the course of your span of duty. You might address verbal, non-verbal, sign, pictorial, written electronic and assisted methods. The means of communication may be personal, organisational, formal, informal or public (information/promotional).
LO2	2.1 In practice (p. 16)	In order to monitor the effectiveness of communication systems and practices you might design a questionnaire to obtain feedback from the following groups of people about your communication systems in place at this time: ● service users ● staff ● visitors ● other professionals you deal with. If you have collected information from personal files and care plans, minutes of meetings, diaries, staff communication systems and emails, ensure that you file them in your portfolio. You may also have gained the views of staff and visitors on how the systems work which need to be shown as evidence of this in your portfolio.

LO	Assessment criteria and accompanying activities	Assessment methods *To evidence coverage of the ACs you could:*
	2.2 In practice (p. 16)	You might compile a report evaluating the quality of the organisation's performance of a particular part of your communication system. Discuss with your assessor how you evaluate the effectiveness, quality and performance of communication systems in your organisation? What standards do you use?
	2.4 Reflect on it (p. 17)	Write a reflective account of the way in which you led the implementation of a revised practice of your communication systems in your setting.
	2.1, 2.2, 2.2.1, 2.2, 2.3, 2.4 Research it (p. 17)	Undertake a small scale study to monitor the communication practice within your own setting and comment upon and evaluate how effective it is. Identify any improvements to the practices and make recommendations for revised systems. Take your evidence to a team meeting.
	2.3 2.4 In practice (p. 17)	Using the information from the questionnaire in AC 2.1 In practice, complete the following and compile a report for evidence of: 1 Which aspects of the communication system in your organisation need to be changed? 2 How did you come to this decision and what methods did you use to collect the information? 3 How did you determine which practices should stay, and why? 4 Who was involved in the decision? 5 What will you do to change the systems and lead the implementation?
LO3	3.1 Research it (p. 18)	Have a look at the Care Act 2014 Go to www.skillsforcare.org.uk/Document-library/Standards/Care-Act/learning-and-development/introduction-and-overview/care-act-overview-factsheet.pdf and research the Care Act 2014. Make a fact sheet for staff showing the main parts of the act.
	3.1 In practice (p. 18)	You could construct a mind map or a flow chart which shows the partnerships which currently exist for your organisation showing how your organisation fits into these. Discuss with your assessor what communication systems are in place to promote partnership working?
	3.1 Reflect on it (p. 18)	Write a reflective piece about the above discussion you had with your assessor and show how the communication systems discussed might be misused or fail.

LO	Assessment criteria and accompanying activities	Assessment methods *To evidence coverage of the ACs you could:*
	3.2 3.3 In practice (p. 19)	You could either compile a questionnaire or set up an action research group to compare and determine the effectiveness of your current working across partnerships with respect to communication. Look at the questions in the activity which may be helpful. The following questions may be helpful: ● Where does communication break down? ● What is good about our communication? ● What needs to be changed? ● Is there anything that we are missing? When you feel you have the information you need, set down some proposals to improve the communication systems for partnership working.
	4.1 In practice (p. 19)	Ask your assessor to attend a team meeting in which you and the team discuss the legal and ethical tensions between maintaining confidentiality and sharing information in your own workplace. You could write a short piece or prepare a hand-out for the staff following the meeting of that discussed.
	4.2 Reflect on it (p. 20)	Discuss with your assessor what the essential features of information sharing agreements within the organisation are and between those you deal with in your workplace? Document the discussion as a professional observation.
	4.2 4.3 In practice (p. 21)	Collect evidence for your portfolio of the information sharing agreements your organisation has in place and undertake an analysis of the essential features of information sharing agreements within and between organisations and show how the information management systems meet legal and ethical requirements.
	4.3 Research it (p. 22)	Prepare a table showing the National Occupational Standards for Managers Unit B8: Ensure compliance with legal, regulatory, ethical and social requirements and then supply evidence of how you meet these standards. You could include documents which show where the standards are set out. Evaluate your own performance against these standards and then ask a colleague or your manager to verify your judgement. Keep the completed work in your portfolio as evidence.

References

Adair, J. (2000) *Effective Teambuilding: How to make a winning team.* London: Pan Macmillan.

Argyle, M. (1978) *The Psychology of Interpersonal Behaviour* (3e). Harmondsworth: Penguin.

Beauchamp, T. L. and Childress, J. F. (1994) *Principles of Biomedical Ethics.* Oxford: Oxford University Press.

Bonham, P. (2004) *Communication as a Mental Health Carer.* Cheltenham: Nelson Thornes.

Burnard, P. (1996) *Acquiring Interpersonal Skills: A handbook of experiential learning for health professionals* (2e). London: Chapman and Hall.

Cole, J. (2011) 'We know why, but do we know how?' Unpublished essay submitted for MSc in Educational Management and Leadership, Worcester University.

Craine, K. (2007) 'Managing the cycle of change,' [Online] *Information Management Journal,* 41, 5, 44–50.

Crawford, P., Brown, B. and Bonham, P. (2006) *Communication in Clinical Settings.* Cheltenham: Nelson Thornes.

Davis, H. and Fallowfield, L. (eds) (1991) *Counselling and Communication in Health Care.* Cirencester: Wiley.

Department of Health (1996) *The Protection and Use of Patient Information.* London: TSO.

Dimond, B. (2008) *Legal Aspects of Nursing* (5e). Harlow: Pearson Education.

DOH (2003) Confidentiality NHS Code of Practice. Crown copyright 2003, alternative? www.gov.uk/government/uploads/system/uploads/attachment_data/file/200146/Confidentiality_-_NHS_Code_of_Practice.pdf.

Donnelly, E. and Neville, L. (2008) *Communication and Interpersonal Skills.* Exeter: Reflect Press.

European Parliament & Council of the European Union (1995) Directive 95/46/EC of the European Parliament and of the Council of 24 October 1995 on the protection of individuals with regard to the processing of personal data and on the free movement of such data. *Official Journal*, L281, pp. 31–50.

Geldard, K. and Geldard, D. (2003) *Counselling Skills in Everyday Life.* London: Palgrave Macmillan.

Givens, D. B. (2000) 'Body Speak: What are you saying?' Successful Meetings, (October) 51.

Goleman, D. (1995) *Emotional Intelligence.* New York: Bantam Books.

Gopee, N. and Galloway, J. (2009) *Leadership and Management in Health Care.* London: Sage.

Graham, R. J. (1991) 'Understanding the beliefs of poor communication,' *Interface*, 11, pp. 80–2.

Hewison, A. (1995) 'Nurses' power in interactions with patients,' *Journal of Advanced Nursing*, 21, pp. 75–82.

Katz, R. (1955) 'Skills of an effective administrator,' *Harvard Business Review*, 33(1), pp. 33–42.

Lord Laming (2003) *The Victoria Climbié Inquiry: Summary report of an inquiry.* Cheltenham: HMSO.

McGrath, J. E. (1985) 'Critical leadership functions' in Hackman, J. R. and Watson, R. E. (1986) *Leading Groups in Organisations.* P. S. Goodman and Associates (eds), San Francisco: Jossey-Bass.

Miller, L. (2006) *Counselling Skills for Social Work.* London: Sage Publications.

NHS Executive (1998) *Information for Health. An Information Strategy for the Modern NHS 1998–2005.* London: NHS Executive.

Porritt, L. (1990) *Interaction Strategies: An Introduction for Health Professionals* (2e) London: Churchill Livingstone.

Rogers, C. (1980) *A Way of Being.* New York: Houghton Mifflin.

Rogers, C. (2002) *Client-Centred Therapy.* London: Constable.

Skills for Care (2006) *Leadership and Management Strategy: Strategy for the social care workforce.* Leeds: Skills for Care.

Tilmouth, T., Davies-Ward, E. and Williams, B. (2011) *Foundation Studies in Health and Social Care.* London: Hodder & Stoughton.

Further reading and useful resources

Alton Barbour, A. and Koneya, M. (1976) *Louder Than Words: Non-verbal communication.* Columbus, Ohio: Merrill.

Bazler Riley, J. (2008) *Communication in Nursing.* Maryland Heights, Missouri: Mosby Elsevier.

Buono, A. F. and Kerber, W. K. (2010) 'Creating a sustainable approach to change: building organizational change capacity.' [Online] journal article: *SAM Advanced Management Journal*, Vol. 75.

Macleod-Clark, J. (1984) 'Verbal communication in nursing' in Faulkner, A. (ed.) *Recent Advances in Nursing 7. Communication.* Edinburgh: Churchill Livingstone.

NHS Executive (2010) *White Paper: Equity and Excellence: Liberating the NHS.* London: NHS Executive.

www.skillsforcare.org.uk/Document-library/Standards/Care-Act/learning-and-development/introduction-and-overview/care-act-overview-fact-sheet.pdf

Unit SHC 52

Promote professional development

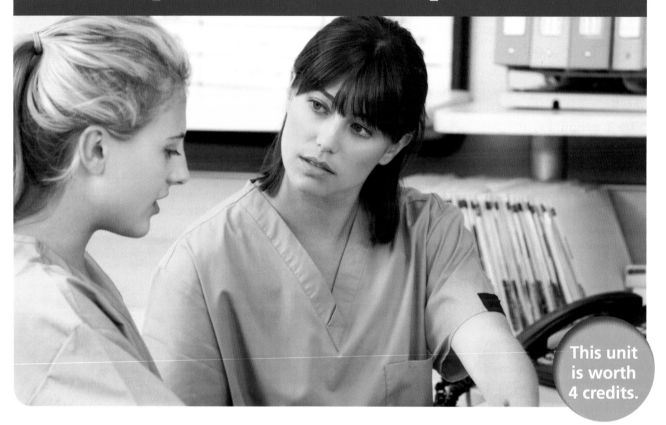

This unit is worth 4 credits.

People receiving care services must be confident that they can trust those who deliver care to not only know what to do but to know how to do it well. This requires you to continually update and extend your knowledge and skills and, as a manager, to ensure that your team is also equipped with appropriate knowledge and skills in order to fulfil their roles effectively. Personal professional development is a journey for the whole of your life; it does not end with the completion of a course or a specific activity but should, ideally, be an 'activity of daily living'. The secret of successful personal development is to learn to be reflective and questioning, both about the things we know and the things we do not know.

This unit will help you to examine and assess your understanding of professional development, professionalism and the responsibilities that these concepts entail as a manager and leader. You will develop your reflective and individual planning skills in order to help you to determine how you can most effectively support your own development and that of others, and you will evaluate strategies to overcome barriers.

Learning outcomes

By the end of this unit you will:

1 Understand principles of professional development.
2 Be able to prioritise goals and targets for your own professional development.
3 Be able to prepare a professional development plan.
4 Be able to improve performance through reflective practice.

LO1 Understand principles of professional development

AC 1.1 Explain the importance of continually improving knowledge and practice

What is professional development? What is the manager's role in developing themselves and promoting the professional development of others?

Care is a complex, multi-dimensional activity and encompasses more than simply performing a skill. While technical competence gained through developing knowledge and skills is important, it is not sufficient on its own. Excellent care can be achieved only when technical competence is accompanied by developing appropriate attitudes, and characteristics that relate to feelings, values and the manner in which activities are carried out.

Professional development is a continuous process and care workers need to ensure they develop newer skills, knowledge and understanding to meet these changing needs and demands. In striving to improve quality of service for service users, only the best possible practice will be acceptable. This can only be achieved with a workforce that continually updates the knowledge and skill in line with any changes that occur.

This is not a new concept but has emerged as changes to the care system have developed. With moves to partnership working and new models of care which value personalisation and individualised health care professionals have had to ensure that upskilling of the workforce has been a top agenda item.

The Leitch review of skills (2006) identified the need for the UK to upskill the workforce in order to be able to compete in a global economy that was undergoing rapid change. This has led to changes in education to ensure that the future workforce is sufficiently skilled in literacy, numeracy and new developments, together with moves to extend training in the workplace to ensure regular upskilling of the current workforce occurs.

Following the serious case review into Mid-Staffordshire NHS Trust, the Cavendish Report (2013) recommended changes to the training of healthcare assistants in hospitals, care homes and service users' own homes, to ensure they provide the highest standard of care. The review recommended that a training course be developed that certificates a care worker in a 'certificate of fundamental care' before they can care for service users unsupervised.

The requirement for professional development is further reinforced in professional codes and standards of conduct, which articulate the standards that the public can expect from those delivering care. These are:

- General Social Care Council Code of Practice for Social Care Workers (GSCC, 2010)
- the Health Professions Council (2008) Standards of Conduct, Performance and Ethics
- Nursing and Midwifery Council (2015) The Code: Professional standards of practice and behaviour for nurses and midwives
- National Occupational Standards.

Additionally, attending mandatory training updates such as Manual Handling and Resuscitation, for example, is important, but it is unlikely to be sufficient to meet the responsibility and breadth of expectations for personal and professional development implied in the law and in codes of conduct. It is important that staff understand the need for change, updates that are made and the reasons for the continual update of knowledge and skill. Further information on change managements is covered in unit SHC 51.

DOH (2013) The Cavendish Review: An Independent Review into Healthcare Assistants and Support Workers in the NHS and Social Care Settings, London HMSO

Professional development and training enables an organisation to keep up to date and to change proactively so that its service is relevant and appropriate. First, it is important to note that to

> **Key term**
>
> **Continuing professional development (CPD)** is the planned process of improving and increasing capabilities of staff and is an ongoing process.

get the most out of investment in professional development it should be planned in line with an organisational vision. Ad hoc training may be useful but may only lead to staff undertaking a disparate set of activities that does not contribute to the greater whole.

Providing staff with a variety of skills-based training and one-to-one support is imperative if staff are to develop in a professional way. They are required to undertake training courses on an annual basis to ensure they remain up-to-date with skills and knowledge and this is all part of professional development.

It is recognised that those organisations that embed personal, professional development into their culture are best able to respond to day-to-day challenges and pressures and are more resilient and able to transform in response to changing situations and requirements (Schon, 1973, p. 28; Harrison, 2009).

Second, professional development is a process. This implies that it is an ongoing activity and needs to be thought about as something that is incremental, with the different elements contributing to a larger whole.

Third, personal, professional development increases the capabilities of staff. If it is tailored to individual needs, it should bring about personal enhancements and opportunities as individuals expand their personal tool box of skills. The image of the 'Knowledge and Skills Escalator' articulated in the *The NHS Knowledge and Skills Framework and Development Review Guidance* (DoH, 2004) is a powerful one. It effectively illustrates the idea of professional development being about continual movement. It generates the image of individuals having access to a range of education and development opportunities at different levels which can be individually selected and packaged in many different ways. It supports the idea that professional development can be undertaken either in a traditional, linear way, starting at the bottom and moving through the levels to the top, but that it is also equally valid for an individual to get off the escalator at any point and move around on that level in order to access a whole package of different activities before re-joining the escalator. The direction of travel may take an individual up a floor to extend previous knowledge, or down a floor to access

In practice

1.1 The importance of continually improving knowledge and practice

What professional development activities have you and your team participated in over the last year?

- How do they reflect the changes that have impacted on your work in health and social care? Make a list.
- Were they planned, and if so, by whom?
- Were they part of a development plan for the organisation or focused on individual needs?
- What is the evidence that they have resulted in positive outcomes?
- Give examples.
- How have they helped to improve knowledge and practice?
- Summarise the importance of improving knowledge and practice.

new learning. It also suggests that there should be no limit to opportunities, that even if you start at the bottom you have the opportunity to move to the top. As a manager it is important that you and your organisation capitalise on the benefits that professional development brings by ensuring that it is purposive and planned to meet the individual needs of your staff and to address organisational needs.

AC 1.2 Analyse potential barriers to professional development

The need for professional development is not contentious and it is not difficult to mount a convincing argument for its integration into organisational culture, yet when times are busy and challenging, it can be the first thing to drop off the agenda. However, staff development is not an optional luxury but rather an essential requirement for any service seeking to provide care for others. The challenge for the manager, therefore, is to find ways of identifying/recognising and overcoming and reducing any barriers to professional development. Barriers are little more than hurdles to get around. While they may seem insurmountable, ingenuity, creativity and a positive attitude may be sufficient to overcome them. Barriers should be viewed as problems to be solved rather than as overwhelming obstacles.

Potential barriers

Barriers may be both internal and external. Internal barriers refer to our own attitudes and thinking, whereas external ones are those that are impacted by the environment around us. These may include other staff, for example, or access to training opportunities. When planning personal professional development, it will be important for you as a manager to engage the expected participants in the process as partners. If the participant is receptive to the development opportunity, they are less likely to think up 'yes, but…' scenarios and will be more likely to find solutions to their own barriers. For example, if attendance at a course is difficult because of someone's personal commitments, a discussion with them about how this could be overcome or different ways of studying could resolve the issue. It is important that individuals are engaged and understand the need for the activity and the benefits and opportunities that might result from it.

Managing time is an important component of developing an effective staff development programme. It takes time to identify individual needs and interests and to assess what things will bring about most benefit to the team and the organisation, but if done effectively, this will be time well spent. It is important to account for interests as well as organisational needs, although the latter may take priority. If staff feel their individual interests are supported, it will help maintain motivation and morale in the team. In addition, staff need to feel that the activity is valued for its own sake and is not just another chore to be squeezed in around more important routine activities. Consequently, staff need the encouragement to put their learning into practice.

Addressing needs of all your staff: as a manager you will be aware that there are never enough resources to meet everybody's needs and wants, and it is important that planning is realistic to avoid disappointment and disillusion. It is also important to ensure that resources are used as efficiently and fairly as possible – time spent researching different means of achieving goals, such as online or blended learning, may substantially reduce costs and increase flexibility.

Reflect on it

1.2 Barriers affecting outcomes for service users

Write a short reflective account of how the potential barriers to professional development affect the outcomes for service users.

In practice

1.2 Analysing potential barriers to professional development

Identify the potential barriers to undertaking professional development in your workplace and then set up an action plan to overcome them. A table has been included to help you.

Potential barrier	Action to overcome barrier	Potential risk if not undertaken

When times are difficult it may be necessary to reduce the amount of development that can be supported. Trying to do too much runs the risk of adding stress on staff and possible loss of good will. It is your responsibility to be able to justify decisions. Sorting your activities into priority categories with identification of associated risks if an activity is not done is one way of prioritising development.

It is important to recognise that individuals' learning styles differ and some development opportunities may suit some individual needs and preferences and not others. Taking time to understand how your staff learn best will help you and them to choose development (training) opportunities that are a good fit.

AC 1.3 Compare the use of different sources and systems of support for professional development

Not all professional development will be achieved by attendance at formal training or education events. There are various forms of informal support that are of significant value in developing others' capabilities.

It has been said that the richest resource that any organisation possesses is the people who work within it. An organisation will evolve and change only if people make it happen. Individuals are interested in, and motivated by, different things and this includes their motivation to learn something. Consequently, everyone's knowledge base and skill set is different, even when similar levels of formal training have been undertaken. If we could pool and share this knowledge, everyone, including the organisation, would benefit. A key role for a manager is to utilise the existing skill set within a team in order to enhance the knowledge and skills of others.

Formal and informal sources of support

Formal support for development is organised and has learning objectives, the intention of which is to gain knowledge and skills. Informal support, meanwhile, may not be organised or planned but may happen as a result of experience in the workplace. Again it is important to understand which style suits the individual. The following paragraphs introduce a few means of achieving this with very limited investment.

Supervision

Supervision is a professional conversation which can be either informal or formal, taking place during a tea break for example, or in a formal meeting. Professionals at all levels of experience need this type of activity to promote their learning and to enable them to reflect on practice.

Appraisal

Requests for and the identification of the need for more formal methods of personal professional development are often generated through formal appraisal processes. **Appraisals** are a key strategy for managers to assess performance and needs against organisational requirements and aims. Appraisals are a formally constituted, annual activity that should be booked with all staff. Appraisals are normally conducted by a manager but can be conducted by peers if their focus is on developmental needs rather than role performance. Whichever model is adopted, individuals need to be warned about what it will involve so that they can prepare. Ideally they should see examples of any documentation that will be used so that they can plan responses to

the questions that will be asked. Appraisal offers a vehicle for structured, personal development planning that can have positive outcomes for both individuals and the organisation. It may help develop a strategy for an individual to meet personal goals and objectives, both short and long term. It will help the manager to match individuals and their training needs against organisational aims and it will also enable managers to assess the fairness of the training and development allocation across the staff team. Where necessary it also provides a process for managing staff performance, as it encourages managers to measure individual performance against role competency criteria.

Appraisal is a shared activity, which takes time and effort and must be planned if it is going to have any significant impact on personal development planning (PDP). PDP can have a number of different purposes and it is important that the method you select for PDP meets your needs as a manager, as well as the individual staff member's needs. It is important that the tool you design or utilise addresses those purposes that you have identified as important for your organisation. If you do not have an appraisal process in your organisation, you may want to consider writing a proposal to implement one.

See AC 1.3 for how to write a personal development plan.

Mentoring

Mentoring is an invaluable tool for supporting staff development and is a powerful means of individual empowerment. Clutterbuck and Megginson (1999, p. 17) describe mentorship as

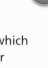

> ### Key terms
>
> **Appraisal**, sometimes referred to as performance appraisal, is the process by which employees and line managers discuss their performance, developmental needs and the support they need in their role. It is used to provide evidence and evaluation of recent performance and focus on future goals, opportunities and resources.
>
> **Mentoring** is a relationship in which an individual with expertise can help another individual to progress in their career.

In practice

1.3 Comparing different sources and systems of support

Think about which of the following functions of personal development planning are important within your organisation.

Function of personal development planning	Tick	Does your PDP enable this function to be realised?
Assessment of competence to undertake a role against predetermined criteria (e.g. role descriptor)		
Opportunity to enhance effectiveness and performance		
Planning for the future (short, medium and long term)		
Clarification of values and behaviours		
Evaluation of service		
Means of enhancing service		
Increase staff motivation		
Opportunity for self-reflection		
Identification of strengths and areas for improvement		
Strategy to solve problems		
Provide a structure for and commitment to staff training and development		
Opportunity to manage and respond to change		
Increase team capabilities		
Manage underperformance		
Provide a structure for individual feedback		

a) Of the systems you use to support your staff, compare the formal and informal training your staff undertake.

b) Which has been the most useful?

'standing in front of a mirror with a trusted other, who can help you see things that you do not know how to see, or that have become too familiar for you to notice'.

Mentoring can be defined simply as a helping relationship between an individual with potential and an individual with expertise. The role of the mentor is to guide the mentee. Knowledge, experience and organisational perspective are shared candidly within a context of mutual respect and trust. It is an effective way of helping people to progress in their careers and is becoming increasingly popular as its potential is realised. A number of roles of the mentor have been listed by Bolton (2010, p. 193): role model, enabler, teacher, encourager, counsellor, befriender, facilitator, coach, confidant, supporter and 'un-learner'.

Coaching

Coaching, although sometimes used interchangeably with mentoring, is in fact a distinct activity, although there are some similarities. Coaching is an activity designed to help individuals fulfil their potential and thus is an ideal strategy for some elements of

Key term

Coaching is a process that supports and enables an individual to unlock and maximise their potential, to develop and improve performance.

professional development. It is a process of helping them to learn rather than teaching them. Coaching requires a belief that individuals are capable of addressing and resolving their issues and needs. Not only are they capable but coaching implies that they are best suited to take responsibility for their decisions and actions and solutions; coaching can therefore be described as a leadership style. Coaches use a range of tools and models to support their coachee. Coaching requires an attitude of positive regard and good communication skills in order to provide the right prompts to enable the coachee to reach their resolutions and conclusions. A coach may or may not have experience or expertise in the coachee's occupation. The skill of the coach is in asking the coachee appropriate prompt questions in order to enable them to think clearly and coherently about their issues.

The 'GROW' model of coaching (Whitmore, 2009) provides a simple and structured model for the coach:

G = Goal setting asks questions to encourage the mentee to clarify what they want and where they want to get to. The coach will encourage the coachee to explore what achievement would look like to them.

R = Reality promotes questions that require reflection now. What is the situation currently? What is stopping you achieving your goals? What do you need to achieve your goals? What is a realistic time scale? What do you enjoy and why? What are the key risks?

O = Options. This stage of the model encourages the coachee to explore different means of achieving the goal. Questions that might be asked include: What are the different ways that you could achieve your goal? What else could you do? What are the pros and cons of different options? What would happen if ...? Which of the options would bring about the best result?

W = Way forward. Finally, the coach will encourage the coachee to make an action plan. Questions that might be useful include: What are you resolved to do, and by when? What support do you need? What commitment do you have? When should we/you review progress?

Coaching enables control and development to remain squarely with the coachee, with the effective coach acting merely as a key to help them unlock their potential.

Presentations and sharing good practice

Formal presentations can be intimidating and time consuming to prepare and deliver. However, creating an opportunity to discuss a 'best kept secret' in an informal, five-minute contribution may be less threatening and an effective way of sharing good practice. Team members can be invited to come to a meeting and be prepared to share with their colleagues an issue of practice, taking only five minutes. This could be something that they think they do well, and should briefly include evidence that demonstrates that this is good practice. They may want to discuss new knowledge, such as highlighting a change in standard treatment. Alternatively, they could present a problem and invite their colleagues to suggest solutions or ways of finding solutions. This type of activity stimulates discussion and provides an opportunity for everyone in the team to learn something new, to reflect on their own practice and knowledge, and to identify those things that should be investigated further, or those things the team would wish to implement and develop. While this activity may not initiate a change of practice, it is an effective way of sharing headlines so that anyone who is interested in taking this further can contact an identified individual. Alternatively, staff can be invited to present to colleagues a summary of knowledge gained at formal training events, or to present and initiate discussion of client case studies to reflect on and evaluate care management. Inevitably the success will depend on the commitment of those involved.

If all members are expected to contribute in rotation and this becomes regular practice in team meetings, it is more likely to be sustained and staff will see it not as an addition to work but as an expectation of everyday work.

While a team is a valuable and often untapped resource, it is also important that staff have access to up-to-date resources that can provide answers to professional questions. Books have their place for reference, for example, but quickly become out of date. Therefore, books need to be purchased judiciously and updated regularly.

Good quality and easily accessible information is increasingly available through electronic means, either through search engines on the internet or through access to electronic and digitised resources and journals. CD training packs which support learning in key elements of your provision are an ideal means of delivering training to a large number of staff without the additional expense of covering attendance and cover for study days.

One strategy that has aroused significant interest in recent years in developing teams and organisations is '**appreciative inquiry**' (Cooperrider *et al.*, 2003). Appreciative inquiry focuses on the positive features of an organisation and its workforce, rather than a deficit model. It directs energy at identifying and building on strengths rather than trying to compensate for or to rectify weaknesses. Appreciative inquiry aims to generate a collective image of a new and better future organisation, in which all of the workforce have an investment and a contribution to make. The aim of appreciative inquiry is to explore best practice, past and present, within the organisation and to concentrate on defining those positive values, practices and processes that improve and enhance best practice.

Cooperrider *et al.* (2003) suggest 4 Ds in appreciative inquiry:

- **Discovery** – seeking that which is 'best', including staff.
- **Dream** – developing a collective vision.
- **Design** – identifying strategies that can achieve the vision and revising these until the vision can be achieved.
- **Destiny** – engendering and supporting new ways of working that can enable the vision to be realised and sustained.

Within and beyond the organisation

While there is much to commend attendance at external training courses to gain knowledge and skills, we should never underestimate the sources of knowledge within the organisation. Staff are often a source of great knowledge and skill that is largely untapped.

AC 1.4 Explain factors to consider when selecting opportunities and activities for keeping knowledge and practice up to date

Funding

Inevitably, investing in opportunities to enable staff to keep up to date is associated with costs and it would be unrealistic and irresponsible not to consider these costs seriously. However, the risk of not engaging in development activities may be very costly in terms of the long-term organisational plan, so it is important to balance these investment costs against this. While it might be tempting to see staff development as a luxury, non-essential activity when times are tight, in an environment in which treatments, practices and expectations are constantly changing, that would be a mistake. It is important to ensure that any development budget is spent appropriately and that key risks are prioritised over other, less important activities.

For example, failing to ensure that staff gain appropriate training in relation to manual handling would leave the organisation vulnerable to litigation and potentially expensive compensation claims from both staff and possibly clients. Given the nature of care work that requires moving and handling to take place, it is highly likely that an incident will occur and it is also likely to have a significant impact. This would result in a high risk score, which should alert the manager that there is a need to do something urgently to rectify the deficit. Risks can be plotted on a chart so that it is easy to get a visual image of where key areas need to be addressed.

Other factors include time and career goals and aspirations. Time is a factor that must be considered if staff need to go off site to attend training, for example. Having a firm career plan in place can be a valuable asset in terms of choosing appropriate training activities.

In practice

1.4 Factors to consider when selecting opportunities and activities
Think about your own organisation and the range of factors to consider when selecting opportunities and activities for keeping knowledge and practice up to date.

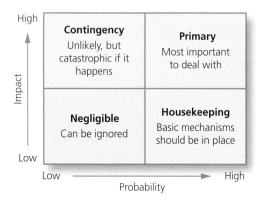

Figure 2.1 Risk assessment chart

In the 'In practice' activity, you may have identified factors such as the employment of new staff; the effective implementation of Care Quality Commission's standards and the effectiveness of evidence to illustrate compliance with these standards; introduction of new care standards or key priorities such as a national focus on infection control, or reduction in pressure areas or increased attention on nutrition; the risk of not sustaining staff motivation and morale; ensuring viability and popularity; and the introduction of new practice or processes.

All of these risks could be lessened by appropriate staff development. In any organisation it is necessary to address priorities. Categorise your risks in the chart in Figure 2.1. Does this provide you with information with which to begin to make choices?

Decision making

In making decisions about priorities, it is important to draw on a range of evidence to ensure that your money and time will be well spent. While this is a time-consuming activity, it can be part of an annual review of quality. Staff development should be

directed towards those areas where there are gaps or where improvements are needed. Consequently, undertaking an analysis of client complaints or staff turnover and individual staff perceptions could indicate areas of underachievement or staff insecurity. More proactively, drawing up a chart of the staff's wish list for development arising from appraisals might be useful.

Keeping knowledge and practice up to date, and responding to change

Managers in the care environment have a professional responsibility to keep up to date. They need to be aware of changes to practice requirements; these could result from changes in government policy or new initiatives, the publication of new standards for practice, or new knowledge that requires different behaviours. Being aware of current issues and practices in your sector enables the manager to be proactive. If a report or publication relating to poor practice is published about another provider in the sector, it gives the manager an opportunity to review practices in their own organisation and address any shortcomings. Ignorance and complacency are not defendable. In situations of rapid change and in competitive markets, it is a fact that only those organisations that are able to be flexible, adaptive and productive will excel. The survival and sustainability of your organisation may depend on its ability to respond effectively and quickly to change, to become what Senge (1990, p. 3) identifies as 'learning organisations', which are:

'organisations where people continually expand their capacity to create the results they truly desire, where new and expansive patterns of thinking are nurtured, where collective aspiration is set free, and where people are continually learning to see the whole together.'

While all people have the capacity to learn, the structures in which they have to function are often not conducive to reflection, engagement and learning. Furthermore, people may lack the tools and understanding to make sense of the situations they face. Organisations that are continually expanding their capacity to control and create their future require a fundamental shift of mind-set among their members. The manager's role is to 'discover how to tap people's commitment and capacity to learn at all levels' (Senge, 1990, p. 4).

LO2 Be able to prioritise goals and targets for own professional development

AC 2.1 Evaluate own knowledge and performance against standards and benchmarks

Individuals working in the care industry will be subject to a range of professional codes, expectations and standards of performance that are set by external organisations and all staff need to demonstrate that they are working to these standards and providing excellent care. The requirement for professional development is reinforced in professional codes and standards of conduct, such as:

- **Code of conduct** for healthcare support workers and adult social care workers 2013.
- **Regulations** such as the acts and laws under which we practise. For example, the Data Protection Act 1998 or the Mental Capacity Act 2005.
- **Minimum/essential standards** refer to the quality and safety of care and identify the experiences individuals are expected to have as a result of the care they receive.
- **National Occupational Standards** describe the skills, knowledge and understanding required to undertake a particular task or job to a nationally recognised level of competence.

- Health Professions Council (2008) Standards of Conduct, Performance and Ethics highlight the standards of practice for individuals to register, as being fit to practise as health care professionals.
- Nursing and Midwifery Council (2015) The Code: Standards of conduct, performance and ethics for nurses and midwives identifies standards for nurses to maintain registration.

These documents articulate the standards that the public can expect from those delivering care. All codes and standards of practice make explicit reference to the need for those providing care to work within their levels of knowledge and experience and to address any knowledge deficits.

Evaluating your own knowledge and performance

Each individual is also accountable for their professional development and you may be required to identify to your managers, to your profession and/or to a legal authority how you have maintained this. You need to be able to evaluate and examine your knowledge with respect to practice so that you are able to identify any gaps in knowledge and your strengths and areas for development. It is most important that you can provide evidence of your knowledge and skills and how you have maintained these. As a manager and leader of others, it is your responsibility to ensure that those you manage are appropriately equipped to effectively fulfil their roles. This requires you to assess each individual's capabilities against their job description to ensure that they have the skills that are necessary to do their job.

As well as identifying the standards of care to be achieved, codes of practice articulate the manner in which care should be delivered. All recipients of care should expect to receive competent care. An organisation that strives for excellence will also ensure that attention is paid to the value base of care provision which facilitates good and excellent practice as opposed to merely competent or safe practice.

Evaluating your own performance requires you to supply an examination of your practice showing that your knowledge and skills are based on sound learning and that you always work within the standards required. You need to show that you are a life-long learner and continually update your practice.

Reflect on it

2.1 Your job description

Look at your job description. Write a list of the essential skills and qualities necessary for someone to fulfil that role effectively.

Are there any requirements in the role for which you feel less confident of your skills to fulfil adequately? These are some areas for professional development.

In practice

2.1 Standards and benchmarks

Make a list of the codes and standards that guide and govern your role.

- When did you last review and reflect on your work against these standards?
- How is your work influenced by these codes and standards?
- Evaluate your performance in the light of these standards, taking into account the standards and benchmarks you are required to work within.

Research it

2.1 Training

Having reviewed your role and reflected upon education and training deficits in relation to this, undertake some research into courses you may wish to embark upon in order to increase your knowledge about an area of your role.

AC 2.2 Prioritise development goals and targets to meet expected standards

The preceding ACs should have provided you with an opportunity to:

- review your role and its requirements according to standards
- review the requirements of those in your team

In practice

2.2 Prioritising development goals and targets to meet expected standards

Think about specific development goals that you have, to meet expected standards.

a What was the timescale you had to achieve these?

b What informed your decision to prioritise these?

- reflect on education and training deficits in relation to roles
- think about a range of different ways of developing the team.

You should now be ready to pull together all of this information in order to draw up a professional development plan for yourself. Once you have done this it is important that you assist members of your team to write their plans. This will then enable you to draw up an organisational plan and assess the viability and the contribution that development activities could make to the enhancement of the organisation. This is covered in AC 3.2.

As a manager it is your responsibility to ensure that staff development both meets organisational needs and priorities and supports and motivates individual team members' personal and professional development. A good development plan will fulfil both requirements. It will identify and prioritise development goals and targets to meet the standards and will address and avert potential risks resulting from knowledge or skills deficits. It will enhance service delivery and develop staff's personal and professional capacities. It should be realistic and recognise any limitations but also strive to be ambitious. It is important to achieve a balance between what can properly be supported and to devise creative strategies to achieve more. It must be fair: opportunities must be fairly distributed across the team and across all levels of staff. It must result in tangible outcomes and consequently staff who are developed must be enabled to share and/or implement their learning. Consequently, when designing your plan, you will need to build in evaluative measures to ensure that you are fulfilling your obligations and objectives.

LO3 Be able to prepare a professional development plan

AC 3.1 Select learning opportunities to meet development objectives and reflect personal learning style

First, what do you know about yourself? How do you like to learn? Individuals learn in different ways and you should think about the method that suits your preferred learning style so that, where possible, you can select appropriate learning activities.

Think about different learning activities you have participated in. Do you like discussion and working with others? Do you prefer tutor guidance? Do you like exploring and learning on your own? Are computer programs a style of learning that you enjoy? If you enjoy the process of learning, you are more likely to stick with it, particularly if it is over a period of time. Your understanding of what development activities suit your learning style means you are likely to get more from your learning.

Having identified your strengths, deficits, training needs and ideas for service enhancements, it is important that these are transformed into tangible actions that can be articulated as objectives. Objectives are statements that describe what the end point of an activity will be. Objectives should be written with the **SMART** acronym in mind; that is, they should be **S**pecific, **M**easurable, **A**ttainable, **R**elevant and **T**imebound. When writing your objectives you should have the end in mind before you start. Think of it as a journey – it is not often that you set out on a journey not knowing where you want to end up. When travelling, you also plan how you are going to get there and you reflect, albeit informally, on how successful your plan was. You may choose a tried-and-tested means of getting to an important occasion, but if you have a lot of time and no specific arrival time, you may be a little more adventurous in selecting your mode of transport. Setting learning objectives is analogous to planning a journey. Your plan must be able to deliver what you set out to do and you must evaluate how successful you have been. Consequently, having more information on which you can base your plan should secure the best chance of success.

What information do you need in order to develop a good plan?

In practice

3.1 Learning styles that meet development objectives and reflect personal learning style

What is your preferred learning style?

Try to remember your most satisfying and least satisfying learning experiences. What was it that made them satisfying or not?

Honey and Mumford (1992) developed a questionnaire that enables participants to distinguish between four key ways of learning. Many have a dominant style, but equally many have more than one.

- **Activists** – prefer to work intuitively, be flexible and spontaneous, generate new ideas and try things out. They like to learn from problem solving, discussion, group work and experience.
- **Reflectors** – like to watch/listen and reflect, gathering data and taking time to consider options and alternatives. They like lectures, project work and information research.
- **Theorists** – prefer to go through things thoroughly and logically, step by step. They like guidelines and prefer to learn from books, problem solving and discussion.
- **Pragmatists** – learn by 'trying things out'. They are practical and realistic, and like work-based learning and practical application in real settings.

Is it helpful to identify your preferred style?

Think about the characteristics of your team. Can you identify their different learning styles?

Now think about the learning opportunities and development objectives that best reflect the preferred styles of learning.

If individuals can be matched with their preferred style it will make learning easier for them. Inevitably, this cannot always be fully accommodated, but knowing one's style will help appropriate planning.

AC 3.2 Produce a plan for own professional development, using an appropriate source of support

Once you understand how you like to learn, you then need to articulate what you need to learn and identify how this can be achieved. Identifying needs and areas for improvement can amount to nothing more than a 'wish list' – 'wouldn't it be nice if ...'. Time spent reflecting on these wishes will help you to prioritise your development needs. Once you have identified your needs these must be articulated as objectives. It is important that objectives are prioritised and committed to paper in the form of a plan.

Developing a formal plan serves a number of purposes. It enables you to:

- structure and prioritise your learning and development.
- set short- and long-term goals (using the SMART model)
- address those things that you must do, such as update your knowledge and skills
- start to devise a more creative and personalised plan.

Remember, the short-term goals may or may not contribute to the longer-term ones. Writing your

In practice

3.2 Producing a professional development plan using sources of support

Use the template below (or one similar) to develop your professional development plan. Ensure that you write objectives that can be measured and evaluated. Clearly articulate the evidence that will demonstrate whether or not you have achieved your objectives.

Overall learning development need	What specifically do you need to know/learn?			
Objectives	Date for achievement	How will you achieve your objective?	Support required	Evidence and outcomes
What specific end or steps do you have in mind? You must include a measurable verb in each objective statement in this column, e.g. *Pass an accredited first aid course.*	When will you assess progress? When will you have achieved your objective? E.g. *dates of course/ training.*	How will you demonstrate that you have met the objective? E.g. *attend a first aid course.*	Human? Financial? Time? Learning resources?	What evidence will you have to confirm your achievement? E.g. *certificate of competence?*
Avoiding barriers and blockers	What positive steps can you take to avoid barriers?			
Objective 1 Example Develop IT skills to enable effective forward planning and publication of staff rotas for off-duty cover.	September this year.	Complete course on using Microsoft Excel.	Either day release to attend course or time to undertake online programme	Publication of all off-duty rotas using computerised support packages. Staff cover will be effective and planned and produced four weeks in advance.

What positive steps can you take to avoid barriers and blockers?

Identify need and actual and potential benefits for the organisation. Research and present different methods of achieving goal, with pros and cons identified. Discuss with and gain commitment from line manager through signed agreement or financial support to enable attendance/completion of the course. Report progress.

objectives in a plan adds weight and structure to them and you are more likely to act on them, especially if the plan is shared with another person, such as a line manager who may commit to supporting it.

When prioritising your objectives, think about how much you want to do something. Before embarking on development activities, you should be clear about what you are prepared to invest in achieving the goals that you set. This may include decisions about your personal motivations, and the time you are prepared to make available, which is likely to be in addition to anything your employer will provide. You must be realistic about resources and in particular the financial burdens and who will be responsible for them. It is also important to acknowledge the potential impact that education and development can have on those around you, both at home and at work. This can be as a result of support that others must provide or in view of the change that may occur in you as a result of the development. You must be realistic about these factors, but that does not mean you should not also have aspirations and set an ambitious plan.

A successful professional development plan will:

- clearly specify how the objectives will be achieved
- identify the timeframes and milestones against which progress can be measured
- suggest criteria against which the activity can be evaluated.

Personal goals for staff should be part of an organisation's goals. Although there may be barriers to developing the staff, plans must be put in place to overcome those barriers and these plans need to be reviewed and changed if necessary. It is a requirement of the CQC that settings have systems in place for staff development.

AC 3.3 Establish a process to evaluate the effectiveness of the plan

Evaluating the effectiveness of staff development enables the manager to assess the value of the investment and make responsible decisions for the future.

First, you should establish whether the objectives you set have been met. Second, what evidence do you have that they have been met? If the activity

was designed to teach the acquisition of a skill, it is relatively easy to assess whether the activity was successful. However, some educational development activities are more intangible, more difficult to assess and may take longer to see any benefit, such as changes in attitude, behaviour and practice. You may be able to assess specific elements of learning, for example an increased knowledge base.

In order to assess the effectiveness of a new practice, there must be an opportunity to use it effectively and its implementation may need to be trialled and supported within the workplace. If the learning requires a change in behaviour or practice, the conditions need to exist to enable that change to be implemented. As a manager you need to think of strategies that can support that change and where relevant, demonstrate to others the benefits of that change.

If the development activity has failed to meet the objectives set, it is equally important to assess why these have not been achieved. Were the objectives realistic? If they were, question why they have not been achieved.

Monitoring and reviewing

Development plans are living documents. Priorities for training and education needs are not static but must be revised and rewritten on the basis of changing requirements, new practice and research evidence and altered expectations, as well as following completion or review of objectives. Plans can be formally reviewed at appraisal meetings but can also be updated to take account of any ad hoc learning opportunities. Many practitioners are required by their profession to keep records of their personal professional development in order to demonstrate their fitness to practise. A well-worked-through plan will provide good evidence of ongoing and simultaneous engagement with continuing professional development requirements.

Key term

Evaluation is to judge the worth or value of something, to make an assessment of it, its importance, or effectiveness.

LO4 Be able to improve performance through reflective practice

AC 4.1 Compare models of reflective practice

Reflective practice is an essential element of personal development. It provides an opportunity to stop and take stock. Bolton (2010, p. 4) identifies a number of applications for reflective practice. Reflective practice enables you to:

- identify what you know but do not know that you know
- identify what you want to know but do not know
- reflect on what you think feel, believe, value
- examine how well actions match up to beliefs
- reflect on barriers to practising the way that you would wish to practise
- think about what you should/can change in your work context and how this could be achieved
- learn how to value others' perspectives even when they differ from your own
- examine your personal behaviours and responses and seek ways to make these more productive.

Jasper, 2006

Jasper (2006, p. 40) sees reflective practice as an essential means of professional growth and development that enables practitioners to develop basic skills and knowledge into expert skills and knowledge. Inevitably, simple repetition of a skill should enable a practitioner to be more competent in its performance. However, reflective analysis about that performance enables you to identify more quickly specific areas for improvement or gaps in your knowledge. A good analogy is to think about the strategies used by elite sportsmen and women – they record, replay and analyse both their own and others' performance in order to identify their strengths and improve them and eliminate substandard practice. Reflection in care work provides a similar opportunity to assist practitioners to improve their performance and that of the teams they work with. While it is not undertaken by video analysis, it can be done by writing a record of events or by analysing current practice against desired practice.

Schon, 1983

Reflective practice is a conscious activity that results in positive decisions. Reflection has gained significant weight in recent years in the health care arena and a number of models have been developed to assist practitioners to reflect. Reflective practice was first coined by Donald Schon (1983). He identified that learning in practice could be enhanced by two different kinds of activity: reflection in-action and reflection on-action:

- *Reflection in-action* requires practitioners to 'think ahead', to critically reflect on what one is doing while one is doing it and to revise actions in the light of that reflection (Greenwood, 1993).
- *Reflection on-action* is a retrospective activity that requires practitioners to interpret and analyse recalled information from activities that they have been engaged with (Boyd and Fales, 1983; Fitzgerald, 1994; Atkins and Murphy, 1994).

Models of reflection are normally illustrated as cyclical activities, such as those depicted in Figure 2.2 and Figure 2.3.

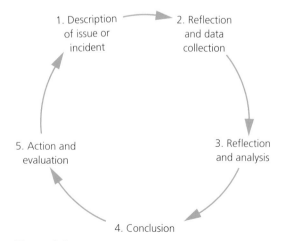

Figure 2.2

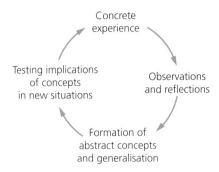

Figure 2.3 (Models of reflection based on Gibbs, and Kolb)

Many models are constructed around the use of structured questions to prompt reflection in a logical and systematic manner (Johns, 1995). These questions are often focused on incident analysis as the key method of reflecting (Gibbs, 1988). This approach entails practitioners selecting a significant incident, writing about it in detail and then analysing what happened, asking why, and identifying what additional knowledge would have enabled the practitioner to behave differently. It requires the reflector to explore what evidence there is that similar things have been addressed by others more effectively and to establish what learning can be drawn from the experience.

It enables practitioners to be better prepared when faced with similar experiences in the future, as well as providing an opportunity to identify shortcomings in knowledge or skills which can be rectified.

Choose a model that suits your learning needs

Different models of reflection suit different learning styles and different purposes. A model is a tool to provide structure to an activity and it is important that you select one that suits your style. The significant thing to remember is that whichever model is selected, it is the learning that results from the activity that is the significant thing. Learning that is either confirmation that behaviour is appropriate or learning that suggests a need to gain more information or change practice.

In practice

4.1 Compare models of reflective practice

Compare different models of reflective practice and reflect on their benefits and drawbacks. Which do you think you would find most useful in your professional context?

Your role as a manager

As a manager of a team, teaching and encouraging staff to be self-reflecting is very important. However, reflection need not just relate to isolated and specific incidents. Reflection in-action can be a powerful tool. It can be used to improve practice by supporting individuals to question their routine work as they carry it out. They may measure their behaviour against their values and the values of the organisation to ensure that these are consistent. Or they may try a new approach to an activity and evaluate its success. Encouraging staff to become self-governing and to take responsibility for their work standards is an important element of a successful learning organisation. Reflective practice provides an opportunity for all practitioners to check their own standards of work and enhance practice.

AC 4.2, 4.3 Explain the importance of reflective practice to improve performance and use reflective practice and feedback from others to improve performance

Reflective practice is invaluable as a staff development tool. Once individuals learn to be reflective they can begin to take responsibility for their learning and to identify their learning needs. That is not to suggest that reflective practice does not need managerial support to enable you to take the outcomes from reflective practice forward; it often does.

Reflective exemplar

During my course I have been told I need to write a reflective journal and to some extent this scares me. It has been explained to us that reflection is important if we are to improve our practice and also the practice of those in the team. As a manager I am a little concerned that I may not be reflecting on the right things and not able to answer questions properly. I wrote a small journal piece about a staff appraisal I did at work and then asked my tutor to read it.

During the appraisal I realised that I was quite concerned about the impact my lack of confidence would have on the member of staff. I have only completed a couple of staff appraisals and so was trying hard to ensure that I had all the relevant paper work and was completing the documents correctly. This led to me not really listening to the member of staff and I missed a lot of what he was saying because I had my head in the writing! I found I was trying too hard to present myself as a confident manager when in fact I felt less worthy than that. Following that particular session I had a bit of a panic! I wondered what the staff would

think of me and if I would ever get this part of my job right.

Feedback from the tutor

This account is descriptive but there is some evidence of reflection. At the start you refer to a past event – a staff appraisal- but you have not considered how other prior experiences such as your own appraisals could have impacted upon your own attempt here. Have you perhaps learned to document appraisals in this way because of your own experience?

You do comment upon how you felt at this time which is good but it might have been useful here to say what the member of staff thought of the appraisal session. Did you ask him? After the session you say you felt panicked and I was left wondering what this was like and what impact it had on you as a team leader? Did you ask the staff member what he felt like at the end of the appraisal? How did you think it might affect the other staff? What made you immediately consider that this part of your job was not right? Did you even consider that this was a good appraisal?

Case study

4.3 Using reflective practice to improve performance

Charlotte is the deputy manager of a domiciliary service. Recently she has noticed that one member of staff seems to be having issues with punctuality and a complaint has been issued by the service user. She undertakes supervision with the member of staff who denies being late and dismissed the allegation as untrue. Charlotte deals with the situation but now feels unsure about how effective she was and is concerned about the decisions she made. She approaches her own manager for some feedback and the manager asks Charlotte to reflect upon the events that led to the decisions she made.

1 Why do you think Charlotte's manager asked her to do this?
2 What would you say is valuable about reflective practice?

Reflective practice is a tool that can be used by all practitioners, individually, to enhance their practice. It can also be used as a management

tool, enabling managers to guide and support staff to reflect on key elements of their role and their performance. Prompts such as 'You did that really well. What was it that made that such a successful activity?' are useful. This approach develops individuals' self-esteem, confidence and a questioning and critical approach to their work. Reflection provides an ideal vehicle of learning that can be shared within the wider team. Teams can reflect as a group, particularly if they are keen to examine or change an aspect of practice which they have in common, and can also share their learning with others.

Reflective practice as a tool to improve performance

Inevitably, when we reflect, no matter how candid we try to be, it is difficult to see the world from anything other than our own perspective. Reflection may require that we seek opinions and information from others to validate our reflections and to help us to see whether any change is required. While information gained in this way can be seen as threatening, if managed and used sensitively, 360-degree feedback can be illuminating and can challenge and refocus our perceptions of reality.

360-degree reflection

360-degree reflection asks us to reflect on our behaviours and performance once we have gathered information from a range of individuals, both those in positions of authority and those over whom you have authority. You contain the threat by selecting those people who will be honest but who can be trusted to feed back responsibly and constructively. It is important that you do not only ask your friends – they are likely to tell you what you want to hear rather than what you need to know. To gain the most from the activity, you need to know how different people experience you and your actions. Learning about how others perceive and experience you, your actions, attitudes and behaviours can be empowering and being self-aware leads to growth both personally and professionally. Getting all-round 360-degree feedback may provide you with insight about the following:

- **A façade** – information that suggests that you are better or worse at something than you think you are.
- **A blind spot** – information that you did not know about yourself.
- **A suggestion** about something that you could easily do which would make a positive difference.
- **An opportunity** to stop doing something.

360-feedback is usually built around a questionnaire as this helps the individual to control the areas on which they want feedback.

The criteria for choosing the wording of questionnaires for 360-feedback reflect general principles when designing performance appraisal systems and criteria, and include the following points:

- Questions should be relevant to the recipient's job.
- Each question should be concise, use plain English and omit qualifiers, such as 'when appropriate' and 'as necessary'. Vague and complex questions rarely produce clear feedback.
- Each question should relate to a clearly defined competency or function to avoid muddled feedback. It must be specific.
- Questions should set clear and appropriate standards. For example, 'makes decisions' is a

In practice

4.2, 4.3 Importance of reflective practice and improving performance

Prepare a PowerPoint presentation to staff to explain the importance of reflective practice to improve performance and demonstrate how you have used reflective practice and feedback from others to improve an aspect of your own performance.

poor criterion as the decisions made could be unclear, late or wrong. A better statement might be 'makes timely and effective decisions'.

Open questions provide the opportunity to add comments in support of the answers to the rated questions and, as such, can be particularly helpful. The recipient is able to look for frequently used words or phrases and for common themes. When wording such questions, it is important to use clear language, for example, 'what does the recipient do well?' and 'what does the recipient need to improve?'

Source: CIPD Factsheet 360 Degree Feedback, www.cipd.co.uk/hr-resources/factsheets/360-degree-feedback.aspx#link_furtherreading

AC 4.4 Evaluate how practice has been improved through reflection on best practice, and failures and mistakes

There is a great deal of emphasis on evidence-based practice and best practice. This is another means of reflection. It has involved somebody identifying an issue and researching it in order to generate evidence. Best practice is to analyse the different ways of doing things in order to identify whether there is a preferred way of undertaking the activity. Access to up-to-date learning resources is important in supporting staff to keep abreast of new evidence and best practice.

Inevitably, identifying mistakes or near mistakes and assessing whether or not these could have been avoided is an important activity. It is important that this is seen as a productive activity and not a punitive or disciplinary one. Its primary focus is about learning from an incident or set of behaviours in order that changes can be made to improve issues. The most significant examples of this are big public and government inquiries, which are called when serious failures and mistakes in public services are identified, such as Alderhay, the Stafford Enquiry, and Baby P. In each case it has been identified that staff failed to follow procedures and protocols, that there were lapses in expected standards of care, and that there was a failure in anyone taking responsibility and reporting these lapses. Ideally, if organisations and individuals practise reflectively then public inquiries of this type should never be needed.

On a smaller scale, investigations into minor mistakes and accidents are designed to enable learning from reflection on the circumstances that allowed an accident or mistake to happen. Importantly, getting the balance between investigation, reflection and assigning blame is crucial. If staff feel they are going to be unfairly blamed or punished for mistakes, it may prevent them from reporting them or coming forward with concerns. An organisation that supports its staff to raise concerns, to acknowledge deficits and to report mistakes is much more likely to be a

Reflect on it

4.4 Raising concerns

Think about the opportunities that exist in your organisation for staff to raise concerns, question practices or acknowledge mistakes. Are these formal or informal?

learning organisation than one where this is not the primary culture. An open organisation provides the conditions for someone to acknowledge and investigate and to reflect on how things can be improved or done differently.

Legislation

Expectations of standards of care are set out in codes of practice and codes of conduct, and codes articulate the standards of care that the public can expect to receive. Revisit relevant codes of practice as well as the Care Quality Commission's Essential Standards of Quality and Safety.

With respect to law, the Data Protection Act (1998) is useful here, as is the Care Act 2014 (see Unit SHC 51).

In practice

4.4 How practice is improved through reflection

Draw on a real example of a failure, a mistake of a standard of practice, or a practice that required change, and write a report that answers the following:

- What happened?
- Was the incident reported to senior staff?
- If the incident was reported to senior staff, who did they (senior staff) report it to and why that individual (or agency)?

- How was the individual perceived?
- What actions resulted from the incident?
- Are policies and protocols fit for purpose?
- If a similar thing occurred again, are you confident that employees feel sufficiently well supported to report the issue?
- What changes could you make in order to make it easier for staff to raise issues that can improve service and help to manage risks?

Assessment methods

LO	Assessment criteria and accompanying activities	Assessment methods *To evidence coverage of the ACs you could:*
LO1	1.1 In practice (p. 30)	Provide a written account answering the questions outlined in the activity. Or you could undertake a piece of research and write a statement about the professional activities you and the team have undertaken over the year. Ensure that you comment upon the changes that have impacted upon your work in Health and Social Care. Make sure you summarise the importance of continuously improving knowledge and practice.

LO	Assessment criteria and accompanying activities	Assessment methods *To evidence coverage of the ACs you could:*
	1.2 Reflect on it (p. 31)	Write a short reflective account of how the potential barriers to professional development affect the outcomes for service users.
	1.2 In practice (p. 31)	Identify the potential barriers to undertaking professional development in your workplace and then set up an action plan to overcome them. A table has been included to help you.
	1.3 In practice (p. 33)	Think about which of the following functions of personal development planning are important within your organisation and complete the table in the activity.
	1.3 Research it (p. 35)	Research Cooperrider et al.'s model. Discuss with your team how useful this would be as a strategy for professional development. Write a short report of the discussion for your portfolio.
	1.4 In practice (p. 36)	Reflect on your own organisation and the range of factors to consider when selecting opportunities and activities for keeping knowledge and practice up to date. Write a piece on factors you need to consider in selecting opportunities and activities for keeping knowledge and practice up to date together with the risk of not sustaining staff motivation and morale.
	1.4 Research it (p. 37)	Research Senge's (1990) five key dimensions for a successful learning organisation and those noted by the Institute of Management Services (www.ims-productivity.com/page.cfm/content/Learning-Organisation). Answer the questions in the activity.
LO2	2.1 Reflect on it (p. 38)	Reflect on your own job role/description and make a list of the essential skills and qualities necessary for someone to fulfil that role effectively. Have a professional discussion with your assessor about any requirements in the role for which you feel less confident of your skills to fulfil adequately?
	2.1 In practice (p. 38)	For your portfolio list the codes and standards that guide and govern your role. Then answer the questions outlined in the activity.
	2.1 Research it (p. 38)	Having reviewed your role and reflected upon education and training deficits in relation to this, undertake some research into courses you may wish to embark upon in order to increase your knowledge about an area of your role.
	2.2 In practice (p. 38)	Write a statement that identifies your learning goals. You could then show how they match the standards you need to meet or answer the questions in the activity.
LO3	3.1 In practice (p. 39)	Complete a learning style questionnaire such as that available at http://www.brainboxx.co.uk/a3_aspects/pages/vak_quest.htm. Alternatively answer the questions in the activity and place the answers into your portfolio.
	3.2 In practice (p. 40)	Following supervision or appraisal, obtain a copy of your professional development plan or if there is not one available compile your own using the template in the activity (or one similar) to develop your PDP. Ensure that you write objectives that can be measured and evaluated. Clearly articulate the evidence that will demonstrate whether or not you have achieved your objectives.

LO	Assessment criteria and accompanying activities	Assessment methods *To evidence coverage of the ACs you could:*
	3.3 In practice (p. 42)	Engage with your assessor and ask for a professional discussion in which you can Evaluate your own development plan and show how you have met your targets. See the activity for further guidance.
LO4	4.1 In practice (p. 43)	You might write a report on two different models of reflective practice and comment on their benefits and drawbacks. Discuss with your assessor which you think you would find most useful in your professional context?
	4.3 In practice (p. 44)	Provide a written account answering the questions in the case study.
	4.2, 4.3 In practice (p. 45)	Prepare a PowerPoint presentation for staff to explain the importance of reflective practice to improve performance and demonstrate how you have used reflective practice and feedback from others to improve an aspect of your own performance. Alternatively, provide a piece of reflective writing from your journal.
	4.4 Reflect on it (p. 46)	Think about the opportunities that exist in your organisation for staff to raise concerns, question practices or acknowledge mistakes. Are these formal or informal?
	4.4 In practice (p. 46)	You might include a reflection on the opportunities that exist in your organisation for staff to raise concerns, question practices or acknowledge mistakes, or a report on a real example of a failure, mistake or required change of or standard of practice, and how it was resolved and discuss these with your assessor. Alternatively, you could draw on a real example of a failure, a mistake of a standard of practice, or a practice that required change, and write a report that answers the questions in the activity.

References

Bolton, G. (2010) *Reflective Practice: Writing and professional development* (3e). London: Sage Publishing.

Bowden, J. (2004) *Writing a Report: How to prepare, write and present effective reports* (7e). Oxford: How to Books.

CIPD (2011) CIPD Factsheet 360 Degree Feedback, www.cipd.co.uk/hr-resources/factsheets/360-degree-feedback.aspx#link_furtherreading

Clutterbuck, D. and Megginson, D. (1999) *Mentoring Executives and Directors*. Oxford: Butterworth-Heinemann.

Cooperrider, D., Whitney, D. and Stavros, J. (2003) *The Appreciative Inquiry Handbook*. San Francisco: Berrett-Koehler.

Department of Health (2004) *The NHS Knowledge and Skills Framework and Development Review Guidance – Working Draft Version 7*. London: Department of Health. www.dh.gov.uk

Department of Health (2013) *The Cavendish Review: An Independent Review into Healthcare Assistants and Support Workers in the NHS and Social Care Settings*. London HMSO.

Duncan, P. (2007) *Critical Perspectives on Health*. Basingstoke: Palgrave Macmillan.

Gibbs, G. (1988) *Learning by Doing: A guide to teaching and learning methods*. Oxford: Oxford Further Education Unit.

Greenwood, J. (1993) 'Reflective practice: a critique of the work of Argyris & Schon,' *Journal of Advanced Nursing*, 19, 1183–7.

Harrison, R. (2009) *Learning and Development* (5e). London: Chartered Institute for Personnel and Development.

Health Professions Council (2008) *Standards of Conduct, Performance and Ethics*. London: HPC.

Jasper, M. (2006) *Professional Development, Reflection and Decision-Making*. Oxford: Blackwell Publishing.

Johns, C. (1995) 'Framing learning through reflection within Carper's fundamental ways of knowing in nursing,' *Journal of Advanced Nursing*, 22, 226–34.

Leitch, S. (2006) *Leitch Review of Skills*. London: HM Treasury.

Nursing and Midwifery Council (2015) *The Code: Professional standards of practice and behaviour for nurses and midwives.* London: NMC.

Senge, P., Kleiner, A., Roberts, C., Ross, R. and Smith, B. (1994) *The Fifth Discipline Fieldbook: Strategies and tools for building a learning organisation.* New York: Doubleday.

Skills for care (2011) *Capable, Confident, Skilled: A workforce development strategy for people working, supporting and caring in adult social care.* Leeds: Skills for Care.

Whitmore, J. (2009) *Coaching for Performance. GROWing people, performance and purpose* (4e). London: Nicholas Brealey.

Further reading and useful resources

Atkins, S. and Murphy, K. (1994) 'Reflective practice,' *Nursing Standard*, 8 (39), 49–54.

Boyd, E. and Fales, A. (1983) 'Reflective learning: the key to learning from experience,' *Journal of Humanistic Psychology*, 23 (2), 99–117.

Fitzgerald, M. (1994) 'Theories of reflection for learning' in *Reflective Practice in Nursing*, Palmer, A. and Burns, S. (eds) Oxford: Blackwell Scientific.

The Skills for Care (2011) *Capable, Confident, Skilled*. London, SfC.

http://www.skillsforhealth.org.uk/standards/item/217-code-of-conduct

Unit SHC 53

Champion equality, diversity and inclusion

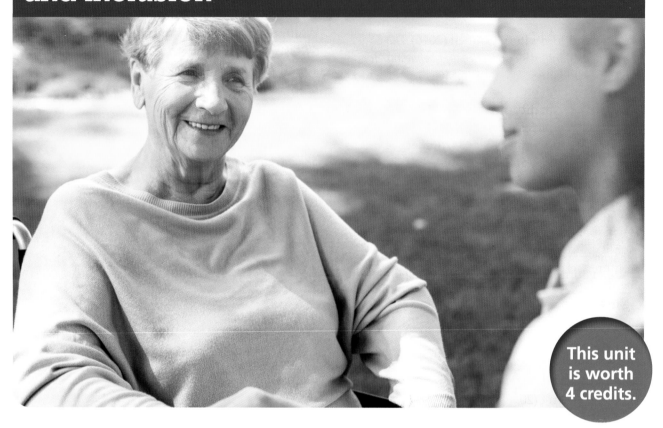

This unit is worth 4 credits.

Understanding and acceptance of others are essential attributes for anyone working within a health and social care setting as you will be supporting people from diverse cultural backgrounds and it is important to ensure that everybody is treated on an equal footing, regardless of their differences. This unit will help you to develop strategies for implementing and leading excellent practice in respect of equality, diversity and inclusion within health and social care contexts.

Learning outcomes

By the end of this unit you will:

1 Understand diversity, equality and inclusion within own area of responsibility.
2 Be able to champion diversity, equality and inclusion.
3 Understand how to develop systems and processes that promote diversity, equality and inclusion.
4 Be able to manage the risks presented when balancing individual rights and professional duty of care.

LO1 Understand diversity, equality and inclusion within own area of responsibility

AC 1.1 Explain models of practice that underpin equality, diversity and inclusion in own area of responsibility

The importance of understanding equality, respect for diversity and inclusion in care work cannot be overestimated. It is important that practice in your setting is reinforced by the principles of equality and diversity and that staff are aware of policies and procedures and it is your responsibility as a manager to ensure all of this. This can be done through training and meetings, for example.

Equality

The manager has a key role in ensuring that equality and anti-discriminatory practice are promoted as a key organisational value and that the law is complied with. Public sector organisations and other organisations that carry out public functions, such as in the health and social care sector, must have 'due regard' to eliminate conduct that is prohibited under the Equality Act.

The Equality Act (2010) provides for the protection of people and their different characteristics, with specific protections in respect of:

- age
- disability
- gender reassignment
- pregnancy and maternity/paternity
- race
- religion or belief
- sex/gender
- sexual orientation.

Legislation will inform practice and this is covered in AC 1.3.

Promoting, implementing and monitoring good equality practices will reduce the likelihood of unlawful discrimination and legal challenge. But what are the models of practice that underpin equality, diversity and inclusion in your area of responsibility?

Value differences

People possess different characteristics – being different is what makes humans so interesting. Some characteristics can pose particular challenges for individuals or can be seen as a challenge by others. The law makes it explicit that these characteristics are not an excuse for substandard treatment of services and requires that reasonable adjustments are made to ensure equality of opportunity. If care workers are to meet needs effectively, they must engage with people as unique individuals and recognise their differences in order to plan to address their specific needs. An aim of good care is that people are treated with equality regardless of their differences.

Treat people fairly

What does equality mean? It does not mean treating everyone the same – treating people with equality means treating people fairly. Fairness requires that individuals receive equally good standards of service and similar consideration and respect. This may mean that actions must be modified to address specific disadvantages in order that the same standard of service is delivered. For example, an individual who has a learning difficulty may need different resources and a different approach to help them understand and consent to a procedure than someone without a learning difficulty. The Equality Act requires both that people understand the procedure they are about to undergo and that the explanation is tailored, or reasonable adjustments are made, to effectively take account of different characteristics.

Ensuring a positive organisational culture

It is important that a positive organisational culture is developed, which reflects and reinforces

Key terms

Equality means treating individuals or groups of individuals fairly and equally irrespective of race, gender, disability, religion or belief, sexual orientation and age.

Diversity in this context is equal respect for people who are from different backgrounds.

Inclusion is positive behaviour to ensure all people have an opportunity to be included and not be unfairly excluded because of their individual characteristics.

a commitment to valuing diversity. The challenge is to ensure that everybody knows what the values and resulting policies of the organisation are and how they are expected to adopt these in their work. Staff cannot be expected to enact values that they are not aware of. An explicit and transparent statement of values must be discussed with staff and made available to the public, thus providing a clear indication of expectations of behaviours. Second, discussion of what this actually means in practice is important in helping staff to make the link from expressed values, which may seem intangible, into real practice. In successful organisations there is a clear correlation between espoused values and the ethical leadership of that organisation's leaders on the successful realisation of values within an organisation (Renz and Eddy, 1996). That is to say, it is essential that the leaders are seen to live and enact the values.

Take an equal opportunities approach

Applying the principle of equality requires practitioners to take a very active stance to ensure that systems, processes and practices do not inadvertently disadvantage anyone. To promote equality it is necessary to understand that all individuals should be afforded equal opportunities to achieve positive outcomes. The equal opportunities approach to equality strives to cancel out disadvantage. This means that barriers must, where possible, be removed, or that positive interventions are implemented to invalidate those things that create disadvantage.

An equal opportunities approach requires that all individuals are offered the same or relevantly similar opportunities. This is known as reasonable adjustment. The law requires that reasonable adjustments are anticipated in advance rather than met only when an issue arises. Legal enforcement of equal opportunity has been very effective in significantly changing behaviours in respect of tolerance and engagement with difference and diversity and has had significant success in improving equality and inclusion.

Key term

Equal opportunity is the principle of having fair and similar opportunities in life to other people and ensuring people are not discriminated against on the basis of individual characteristics.

Diversity

Diversity and equality can be seen as two sides of the same coin. Equality involves fairness and diversity involves valuing difference (Thompson, 2011, p. 9). Thompson points out that what connects equality and difference is not the level of equality or the fact that something is different, it is the discriminatory response that the inequality or difference provokes in others. For example, different and diverse characteristics should not matter – it should not matter if someone has differently coloured hair, unless someone takes issue with the person on the basis of their hair colour. Difference matters only when you are treated differently purely because of that difference. Anti-discrimination legislation anticipates that individuals' differences may cause them to be unlawfully discriminated against and puts in place penalties for breaches. Equal opportunities takes a more proactive and positive approach. So, the legislation punishes the breach whereas equal opportunities encourages people to see difference as something to celebrate rather than something to be tolerated or enforced by law.

Walker (1994, p. 212, adapted) identified that the difference and diversity model for promoting equality is based on four key principles:

- People function best when they feel valued.
- People feel more valued when they believe their individual and group differences have been taken into account.
- The ability to learn from those who are different is the key to becoming empowered.
- When people are valued and empowered they can work independently and together to build relationships and build capacity.

Reflect on it

1.1 Equality, diversity and difference

Think about the approach taken to equality, diversity and difference in your own organisation. Is it a model based on rules that see inequality as barriers to be overcome, or does it frame equality as a celebration of difference?

What do you think are the advantages and disadvantages of the two approaches in your organisational context?

1.1 Models of practice that underpin equality, diversity and inclusion

What models of practice underpinning equality, diversity and inclusion do you favour and why? Write a short piece to show your understanding.

In tackling inequality, there is a danger that we may focus on the celebration of difference yet fail to address the underlying social inequalities and barriers that construct difference as a problem.

Inclusion

Inclusion ensures that people feel they belong and are connected irrespective of race, gender, disability or other attributes which can be perceived as different. It includes being valued and respected and removing discriminatory practice.

In order to uphold the law and to practice ethically, the equality, diversity and inclusion policies and procedures you have in place can be used to provide guidance.

AC 1.2 Analyse the potential effects of barriers to equality and inclusion in own area of responsibility

Ensuring that equality, diversity and inclusion are effectively embedded within an organisation requires that all staff in all roles embrace and implement these principles. The role of the manager is crucial in identifying and removing barriers to the implementation of these principles.

All organisations have their own culture or, as Thompson (2011, p. 199) suggests, a 'symbolic universe' in which a shared set of meanings, beliefs, values, norms and practices is based. More simply, 'the way we do things'.

Barriers and their effects
Values, beliefs and attitudes
People's values, beliefs and attitudes are often deeply ingrained and are acquired through learning and our upbringing. We are encouraged to believe that certain attitudes and behaviours are acceptable. It is only when these values, beliefs and attitudes are challenged, either by new information

or different experiences, that they may be seen to be flawed. Even when individuals' views can be shown to be discriminatory, deeply held beliefs may be resistant to change and this is termed prejudice.

Prejudice
A prejudice is an attitude or belief that is based on a faulty and inflexible generalisation/belief which can lead to negative emotions and discriminatory actions. Prejudice does not necessarily cause someone to discriminate unfairly, but examining such beliefs and values and questioning them is a first step in recognising and tackling prejudice.

There is more information on discrimination and challenging this in LO2 and on exclusion in AC 2.2.

The second step in eliminating prejudice is to redefine beliefs and attitudes in the light of new information. The third is to change behaviour in the light of that information, and the fourth is to challenge others who articulate similar prejudices.

None of these steps is easy, particularly the latter; however, challenging others can have a significant impact on breaking down discrimination and prejudice. Often prejudice is not only an individual issue but represents views that might be more widely held within a group or specific context. When a strong, widespread belief is apparent, challenge is difficult and individuals who try to challenge it may fear ridicule, victimisation or reprisals if they stand up against the prevailing beliefs and practices. In an organisation it is important that everyone is aware that prejudice and discriminatory practice cannot be tolerated. Individuals who become aware of such practice must be supported and protected to speak out. Creating a culture of discussion and tolerance is important in developing an open-minded community and in preventing abusive practice.

Prejudice can lead to unacceptable behaviours, including harassment, bullying and victimisation, as well as poor standards and abuse of power over others. Harassment, bullying and victimisation are all behaviours that individuals are protected against under the Equality Act (2010); it is important to remember that it is not just individuals and groups that can be prejudiced and discriminatory.

Structural, institutional and physical barriers

Thompson (2011, p. 32) points out that significant structural barriers exist that discriminate negatively on individuals. For example, there may be an unfair unwritten policy and agreement that women in their 20s and 30s are not employed in managerial posts because of the potential for them to leave or take maternity leave. Alternatively, the organisation that fails to provide accessible facilities for those in wheelchairs is discriminatory and in breach of the law.

Many organisations are constrained by the premises and resources available to them in developing completely fair facilities. However, this is not an excuse for doing nothing. The expectation is that reasonable adjustments must be made and while these adjustments may not be perfect, they must be fit for purpose. Failure to address such issues may oppress certain groups in society simply because they cannot access a building or a service, thus undermining confidence and self-esteem.

Key term

Prejudice is an unreasonable, pre-conceived judgement or conviction that is not based on knowledge, evidence or experience.

In practice

1.2 Potential effects of barriers to equality and inclusion

Identify the potential barriers to equality and inclusion in your own area of responsibility and analyse how they affect the service users and staff in your setting.

Research it

1.1, 1.2 Diversity, equality, inclusion

Carry out a small-scale research study in your own setting which looks at diversity, equality and inclusion. Identify the strengths and limitations within your area of practice and make recommendations for improvement.

AC 1.3 Analyse the impact of legislation and policy initiative on the promotion of equality, diversity and inclusion in your own area of responsibility

Legislation

The Equality Act (2010) clearly identifies that if a health or social care organisation provides goods, facilities, services or functions to the public then it must make sure that it does so within the requirements of the law. The Act brings together a number of individual pieces of legislation into one law in order to make the law on equality, diversity and discrimination much clearer and simpler.

The Equality Act 2010 applies to any organisation that provides goods, facilities or services to the public, or to a section of the public. The act applies to private, statutory and voluntary organisations, no matter what the size. Equality law affects everyone running an organisation as well as applying to the staff and volunteers that might do something on behalf of the organisation.

Additionally the Mental Capacity Act (MCA) 2005 empowers individuals who may lack the mental capacity to make their own decisions. The impact of this act for service users has been to liberate them for previous restrictive practices in which they had no say over their care or treatment. Forward planning can now be undertaken and advance statements about what will happen when the service user no longer had capacity to speak for themselves are put into place. There is more on this in AC 4.3.

In practice

1.3 Impact of legislation and policy

In your setting, analyse which law has had the most impact upon the care you give to your service users. For example, you may comment on how the MCA has changed the way you undertake assessment for care.

Case study

1.3 The Equality Act 2010

In each of the following cases identify whether you think discrimination has occurred and whether there is a case to appeal to the law through the Equality Act (2010).

- Mary, 62, applies for a job as a care assistant. Despite having previous experience in this area of work, she is not offered an interview. She is told that she has not been shortlisted for the position because of her age.
- Parminder attends a day centre. She overhears another attendee making comments about her skin colour and dress to a member of staff.
- Gemma has a long-standing disability and uses a wheelchair. She is required to attend meetings for the care company she works for, but these meetings are always held in an upstairs room in an old building with no lift. She finds being carried upstairs humiliating and has stopped attending the meetings. Her manager is adamant that she must attend.
- John has had a stroke and lives in a care home where he depends on care from others for his daily activities. He has cross-dressed for many years. Since his stroke, the care staff have refused to dress him in (his own) women's clothing, because they feel it will cause upset to the other residents.
- Wendy, a white, middle-class woman aged 40, has applied for a post in a women's refuge set up specifically to cater for young Asian women. The refuge is funded by the local Asian community. The advertisement specifically identified being Asian as a necessary characteristic.
- Julie has been off sick with depression for five months. While on sick leave and a week before she is due to return to work, Julie is invited for an interview with her manager, who suggests that she should hand in her resignation.

LO2 Be able to champion diversity, equality and inclusion

AC 2.1 Promote equality, diversity and inclusion in policy and practice

The culture of an organisation will have a powerful and pervasive influence over the behaviour and practices of the people within that organisation (Mullins, 2009).

Organisations are complicated places, where complex interactions occur between individuals. The complexity and interdependency of relationships support an environment in which conflicts of interest and power differentials can be abused if appropriate policies, practices and guards are not in place to counteract this.

Formal power structures are necessary in most organisations. These structures are supported by policies and procedures which provide a framework to help everyone to understand expectations and responsibilities. Power is exercised through management structures and is evident in an organisational hierarchy, role and position and sometimes by virtue of specialist knowledge or experience. Within this system, each layer has some exercise of power over those below them and this is acknowledged and understood by both those in leadership roles and those who are subordinates. Where individuals step outside the responsibilities of their role, those in leadership positions are legitimately empowered to take appropriate sanctions to ensure the smooth and effective running of the organisation. This type of power is legitimate and provides a framework for keeping the organisation running effectively. However, power operates also on an informal level.

Informal power is more difficult to understand because it is insidious, operates beneath the surface and is not formally acknowledged. Such power is not related to role or position – some people are natural leaders and have an innate ability to influence others, and this may be entirely independent of their position within the organisation. Where this is a positive, value-based influence it can be invaluable to the manager in spreading good practice. As manager you might use your position to encourage your staff to adopt anti-discriminatory and non-judgemental attitudes in their work by challenging discrimination that may come to your notice.

Research it

2.1 Championing equality, diversity and inclusion

Research an organisation other than your own and comment upon how it has championed diversity, equality and inclusion.

In practice

2.1 Promoting equality, diversity and inclusion

Write a short piece that shows how you as a manager promote equality, diversity and inclusion in policy and practice.

This can be accomplished through the manager providing a good role model demonstrating fairness and anti-discriminatory practice to all staff and service users. Discrimination should be challenged at all levels of the staff structure and staff need to feel that they are able to report practices they believe to be wrong. Though training sessions and supervision as well as clear job descriptions, staff will understand their role in relation to equality, diversity and inclusion.

Powerful personalities on the team may lead others negatively, encouraging them to cut corners, bend rules or manipulate situations for their own advantage. The impact of this may inevitably mean that service users and other members of staff are treated in an unfair manner and this will compromise the equality, diversity and inclusion of the service and the manager must then find strategies to minimise their influence.

Training and supervision

You may need to remind your staff about issues surrounding equality, diversity and inclusion at team meetings and update them on the policies and procedures. You can also recommend training to remind them of their duty with respect to equality, inclusion and diversity.

AC 2.2 Challenge discrimination and exclusion in policy and practice

Exclusion refers to the barring of somebody from a service or an activity or not allowing a group or an individual to join in due to a barrier of some sort.

In practice

2.2 Challenging discrimination and exclusion

1 Define what these forms of discrimination mean and identify examples of discrimination that could occur in your own context in each of these categories.
2 How would you go about challenging these?

Whatever way it occurs, it is disabling and a form of discrimination. Discriminating against someone generally implies conferring disadvantage or oppression on that individual which impacts negatively upon their self-concept, their dignity, their opportunities or their ability to get justice.

Discrimination takes many forms:

● stereotyping
● marginalisation
● invisibilisation
● infantilisation
● medicalisation
● dehumanisation
● trivialisation.

Organisations must develop, implement and monitor policies and practice that support anti-discriminatory practice and exclusion. These policies help to raise awareness about unacceptable behaviours and provide a structure for individuals to challenge such behaviours. This includes the responsibility of management to ensure that all staff work within the policy and respect the difference of others. Most organisations will have equality and diversity policies which should also explicitly identify how staff seek redress when they believe there is non-compliance with the policy or law. This can be accomplished through staff meetings and in supervision, for example.

AC 2.3 Provide others with information about the effects of discrimination, the impact of inclusion and the value of diversity

The effects of discrimination

Discrimination causes people to feel devalued, worthless, angry, hopeless and powerless, and undermines confidence. From an organisational or managerial perspective, this can have a

Key term

Discrimination is the practice of unfairly treating a person or group differently from other people or groups of people, usually on the basis of an individual characteristic or difference.

significant impact on the effectiveness of your workforce as well as the individuals they care for. Discriminatory practice is likely to result in poor performance, poor staff relations and a missed opportunity to benefit positively from the different attributes and potential of the staff employed.

As discussed in LO1, discrimination may be a result of individual prejudice or cultural or structural causes. Prejudice is a belief that one group of people, or one person, is better or worse than others on the basis of particular characteristics.

False beliefs may be widely held and deeply ingrained; they are not easily changed, even in response to evidence to their contrary (Thompson and Thompson, 2008). If the false belief is not successfully challenged, it may be accepted as a fact and this may invoke an emotional response, which may be dislike or dismissal of the person or individuals associated with the belief.

Discriminatory, unfair behaviour often follows – inequitable treatment, exclusion, dismissal, becoming the butt of humour, being ridiculed or deliberately being marginalised may be common outcomes. Threats and violence are extreme forms of discriminatory behaviour. Importantly, in the workplace much discriminatory behaviour may be covert and dressed up in the form of humour. Perpetrators may justify and trivialise the action with statements such as 'It's just a bit of fun', 'She's got no sense of humour', 'He's so sensitive'. This trivialisation may make it difficult to address; individuals or staff may not want to be seen to be making a fuss or unable to take a joke. This requires a clear policy that is carried forward into practice stating that singling out an individual's characteristics and using these to ridicule or humiliate them is completely unacceptable.

As a manager your role is to ensure that you are well versed in the effects of discrimination and have at your disposal information about how you deal with or meet the needs of individuals in your care and workforce. You should also be aware of the effects of oppression.

The main outcome of inappropriate use of power is oppression. Oppression as a result of discriminatory practice results in significant harm. It may manifest as another's loss of confidence, or undermining of one's self-belief and self-esteem; it may cause stress anxiety or depression, all of which impact on work performance and subsequent work opportunity. If the individual is unable to successfully challenge the oppression, there is a risk that the prejudicial belief or disabling structure takes on the significance of 'fact' which then results in the oppressed person responding defensively by avoiding situations and people that discriminate against them by trying to keep a low profile, and a negative cycle begins. If nobody stops or challenges the above, then the perpetrators continue and the victimised learn strategies to cope. However, this is clearly unfair.

The impact of inclusion

So far much of the discussion has been focused on the impact of discrimination and strategies to redress unfairness. While this is extremely important, anti-discriminatory approaches are focused on the negative acceptance that discrimination is a fact of life and that energy should be spent on mitigating the effects. Inclusion, however, takes a more positive approach. A philosophy of inclusion is concerned with how things should and could be. Energies are spent on becoming better members of a community, by creating new visions for the community. The emphasis for inclusion is not on justifying reasons for why someone should be included and developing policies and procedures to support this; inclusion starts from an assumption that everyone has equal rights and opportunities and that these should differ only when there is an appropriate reason to do so.

The value of diversity

No two people are alike – even identical twins will have different skills and attributes. When building a team, Belbin (2010) suggests that the most effective teams are those in which the participants have different and complementary skills and attributes in order that the team is balanced and able to effectively fulfil all of its responsibilities. Belbin (2010) described a team inventory against which different team members' skills and attributes could be measured in order that they could be used most effectively; additionally, the

In practice

2.3 Providing others with information

Access your organisation's equality policies. What categories does the policy cover? How well publicised is it?

Undertake a small pilot study and ask different staff members in different levels of the organisation how familiar they are with the policy and what this means for them and their behaviour.

a How well do the policies provide information about the effects of discrimination, the impact of inclusion and the value of diversity?

b Do you need to make changes to include all of these things?

inventory enables the team to identify gaps that may need to be filled.

You can use Belbin's model to analyse your team, as a basis for developing your team's strengths, managing its weaknesses, and for gaining new or absent skill sets when you have an opportunity to recruit. While teams are unlikely to be perfectly balanced, developing a team with diverse skills, attributes and strengths makes a more effective team. Diversity is a strength and if we appreciate and harness its potential rather than fear it, there is an opportunity to capitalise on it. You can found more information on Belbin in unit LM1c.

Celebrating difference and diversity is not something that is just desirable but rather is something that is essential for an organisation to grow and develop. Organisations need to employ a diverse workforce to maximise their potential. There are many benefits to this. The organisation benefits in terms of having the right skill mix but also from the fact that introducing a diverse range of perspectives creates opportunity for innovation, different and possibly enhanced ways of doing things. Increasingly the client base that any organisation serves is diverse and it is necessary to be able to understand and reflect the needs of the whole population that is served.

AC 2.4 Support others to challenge discrimination and exclusion

The first step in supporting others to challenge discrimination and exclusion is to accept that it

exists and to acknowledge that discrimination is a significant factor in inhibiting equality. As managers it is necessary to communicate to staff that discrimination is fundamentally wrong and that it cannot be tolerated within an organisation. We should also be quick to challenge any sort of discriminatory behaviour in order to send out a strong message of zero tolerance. However, challenging discrimination is not easy.

Few people are exempt from prejudice or exclusive practice. What is important is that individuals are open to recognising their prejudices and are committed to change. It takes practice and time. It will be helped by promoting policies that set out expectations of behaviour to others and that remind staff of disciplinary sanctions should they breach the policy. However, while it might be possible to get staff to comply with policies, that is only part of the picture. Policies alone do not change hearts and minds. The risk is that if only compliance is achieved, when not observed the behaviour will revert to that which perpetuated inequality. For many people, understanding the consequences and impact of their actions will cause a change in behaviour and encouragement for others to change, but we cannot assume this will be universal and managers must be vigilant.

We are all products of our culture, our experiences and our education. Discrimination and exclusion may not be intentional but may be the result of the belief that everyone experiences life in the same way. If we have never consciously experienced discrimination, we may not see it when it happens to others. Alternatively, we may be very conscious of discrimination and attitudes. A working mother, for example, may be very sensitive to individuals who make value-based assertions about the negative effect of working mothers on their children. One often needs to be able to relate to another person's experience in order to appreciate the injustice that is felt by others. It is not possible to be somebody else, but it is possible to ask them how it feels and to try to imagine what that must be like. Sometimes it is useful to assume the role of the impartial observer, setting aside emotion and experience and asking whether something is right or not.

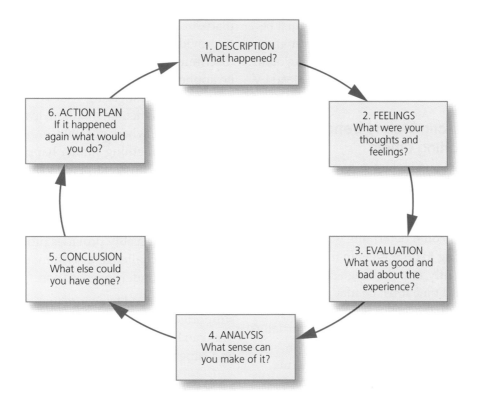

Figure 3.1 Gibb's Model of Reflection

Encourage reflection

It is imperative that we reflect critically on ourselves, our values, attitudes and behaviours towards others. Where do these come from? Are they consistent with the values that one would choose to have? Reflective practice is an excellent vehicle for critical self-reflection and as managers we need to be encouraging our staff to complete this task on a regular basis. By reviewing practice in this way you can help staff to feel supported in their efforts to change practice. They will also feel empowered to challenge bad practice.

The most simple reflective model asks the participant to engage in three critical reflections:

● A detailed interrogation of the issue or situation.
● Why is this so or why did it happen?
● So what does this mean?

Gibb's (1988) Model of Reflection (Figure 3.1) is particularly useful in reflecting on values because it requires the reflector to engage with their feelings and to consider and evaluate the morality of their thoughts and feelings.

Reflect on it

2.4 Labels and assumptions

Using an incident analysis model of reflection, reflect on thoughts, feelings and behaviours from a situation where you may have, or have been tempted to label someone, or make assumptions about their capabilities or trustworthiness, or when you have felt anxious or threatened by someone you did not know.

Reflect on what caused you to respond in the way that you did. Was your response reasonable? Could you have behaved differently? What risks would there have been if you had behaved differently? Can you think of strategies to prompt you to behave differently in the future?

Model good practice

Discriminatory behaviour is often hidden, even from ourselves, and unless we take the time to reflect and be sensitive, question and change our responses to others, evaluate the impact of our behaviours, service users will continue to be treated unjustly.

Managers must model good practice. You must be someone who positively challenges discrimination and supports others to do this. This requires you to be conscious of your own behaviour and to lead by example.

Dealing with discriminatory behaviour in staff and supporting others

Promoting equality and inclusion as positive concepts that are everybody's responsibility helps others to challenge discrimination when they encounter it. However, the way that the manager responds could determine whether the individual is willing to do this again in any future situation. Importantly, any challenge should be taken seriously and time must be made to listen to what the individual believes is occurring. The manager must investigate the situation impartially, trying to gain as much evidence as possible in order to ensure that they have the whole picture before they make any decisions. This includes talking to everyone involved, or to someone who has witnessed the potentially discriminatory behaviour, and taking statements.

Confidentiality should be maintained as these issues are often very sensitive. If the discrimination is found to be a reality, it is important to put in

place an action plan to improve the situation and to provide managerial support to those affected. If discrimination has been proven, sanctions should be applied appropriately and proportionally. One purpose of investigating issues of concern is to resolve the particular situation, learn from the situation and, where possible, implement strategies to prevent something similar happening in the future. Where possible, actions should primarily be focused on enhancing and improving practice rather than on retribution or vengeance. Having clear processes that support individuals to raise concerns responsibly provides protection for those who wish to challenge discrimination and for those who may be under investigation.

You will also need to ensure that staff feel supported and are able to challenge issues safely. This can be achieved through staff meetings, CPD and supervision.

LO3 Understand how to develop systems and processes that promote diversity, equality and inclusion

AC 3.1 Analyse how systems and processes can promote equality and inclusion or reinforce discrimination and exclusion

The appropriateness and 'usability' of systems and processes that exist within an organisation determine whether those systems and processes help to dispel and reduce discrimination or whether they support and promote it. The first step is to ensure that clear and well-understood systems and policies exist that set the standards of the behaviours expected of all employees in the workplace. When designing policies there are three requirements.

1 The policy with regard to diversity, equality and inclusion must be clear.
2 There should be no possibility of misinterpretation of what is intended.
3 It must address the issue directly and it must reflect current legal requirements.

Policies can promote equality and inclusion by setting out the organisation's commitment to tackle discrimination in areas such as recruitment, training, management and pay.

In practice

2.4 Challenging discrimination and exclusion

Imagine yourself in a world in which you are seen as an inferior being. You have similar capabilities to others and yet these are dismissed because your characteristics mark you out as being of lesser value. You are constantly overlooked, marginalised and given the worst and dirtiest jobs to do. You do not have access to the developmental opportunities afforded to others. You are good humouredly ridiculed for the amusement of others. If anything goes wrong, it is assumed that you are responsible.

What sanctions do you think are appropriate to improve the situation and bring about a more equal environment? What are the risks, if any, of imposing sanctions? How could you support others in a similar situation to challenge discrimination and exclusion?

Policies provide a framework for promoting equality and inclusion but if they are not monitored or staff are in any way unclear about how they should be practising, then it may be that your service is in some way reinforcing discrimination and exclusion. Staff who are not challenged about behaviours that may be seen as discriminatory or exclusive, however small, may be condoning practices that are reinforcing discrimination and therefore excluding members of staff or service users.

You must ensure that there have been no amendments, extensions or changes to equality laws. A well-designed policy is essential in addressing discrimination and promoting a positive culture that celebrates diversity. All new policies should be agreed or designed in consultation with unions or employee representatives.

Policies should:

- give examples of what constitutes discrimination, harassment, bullying and intimidating behaviour, including cyber-bullying, work-related events and harassment by third parties
- explain the damaging effects of discrimination and why it will not be tolerated
- state that if discriminatory behaviour has occurred it will be treated as a disciplinary offence
- clarify the legal implications and outline the costs associated with personal liability
- describe how individuals can get help, raise a concern, make a complaint, formally (complaints and grievance procedures) and informally (advice and counselling)
- promise that allegations will be treated speedily (including expected timeframes), seriously and confidentially and to prevent victimisation
- clearly identify steps in the process – who will investigate, how this will be escalated if necessary, what other actions could result (for example, no action taken as there is no case to answer, implementation of action plans rather than escalation)
- clarify the accountability of investigators and managers and the role and responsibilities of union or employee representatives (investigators should be independent of the issue and staff involved)

- identify requirements for documentation and record keeping
- require supervisors/managers to implement policy and ensure it is understood
- emphasise that every employee carries responsibility for their behaviour.

The policy should be monitored and regularly reviewed for effectiveness, including:

- records of complaints, why and how they occurred and who was involved – an analysis of trends will help you to identify if the policy is working or if there are any systemic problems
- individual complaints to ensure that action plans were implemented as intended, to identify resolution and to identify whether there was any evidence of victimisation for those involved.

Communication

When designing or updating a policy, it is important that a communication strategy is designed at the same time. A policy that nobody knows about is of no value. It is important that it is tailored to the different networks within the organisation to ensure all staff are alerted. It also needs to be clear as to who the policy is aimed at – staff in general, individuals or service users and visitors.

Many organisations have staff intranet sites, so a pop-up alert is a good way of raising awareness. This allows you to add a link to the policy and to highlight changes to existing policies. You can add information here, for example you could add a 'Frequently Asked Questions' page or examples of cases to illustrate how this policy may be applied in practice. You can also check out the effectiveness of your communication by doing informal and random checks to see whether staff are aware of the policy.

Training

Raising awareness, although crucial, is not enough. Equality, diversity and anti-discrimination policies need to be supported by staff training. This helps people to really think about their responses to different situations and assists people with different ways of responding to situations. It also ensures that staff are up to date with latest legislation and practice. Training can be provided as part of the staff development programme or via an online package.

Provide advice and support for staff when complaints are made

A reflective, learning organisation tries to identify issues before they become grievances or complaints. Consequently, a well-publicised and confidential opportunity to access advice, support and counselling should be a feature of how organisations engage with diversity and equality. One way is to recruit a number of advisers, trained to provide initial informal advice to any person who believes they are being discriminated against. They can talk through their situation and look at all the options before they take action. Often talking through the issue and being believed and supported is enough to enable the individual to draw on their own reserves and tackle the issue directly or change the situation indirectly. This level of support must be independent of line management, which involves a different level of formality and responsibility, and independent of anyone who may subsequently be asked to investigate an issue if it is escalated. It must also utilise individuals who can be relied on to be impartial to provide information and options but not to make decisions on behalf of the complainant. Confidentiality is essential. The decision whether or not to progress a complaint should normally rest with the individual; however, managers may need to do so on behalf of another when the complainant is in a subordinate role.

Having champions for diversity will help to keep issues about equality on the agenda. Reflecting on best practice in your own and other organisations is valuable. It is not necessary for the manager to take on this role – it can be an opportunity for someone interested in this area to extend their skills and develop their role.

The aim of any activities that you instigate is to support compliance with equality legislation and to eliminate discriminatory behaviour.

All policies

If it is communicated that equality and diversity are everybody's responsibility, it confers an **obligation** on employees to challenge or report discrimination if they encounter it. This can be daunting for employees who have to continue to work in an organisation in which an investigation, suspension or prosecution occurs as a result of the challenge. While the expectation is that individuals should raise challenges and concerns, it is imperative that

they can do this in a supportive and protective environment. Most challenges should be able to be dealt with inside the organisation, which should, with appropriate guidance, allow you to resolve the situation or support sanctions. However, there are occasions when a practice is so widespread and resistant to change, or of such a serious nature, that a more radical approach is required. In such circumstances, staff who witness such activities will be protected by law for making this public. However, this does not mean that the individual has a right to go to the press or other public forum to expose an organisation without trying to resolve issues internally first.

The policies and systems discussed apply to staff as well as service users.

Protection for 'blowing the whistle'

A **whistle-blower** is protected by law for disclosure if they:

- are a 'worker'
- believe that malpractice in the workplace is happening, has happened in the past or will happen in the future
- are revealing information of the right type (a 'qualifying disclosure'), which refers to information that the worker believes is a criminal offence, a miscarriage of justice or failure to comply with a legal obligation. This may have taken place in the past, or may happen in the future
- reveal it to the right person and in the right way (making it a 'protected disclosure'). This is where workers bring information about a wrongdoing to the attention of their employers or a relevant organisation, and in doing so they are protected in certain circumstances under the Public Interest Disclosure Act 1998.

Key terms

Whistle-blowing means making a disclosure or revealing information that is in the public interest.

Disclosure is the release of information about something.

Obligation is an action or restraint from action that a person is morally or legally bound to owe to (an) other(s).

Protected disclosures

For a **disclosure** to be protected by the law, it should be made to the right person or authority and in the right way. Disclosure must meet the following criteria:

- The disclosure must be in good faith (honest intent and without malice).
- The whistle-blower must reasonably believe that the information is substantially true.
- The whistle-blower must reasonably believe they are making the disclosure to the right 'prescribed person'.

If a qualifying disclosure is made in good faith to an employer, or through a process that the employer has agreed, the whistle-blower will be entitled to protection.

If a worker feels unable to make a disclosure to their employer, there are other 'prescribed people' to whom a disclosure can be made. Disclosure can be made to the person responsible for the area of concern such as a team leader or mentor.

To make a protected disclosure to 'others' rather than the employer, the whistle-blower must:

1 Reasonably believe their employer would treat them unfairly if the disclosure was made to the employer or a prescribed person.
2 Reasonably believe that the disclosure to the employer would result in the destruction or concealment of information about the wrong-doing.
3 Have previously disclosed the same or similar information to the employer or a prescribed person.

If an employee loses their job and wants to claim compensation, an employment tribunal must be satisfied that the employee's actions to whistle-blow and make the disclosure were reasonable. The employment tribunal will take into account the following:

- the identity of the person the whistle-blower made the disclosure to (e.g. disclosing to a relevant professional body may be more likely to be considered reasonable than, say, one made to the media).
- the seriousness of the wrong-doing
- whether the wrong-doing is continuing or likely to occur again
- whether the disclosure breaches the employer's duty of confidentiality (e.g. if information was made available that contains confidential details about a client)
- if the whistle-blower made a previous disclosure, whether they followed any internal procedures then.

It is important to note that the term 'worker' includes agency workers and people who aren't directly employed but are in training with employers. Some self-employed people may be considered to be workers for the purpose of whistle-blowing if they are supervised or work off-site.

Whistle-blowers should not become the subject of an internal investigation, or be ridiculed or dismissed as a result of raising concerns. In health and care organisations, the law requires a Duty of Candour, which protects individuals from poor or unsafe care. The Duty of Candour (2014) requires transparency about failures or lapses in respect of care.

AC 3.2 Evaluate the effectiveness of systems and processes in promoting equality, diversity and inclusion in own area of responsibility

It is important that you are not complacent about the effectiveness of policies and procedures that have been designed to support a culture that promotes and assures equality and respect for diversity and inclusion. Occasionally, a policy may be reinforcing discrimination and exclusion accidentally (without meaning to), or because of the language being used or out-of-date practices being continued. An annual audit of effectiveness is a good way of checking whether this issue remains at the forefront of people's minds and practice.

In practice

3.1 How systems and processes promote equality and inclusion, and reinforce discrimination and exclusion

1 Look at the systems and processes that promote equality and inclusion or reinforce discrimination and exclusion in your workplace and comment on how effective they are.
2 Check whether you have a whistle-blowing policy in place and identify whether the responsibilities contained within it clearly identify for the worker what is expected of them in this situation.

The types of activities that can be used to monitor the effectiveness of your policies include:

- User surveys – you can use a quick questionnaire to assess how well the users of your service feel their differences are respected and equality is promoted by your staff.
- When you work alongside others and have an opportunity to witness staff interactions, you can use this as an opportunity to observe how well staff promote equality and respect diversity.
- Reflective practice, including incident analysis (where we analyse an incident by considering what happened, how and why it happened, what might reduce the risk of it happening again and what we learned), allows you and your team to reflect on behaviours, interactions and incidents and to identify ways of enhancing or improving practice. Do not forget that reflective practice also allows you to identify good practice and share this more widely.

AC 3.3 Propose improvements to address gaps or shortfalls in systems and processes

The results gained from your audit should enable you to determine whether staff are knowledgeable about and compliant with equality and diversity policies and procedures. It should help you to assess the extent to which equality is embedded within the organisational culture and will also identify gaps in the provision for which improvements can be proposed and on what sort of time scale. Action plans can then be drawn up based on firm and reliable evidence. Possible actions may be raising awareness, further staff development and transforming practice, and in some cases may lead to disciplinary action.

LO4 Be able to manage the risks presented when balancing individual rights and professional duty of care

Rights of individuals

Health care environments are believed by both service users and workers to exist on the premise that they are primarily concerned with 'doing good' and supporting and promoting individuals' health and well-being. In fact, all care professionals are legally bound to provide a 'duty of care' to their service users which requires them to adhere to standards of 'reasonable' care on the services they provide. However, this assertion can be interpreted differently by different stakeholders (i.e. individuals, and groups or organisations that have an interest in your organisation or business) and can be the subject of a dilemma. Health care workers owe a responsibility and are accountable to various people: their patients or clients, their employers, their professional or regulatory body, and the law. At times the duties owed to different stakeholders come into conflict. It is widely accepted that those in receipt of care, and those providing care, have both rights and responsibilities; rights do not exist without a correlating responsibility to protect or action that right. Rights are often referred to as entitlements (Buchanon, 1984).

These entitlements may be universal (applicable to all) or may refer to a defined group on the basis of specified criteria. Universal rights are those that have been agreed by the international community and are protected under the Human Rights Act (1998), which sets out 16 basic rights owed to any citizen in the UK. Where these rights are violated or restricted, an individual has a legal entitlement to challenge the infringement.

A number of rights relate specifically to those receiving care. These rights are articulated in health policy, the NHS Constitution (2011) care standards documents, patients' charters and professional codes of conduct. Responsibilities for upholding rights are placed on care practitioners to ensure that entitlements are met.

AC 4.1 Describe ethical dilemmas that arise in own area of responsibility when balancing individual rights and duty of care

The dilemma that the practitioner must reconcile is how far someone's right to make decisions for themselves can be supported when it is in conflict with a professional obligation. The duty of the care worker is not to control others' lives but to inform them and support them in order that they can make good decisions for themselves.

When an accident occurs which goes against your own values and beliefs, you are faced with an ethical dilemma. For example, a dilemma may arise when you feel you are obliged to break confidentiality. You may feel an individual is at harm from a family member but the person has asked you not to say anything. This is the individual's choice and they are entitled to that choice. But to safeguard them you will be required to follow your organisation's vulnerable adults' procedure. The Mental Capacity Act may also be accessed in such cases to ensure that the person involved does have capacity to make such decisions.

Another example may include actions taken when you observe poor practice in the setting. Whilst it is the correct course of action to report such matters, it may be difficult to do so if you believe somebody may lose their job as a result of this.

Key term

Duty of care refers to the professional's legal obligation as well as ethical responsibility to safeguard and protect the well-being of others and to perform to a standard of reasonable care when performing any acts that could harm others. Failure to do so may be termed negligence.

In practice

4.1 Rights of individuals

Review a range of documents, e.g. policies, standards, codes of practice, relevant to your work context. What rights are articulated in these?

In practice

4.1 Ethical dilemmas and balancing rights and duty of care

Here are some other examples of activities where duty of care and responsibilities come into conflict. Should they be supported and on what basis is this justified?

- An individual who does not want confidential information to be shared with their daughter.
- An individual who you see being treated disrespectfully by one of your colleagues does not want the incident reported.
- A staff member who wants time to attend mass when on duty on a Sunday.
- A service user who does not want to be supported to meet their hygiene needs.

Reflect on it

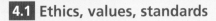

4.1 Ethics, values, standards

Reflect on what checks you could implement in order to reassure yourself that values and standards are being met. How frequently is it necessary to implement these?

These could, for example, involve discussions with clients, self-assessment by staff or observations of practice in relation to a particular standard.

Finding a solution to balancing individual rights and duty of care

A useful 'rule of thumb' is to encourage and support individual decision making as far as is reasonably possible, as long as this does not infringe the rights of others. The reason that these kinds of situations are called dilemmas is that there are often no wholly satisfactory solutions that will appease all parties; rather, it requires a workable compromise that all parties feel is acceptable to them. The challenge for practitioners when there are no clear and obviously right answers lies in intelligently applying good judgements, based on strong values which support good principles of practice. These principles should underpin all care practice: respect for dignity and autonomy, promotion of equality and diversity, fairness and justice, management of risk and protection from harm, and sound judgement and compassion.

AC 4.2 Explain the principle of informed choice

Informed choice is the ability to make decisions based upon information received and this is supported by the principle of autonomy, which can be defined as:

'Self-rule that is free from both controlling interferences by others and from personal limitations that prevent meaningful choice, such as inadequate understanding.'

(Beauchamp and Childress, 2013, p. 58)

There are at least four elements necessary for autonomous decision making:

- Understanding the value of respect for persons and their differences.
- The ability to be self-governing and being able to determine one's personal goals, desires and preferences.

- The capacity or competence to make choices or decisions based on deliberation and reason.
- The freedom to make choices for oneself and then to act on these.

(Cuthbert and Quallington, 2008)

Your role as a manager

In terms of your role in a health and social care context, 'informed choice' means supporting individuals to make decisions. Informed choice and autonomous decision making require more than the simple articulation of preferences in order to meet the requirement for informed choice. In making an informed choice, an individual must be given alternatives, even if that choice is simply to do or not to do something. Making a meaningful choice entails that a person understands what those choices mean and what the impact of those choices could signify. It is the responsibility of the practitioner to ensure that the individual has sufficient information which is unbiased, based upon facts and provided in a coherent and understandable way, to enable them to make informed choices. If the individual does not understand the information, the onus is on the practitioner to find an alternative way to explain it. It is not sufficient to claim that because you told them something, they were adequately informed. Checking understanding about what they think they are being told by asking questions and getting them to summarise what you have said is a useful way of assessing understanding. You may need to involve family or advocates to ensure that everyone concerned in the care of the person feels included.

The individual's capacity to make an informed choice

Informed choice requires that an individual has the capacity to manipulate the information that they have been given in order for them to reach a decision. However, capacity should be assumed unless there is evidence to demonstrate that it is compromised. A further requirement is that the choice is made by the individual and should not be unduly influenced by those around them. That does not preclude guidance, but guidance should be in the form of benefits, risks and questions rather than directives telling individuals what to do.

Allow the individual time to reflect

Another condition of informed choice is the requirement for opportunity for deliberation and time for reflection. This condition is often overlooked. Given time to reflect on various risks and potential outcomes, individuals may decide on a choice that is quite different from the one they originally thought they might select.

Allow individuals to implement their choices

The final condition of informed choice is that individuals must be able to implement the choices they have been given. Being offered a choice means that this should then be respected and actioned as this is an essential element of trust in any therapeutic relationship. It is this element of informed choice that can make practitioners nervous, as it requires individuals to balance risks and their own responsibilities against the rights and choices of those in their care.

AC 4.3 Explain how issues of capacity may affect informed choice

Anything that affects an individual's capacity to weigh up information and make choices may compromise their ability to make choices. Decisions about capacity are judged on the basis of competence. Factors that compromise an individual's ability to make decisions may be internal to that individual – they may be affected by

things such as mental or physical ability, intellectual capacity, anxiety or pain, or factors such as ability to communicate, age, or culture – or they can be as a result of external factors, such as control or protective behaviour of others, lack of adequate information, or not being presented with real choices.

Competence is not easy to define or assess and yet it is an important element of determining the level of decision making that should be supported. One definition of it is the measure of the 'fitness' of an individual to act or behave in certain situations. In health and social care, standards of competence tend to focus on the ability to make choices. Assessment of competence then is not dissimilar from assessing the conditions required for informed consent. Beauchamp and Childress (2013, p. 73) present a table aimed at identifying abilities and inabilities, which can be used as a basis for determining competence – see Table 3.1.

The values and duties expected in care practice regarding the standards and assessment of capacity have been set out in legislation. The Mental Capacity Act (MCA) (2005), which was enacted in 2007, is designed to protect and empower individuals who may lack the mental capacity to make their own decisions about their care and treatment.

The MCA sets out five statutory principles that underpin the legal requirements. These are

Table 3.1 Identifying abilities and inabilities

Type of ability or skill	Inabilities used to judge competence
Ability to state a preference	● Inability to express or communicate a preference or choice.
Abilities to understand information and appreciate one's situation	● Inability to understand one's situation and its consequences. ● Inability to understand relevant information.
Abilities to reason about a consequential life decision	● Inability to give a reason. ● Inability to give a rational reason. ● Inability to give risk/benefit-related reasons. ● Inability to reach a reasonable decision (as judged by the Reasonable Person's Standard).

the values that care managers must ensure are embedded within the practices in their organisation:

1 A person must be assumed to have capacity unless it is (formally) established that they do not have capacity.
2 A person is not to be treated as unable to make a decision unless all practicable steps to help him/her do so have been taken without success.
3 A person must not be treated as unable to make a decision merely because he/she makes an unwise one.
4 An act done, or decision made, under the Act for and on behalf of a person who lacks capacity must be done or made in his/her best interests.
5 Before the act is done, or the decision is made, regard must be made to whether the purpose for which it is needed can be as effectively achieved in a way that is less restrictive of the person's rights or freedom of action.

AC 4.4 Propose a strategy to manage risks when balancing individual rights and duty of care in own area of responsibility

Balancing individual rights and the duty that is owed to protect those in your care from harm is complex. In focusing on the duty to protect, it is all too easy to focus on the negative and be unduly swayed by potential risks that can befall someone, rather than concentrating on the benefits from supporting and managing an activity. The fear of harm and resulting disciplinary action or public investigation means care practitioners tend to err on the side of caution in managing risks and this 'over protection' can take precedence over individual rights.

The policies and procedures in your organisation should cover risk assessment as well as processes that consider the potential for harm against the actual benefits of an activity for a service user.

Practitioners have an obligation to 'do good and promote the interests' of their patients and clients,

and avoid and protect those in their care from harm. However, the law is equally clear that this does not involve acting 'paternalistically' and overriding an individual's rights and opportunities to make choices for and about themselves, even when the motives of those wishing to impose their decisions on another are beneficially motivated and intended to be in the best interests of the client. The only person who should judge what is in their best interest is the individual themselves.

It is important to remember that the risk that is taken belongs to the individual and this is why informed consent is such an important element of care decisions.

A strategy to manage risk

As a manager you will be familiar with the need to conduct risk assessments. When these concern individuals, it is important that they are conducted specifically in relation to individual service users. It is only in this way that differences, choices and preferences can be properly accommodated. A risk assessment and subsequent action plan to manage risk do not require that all potential and actual risks be eliminated; it means that all serious risks must be considered and, where possible, a plan to reasonably manage the degree of risk be designed in partnership with the person affected.

Predicting or anticipating risk is not a precise art and is influenced by many things, including personal experience, particularly negative experiences, whether a similar event has occurred recently, the degree of damage if the risk comes to pass, the degree of fear or anxiety generated by the potential risk, the personality of the individual analysing the risk, and whether they are naturally risk averse or welcome risk taking (Cuthbert and Quallington, 2008, p. 130).

Balancing risk of harm with individual choice and rights

When practitioners enter into a contract of care with an individual, they assume duties and obligations in relation to that contract. These obligations include those issues that have been discussed in this unit, such as respect for dignity and diversity and promotion of equality and fairness.

Duty of care and promoting culture of mutual accountability

Management of care is inherently unpredictable and risky. It is not always possible to anticipate the outcome of interventions and therefore the requirement for safe and effective care cannot be focused on outcome alone. If called to account, the practitioner must be able to demonstrate that the activity was within their scope of knowledge and responsibility, that they had performed the activity based on best or accepted practice standards, that they had assessed the individual risks in this situation and tried to manage these appropriately, and had, wherever possible, involved and sought informed consent from the individual affected by the activity. Accidents and unfortunate outcomes still occur, but all reasonable action must have been taken to try to avoid them.

Legislation

The Equality Act (2010)

The Equality Act (2010) came into force on 1 October 2010. It brings together more than 116 separate pieces of legislation into one single Act. Combined, they make up a new Act, which provides a legal framework to protect the rights of individuals and to advance equality of opportunity for all. The Act simplifies, strengthens and harmonises the previous anti-discrimination legislation to provide Britain with a new discrimination law.

> ## Research it
>
> **4.4** Balancing individual rights and duty of care
>
> Identify the most prevalent risks associated with your own work setting and undertake a small-scale study to show how you balance individual rights and professional duty of care.

The nine main pieces of legislation that have merged to form the new Equality Act are:

- Equal Pay Act 1970
- Sex Discrimination Act 1975
- Race Relations Act 1976
- Disability Discrimination Act 1995
- Employment Equality (Religion or Belief) Regulations 2003
- Employment Equality (Sexual Orientation) Regulations 2003
- Employment Equality (Age) Regulations 2006
- Equality Act 2006, Part 2
- Equality Act (Sexual Orientation) Regulations 2007.

The Mental Capacity Act (2005)

The Mental Capacity Act 2005 is a law that protects and supports people who do not have the ability to make decisions for themselves. The act applies to people aged 16 and over in England and Wales and makes provision in a number of different conditions for those whose capacity is affected.

To have capacity a person must be able to:

- understand the information that is relevant to the decision they want to make
- retain the information long enough to be able to make the decision
- weigh up the information available to make the decision
- communicate their decision by any possible means, including talking, using sign language, or through simple muscle movements such as blinking of an eye or squeezing a hand.

Making decisions in a person's 'best interests'

Anyone making a decision on behalf of a person they believe to lack mental capacity must do so in that person's best interests.

Lasting Power of Attorney

The Mental Capacity Act introduced a new type of power of attorney known as a Lasting Power of Attorney (LPA). An LPA allows people to choose someone who can make decisions about their health and welfare, as well as their finances and property, if they become unable to do so for themselves. See page 72 for information on advance decisions, deputies and the Court of Protection.

Assessment methods

LO	Assessment criteria and accompanying activities	Assessment methods To evidence coverage of the ACs you could:
LO1	1.1 Reflect on it (p. 52)	Write a short essay which argues the case for the advantages and disadvantages of the two approaches in your organisational context.
	1.1 In practice (p. 53)	Write a short piece stating what your responsibilities are with respect to implementing them or discuss them with your assessor. Or Discuss with your assessor how the Equality Act impacts on your own setting by describing how you demonstrate good practice. Practise applying the Equality Act to a number of different scenarios to assess whether you think that an organisation is demonstrating good practice within the law.
	1.2 In practice (p. 54)	Prepare a table to show what the barriers and the effects are.
	1.1, 1.2 Research it (p. 54)	Undertake the study and then make a presentation for findings to management and staff.
	1.3 In practice (p. 54)	Prepare a spider diagram which shows the function of the MCA and the effects it has had on your setting.
	1.3 Case study (p. 55)	Prepare a short staff training session using the case studies and ask staff to identify whether you think discrimination has occurred and whether there is a case to appeal to the law through the Equality Act (2010).
LO2	2.1 Research it (p. 56)	Research an organisation other than your own and comment upon how it has championed diversity, equality and inclusion. Write a short description of the organisation and then a couple of examples of how they have championed equality and diversity.
	2.1 In practice (p. 56)	Discuss with your assessor how you as a manager promote equality and diversity in policy and practice. You could provide a list of the ways which shows how you champion equality, diversity and inclusion in order to lead the development of a positive culture for your portfolio. You could write a short piece as evidence.
	2.2 In practice (p. 56)	Write a short piece answering the questions in the activity. Discuss with your assessor the means by which you challenge discrimination in your setting.
	2.3 In practice (p. 58)	You could place copies of the policies within your portfolio which highlight the categories. Interview staff about the policies to ascertain their knowledge. Write a short piece which identifies your findings from the interviews then discuss with your manager what needs to change.

LO	Assessment criteria and accompanying activities	Assessment methods To evidence coverage of the ACs you could:
	2.4 Reflect on it (p. 59)	Using the questions and the model of reflection prepare a mind map which shows your responses. Role-modelling of good practice is very important in embedding values and setting a culture. Think about ways in which you may be able to be an advocate or role model being able to champion equality, diversity and inclusion in order to lead the development of a positive culture.
	2.4 In practice (p. 60)	Prepare a presentation for a staff meeting which uses the above scenario and gain their views on how they would challenge discrimination. Write a short piece for your portfolio.
LO3	3.1 In practice (p. 63)	You might prepare a staff agenda item discussing this with the team. Place the minutes of the meeting in your portfolio.
	3.2 In practice (p. 64)	Discuss with your assessor the tool you are developing and record your findings. Access the policies and highlight the areas that identify the responsibilities. Discuss with your assessor the effectiveness of the policies
	3.3 Research it (p. 64)	Use the information you have gathered from the research, prepare a paper for management which identifies areas for improvement.
	3.3 In practice (p. 64)	Provide a written account answering the questions in the activity.
	LO3 Reflect on it (p. 64)	Provide a written account answering the questions in the activity. Ask your assessor to record a professional discussion about your thoughts on this.
LO4	4.1 In practice (p. 65)	Review a range of documents, e.g. policies, standards, codes of practice, relevant to your work context. What rights are articulated in these? Provide a written piece.
	4.1 In practice (p. 65)	Discuss the questions in the activity with staff members to ascertain their thoughts then write a short piece to show your understanding.
	4.1 Reflect on it (p. 66)	Prepare a table or checklist.
	4.2 Reflect on it (p. 67)	Write a short essay to show your understanding of this.
	4.2 In practice (p. 67)	Check your understanding about the principle of informed choice by explaining it to a member of staff.
	4.3 In practice (p. 68)	Give an example of how issues of capacity may affect informed choice. Discuss these with your assessor.
	4.4 In practice (p. 68)	Construct a table which shows the differences.
	4.4 Research it (p. 69)	Ask your assessor to accompany you on an observation of the workplace to undertake this activity.

Advance decisions

An advance decision allows someone to specify the types of treatment that they do not want, should they lack the mental capacity to decide this for themselves in the future.

Deputies and the Court of Protection

Deputies are appointed to make decisions for people who lack the capacity to do so themselves. This applies particularly in situations where formal arrangements have not been made – for example, if a person loses capacity and has not set up a Lasting Power of Attorney or an advance decision.

References

Beauchamp, T. and Childress, J. (2013) *Principles of Biomedical Ethics* (7e). Oxford: Oxford University Press.

Belbin, R. (2010) *Management Teams: Why they succeed or fail* (3e). London: Butterworth-Heinemann.

Buchanon, A. (1984) 'The right to a decent minimum of health care,' *Philosophy and Public Affairs*, 13(1), 55–78.

Care Quality Commission Report (2011) *National Report on Dignity and Nutrition Review*. 13 October. London: CQC.

Cuthbert, S. and Quallington, J. (2008) *Values for Care Practice*. Exeter: Reflect Press.

Department of Education (2010) *Working Together to Safeguard Children*. London: The Stationery Office.

Department of Health (2000) *No Secrets: Guidance on developing and implementing multi-agency policies and procedures to protect vulnerable adults from abuse*. London: The Stationery Office.

Directgov website (2011) *Protection for Whistleblowers*, www.direct.gov.uk/en/ Employment/ResolvingWorkplaceDisputes/ Whistleblowingintheworkplace/DG_10026552

Gibbs, G. (1988) *Learning by Doing: A guide to teaching and learning methods*. Oxford: Oxford Further Education Unit.

Mullins, L. (2009) *Management and Organisational Behaviour* (8e). Harlow: Prentice Hall.

Ombudsman's Report (2011) 'Care and compassion,' *Report of the Health Service Ombudsman on Ten Investigations into the Care of Older People*. London: Parliamentary and Health Service Ombudsman.

Renz, D. and Eddy, W. (1996) 'Organisations, ethics and healthcare: building an ethics infrastructure for a new era,' *Bioethics Forum*, 12(2), 29–39.

The Mental Capacity Act (2005) Department of Constitutional Affairs at http://webarchive. nationalarchives.gov.uk

http://www.dca.gov.uk/legal-policy/mental-capacity/mca-summary.pdf (accessed October 2011).

The Francis Report (2013) *Inquiry Report into Mid-Staffordshire NHS Foundation Trust*. London: Department of Health.

Thompson, N. (2011) *Promoting Equality: Working with diversity and difference* (3e). Basingstoke: Palgrave Macmillan.

Thompson, N and Thompson, S. (2008) *The Critically Reflective Practitioner*. Basingstoke: Palgrave Macmillan.

Titterton, M. (2005) *Risk and Risk Taking in Health and Social Welfare*. London: Jessica Kingsley Publishing.

Walker, B. (1994) 'Valuing differences: the concept and a model' in Mabey, C. and Iles, R. *Managing Learning*. Buckingham: Open University Press.

Further reading and useful resources

Care Quality Commission:
www.cqc.org.uk

Equality and Human Rights Commission:
www.equalityhumanrights.com

Nursing and Midwifery Council:
www.nmc.org.uk

Skills for care:
www.skillsforcare.org.uk

Unit M1

Develop health and safety and risk management policies, procedures and practices in health and social care settings

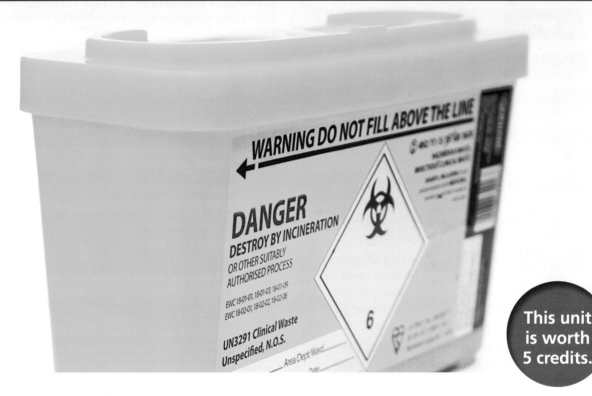

This unit is worth 5 credits.

The health and safety of all individuals who work in or visit your setting is of paramount importance. As a manager you are required to take responsibility for this and to practise the legal aspects of health and safety in order to deal with staff and service users in a safe manner. Creating a culture where risks are balanced with health and safety requires you to have knowledge of the legislation that informs policies and procedures to manage risk and safeguard service users. This unit will help you to understand how to assess your knowledge, understanding and skills required for health and safety and risk management, including the development of policies, procedures and practices in health and social care. You will also learn how to improve health, safety and risk management policies, procedures and practices.

Learning outcomes

By the end of this unit you will:

1 Understand the current legislative framework and organisational health, safety and risk management policies, procedures and practices.
2 Be able to implement and monitor compliance with health, safety and risk management requirements.
3 Be able to lead the implementation of policies, procedures and practices to manage risk to individuals and others.
4 Be able to promote a culture where needs and risks are balanced with health and safety practice.
5 Be able to improve health, safety and risk management policies, procedures and practices.

LO1 Understand the current legislative framework and organisational health, safety and risk management policies, procedures and practices relevant to health and social care settings

AC 1.1 Explain the legislative framework for health, safety and risk management in the work setting

Key terms

Policy is a plan or principle of action proposed by an organisation, also known as guidelines or codes.

Procedures state how policies will be carried out or actioned in the setting.

Health and safety is ensuring people are safe and come to no harm in the workplace. This will inform policies such as Control of Substances Hazardous to Health (COSHH), infection control, safe handling of medicine, moving and handling, and fire safety, for example.

Risk management is the forecasting of potential risk and minimising them or avoiding them altogether. Your policies should identify how you undertake risk assessment in your area and how you intend to manage risks that arise.

The Health and Safety Executive (HSE) is the regulator or official supervisory body for the health, safety and welfare of people in work settings in the UK.

Health and safety and regulation in health and social care

Florence Nightingale famously stated: 'The very first requirement in a hospital is that it should do the sick no harm' (Nightingale, 1859). Yet we are frequently confronted with headlines that state otherwise. Incidents of service users failing to receive treatment in line with their care plan and being severely harmed as a result include ill-treatment or wilful neglect of a patient/service user, employees developing dermatitis related to incorrect glove use, or suffering a manual handling injury from moving ill-maintained and failing equipment.

Case study

1.1 Healthcare provider fined over death in its care (October 2015)

In 2010 a man was found hanged in the A&E department of a hospital. Despite being resuscitated he suffered brain damage and subsequently died. The Trust was fined £67,000 for its failure to follow its own procedures which highlighted the risk of leaving known psychiatric patients alone. The patient called for an ambulance clearly stating his suicidal thoughts and admissions of previous attempts to hang himself. He had a history of depression.

Despite the trust having policies in place these had not been followed on this occasion and the trust had therefore been found guilty of breaching the Health and Safety at Work Act (1974).

[You can find the full story at http://press.hse.gov.uk/2015/healthcare-provider-fined-over-death-in-its-care

Contains public sector information licensed under the Open Government Licence v3.0.]

a What might have been the cause here of the breach of the policy?
b What lessons can you learn from this incident and how might you ensure staff are aware of their duty with respect to adhering to policy?

Tragic incidents can happen when the legal aspects of care work are either not followed correctly or ignored altogether. Health and safety in the workplace is a legal requirement and monitored regularly by the **Health and Safety Executive**. Failure to uphold the law will inevitably lead to consequences not only to service users but also to staff and the care establishment as a whole. As a manager you are required to have in place policy and procedure to protect service users, staff and visitors from breaches of health and safety law. The Francis Enquiry, published in 2013, reported on the Mid Staffs hospital trust where a major failure in patient care was uncovered. As a result, an important change was introduced in April 2015, giving new enforcement powers to the Care Quality Commission (CQC) with respect to health and safety in the care sector. The main purpose of the group is to monitor, inspect and regulate services to ensure standards of quality and safety are being met. Failure to do so would result in prosecution.

The change ensures that there is effective and coordinated regulation of health and safety for service users, workers and members of the public and a shared responsibility between the CQC, the HSE and local authorities to ensure safety.

Care Quality Commission (CQC), Health and Safety Executive (HSE) and local authorities (LAs)

Under the Health and Social Care Act 2012 (and mentioned in the 2014 Care Act) the CQC is the lead inspection and enforcement body for safety and quality of treatment and care matters involving service users in receipt of a health or adult social care service from a provider registered with the CQC.

The HSE/LAs are the lead inspection and enforcement bodies for health and safety matters involving service users who are in receipt of a health or care service from providers not registered with the CQC.

The process recognises that certain bodies may be more appropriate to deal with specific cases. So, for example, the CQC will be called to investigate an incident where a service user is seriously injured or dying after being physically restrained by staff, but the HSE and LA may be asked to investigate a manual handling injury to an employee.

Key term

Regulation is a rule or order which is underpinned by law. In health care settings, apart from those concerned with health and safety care, regulations with respect to health protection and control of disease are also available.

Research it

1.1 The Care Quality Commission (CQC)

The CQC highlights a number of regulations for dealing with person-centred care, dignity and respect, and safe treatments, among other things. You can see more at:

www.cqc.org.uk/content/regulations-service-providers-and-managers

Where there is uncertainty about jurisdiction, the relevant bodies will work collaboratively and come to a joint decision about the action to be taken.

Your role as a manager or leader

For you as a manager and leader in health care, your knowledge of the law and how it is translated into practice through policy and implemented by your staff must underpin your practice. Undoubtedly you will already have a good working practice of the legal aspects of care work, but it is wise to revisit this from time to time.

In your role as manager you will need to ensure you offer strong induction activities and training for staff. Staff need to understand their roles and responsibilities with regard to health and safety record keeping and reporting and must also be aware of the necessity of complying with policies and procedures and practice. Any breaches must be dealt with effectively and quickly to avoid unsafe practice. By monitoring compliance to the policies and procedures and ensuring that checks/audits take place and that risk assessments are updated you will be practising safely with respect to this part of your management role.

Legislation

The legislation you will be familiar with is the Health and Safety at Work Act 1974, or HASAWA, which is the main piece of UK health and safety legislation. It places a duty on all employers 'to ensure, so far as is reasonably practicable, the health, safety and welfare at work' of all their employees. Additionally, it requires:

- *'The safe operation and maintenance of the working environment, plant (equipment) and systems*
- *maintenance of safe access and egress to the workplace*
- *safe use, handling and storage of dangerous substances*
- *adequate training of staff to ensure health and safety*
- *adequate welfare provisions for staff at work.'*

Source: www.hse.gov.uk/legislation/trace.htm

The Management of Health and Safety at Work Regulations 1999 (the Management Regulations) further highlights and details in greater depth what employers are required to do to manage health and safety under the Health and Safety at

Work Act. The main requirement is the need to carry out a risk assessment. Employers with five or more employees need to record the significant findings of the risk assessment.

All the laws will be enshrined in the policies and procedures you are required to have in your workplace and these will cover a variety of laws. In this unit we will be addressing the health and safety policy.

Policies set out the arrangements you have for complying with the law and procedures identify the activity surrounding practice in order to implement the policy. As a manager, one of your roles is to ensure that staff are aware of the importance of carrying out practice according to policy. Failure to do so can have major consequences for the client, the organisation and the member of staff, as we shall see in the next section.

In practice

1.1 Legislative framework for health, safety and risk management

You are to give a lecture at the local college about the legal aspects of health care and how they apply to the health and social care settings.

To make a start, see if you can list the laws you are familiar with and explain their purpose and your responsibilities with respect to implementing them. Now see if you can add to your list from a sector you are unfamiliar with.

Table 4.1 shows the purpose of the laws and your responsibility with respect to each – you can check your answers here.

Table 4.1 Legislation, purpose, practice and examples of your responsibilities

Legislation	Purpose	Practice: Examples of your responsibilities
The Care Act 2014	The act will help to improve people's independence and well-being.	Local authorities must provide or arrange services that help prevent people developing needs for care and support, or delay people deteriorating such that they would need ongoing care and support.
Health and Safety at Work Act 1974 (HASAWA)	Anyone affected by work activity must be kept safe.	To ensure all staff are aware of their part in health and safety and to regularly check that the policies in place meet all needs. Also to ensure that written policies are in place.
Health and Safety (First Aid) Regulations 1981	To ensure that everybody has access to immediate first-aid care in the workplace.	To maintain first-aid training of designated first aiders and to supply resources for first aid.
Mental Health Act 1983	This act allows compulsory action to be taken, where necessary, to ensure that people with mental health disorders get the care and treatment they need for their own health or safety or for the protection of other people.	Staff need to be aware of the rights of individuals under this act and the choices the service user has.
Mental Capacity Act 2005	Provides a legal framework for acting and making decisions on behalf of adults who lack capacity to make particular decisions for themselves.	To ensure that staff are fully informed of issues such as informed consent and of respect to the law. This should be clearly stated in job descriptions and contracts of work.
Electricity at Work Regulations 1989	To minimise the risk due to electricity in the workplace.	To maintain upkeep and ensure regular safety checks are made.

Legislation	Purpose	Practice: Examples of your responsibilities
Food Safety Act 1990	To minimise the risk due to food handling in the workplace.	Ensure any hazards are identified and controlled.
Food Hygiene Regulations 2006	To minimise the risk due to moving and handling food. To show how to identify and control food safety risks in the process of preparing and selling food and set out basic hygiene principles.	Ensure good personal hygiene procedures are upheld.
Food Information Regulations (FIR) 2014	To combine existing rules on general food labelling and nutrition into a single regulation to enable consumers to make an informed choice.	All staff must be trained in checking for any allergens contained in the food served in the setting.
Manual Handling Operations Regulations 1992 (MHOR)	To reduce the risk of injury for manual handling.	Ensure staff are trained in moving and handling protocols. A risk assessment for manual handling, moving and handling must be in place and monitored.
Workplace (Health, Safety and Welfare) Regulations 1992	To minimise the risk due to working conditions in the workplace.	Ensure that standards for heating, lighting, sanitation and building upkeep are maintained.
Personal Protective Equipment at Work Regulations 1992 (PPE)	To minimise the risk of cross-infection in the workplace.	To ensure staff are aware of infection-control procedures and are trained in dealing with potential cross-infection. To supply work wear and PPE.
Reporting on Injuries, Diseases and Dangerous Occurrences Regulations 1995 (RIDDOR)	Ensure that procedures are in place for the reporting of injury and illness to the HSE or local authority where appropriate.	Maintain the policy in the workplace and ensure that accident forms and reports are in place.
Provision and Use of Work Equipment Regulations 1998 (PUWER)	Risks due to the use of equipment must be minimised.	Train staff in use of equipment and ensure equipment is maintained and safe to use.
Data Protection Act 1998	Ensure that personal information is kept private and safe.	Check policy on confidentiality and arrange to undertake regular risk assessments.
Management of Health and Safety at Work Regulations 1999 (MHSWR) Amended 2003 and 2006.	This revokes and replaces the 1992 Regulations of the same title. The 2003 amendment allowed claims to be brought against employees by third parties who were affected by their work activity, e.g. members of the public. The 2006 amendment changed the civil liability provisions in the regulations so as to exclude the right of third parties to take legal action against employees for contraventions of their duties under these Regulations.	Carry out risk assessments to minimise any risks to safety with respect to fire and safe handling of substances hazardous to health.

Table 4.1 *(Continued)*

Legislation	Purpose	Practice: Examples of your responsibilities
Control of Substances Hazardous to Health Regulations 2002 (COSHH)	Minimise the risk from the use of substances that may be hazardous to health.	Carry out risk assessments and ensure staff are trained in use of hazardous substances.
Regulatory Reform (Fire Safety) 2005	Minimise fire hazards.	Regular checks of fire-safety procedures in the workplace.
Corporate Manslaughter and Homicide Act 2007	If the death of somebody occurs in suspicious circumstances, then an organisation may be convicted of negligence.	Ensure staff are aware of duty of care and are following policy.
Health and Social Care Act 2008, 2012	Highlighted significant measures to modernise and integrate health and social care.	The changes that were introduced in 2012 mean that practitioners need to understand the reforms and how these may impact them and their service users. As a manager you need to be aware of the changes and be able to direct staff to better understanding.
Human Medicines Regulations (2012)	Replaced most of the Medicines Act 1968 and 200 statutory instruments with a simplified set of rules. The new regulations set out a regime for the authorisation of medicinal products for human use; for the manufacture, import, distribution, sale and supply of those products; for their labelling and advertising.	Ensure a medicines policy reflects the law and staff are continually trained and updated in this role.
Equality Act 2010	Brought together over 116 separate pieces of legislation into one single act that provides a legal framework to protect the rights of individuals and advance equality of opportunity for all. The main pieces of legislation that have merged are: ● Equal Pay Act 1970 ● Sex Discrimination Act 1975 ● Race Relations Act 1976 ● Disability Discrimination Act 1995 ● Employment Equality (Religion or Belief) Regulations 2003 ● Employment Equality (Sexual Orientation) Regulations 2003 ● Employment Equality (Age) Regulations 2006 ● Equality Act 2006, Part 2 ● Equality Act (Sexual Orientation) Regulations 2007	To ensure policies and procedures reflect the Act and staff are aware of duties of care with respect to equality and diversity.

Table 4.1 *(Continued)*

Legislation	Purpose	Practice: Examples of your responsibilities
Health and Safety Information for Employees Regulations (1989)	The Act sets out the general duties which employers have towards employees and members of the public, and employees have to themselves and to each other.	Ensure that staff are aware of the arrangements for implementing the health and safety measures identified by the risk assessment. Be aware of emergency procedures. Have clear information and training. Be aware of the need to work together with other employers in the workplace. HASAWA risk assessment-managing health and safety requires you to control the risks in your workplace. There should be audits and reviews of the risk assessments. See LO2 for more information on risk assessments.

Table 4.1 (*Concluded*) The table outlines some examples of responsibilities. It will be up to you and your setting to be aware of your full duties and responsibilities with regard to legislation.

Research it

1.1 Legislation, policies and procedures

Look at the legislation listed in Table 4.1 and for each one think about your setting. Find out the purpose and related policies and procedures in your setting; the practice of your responsibilities and examples of how legislation is implemented in your setting.

AC 1.2 Analyse how policies, procedures and practices in own setting meet health, safety and risk management requirements

If you work in a setting where there are more than five employees, you are required to have a written health and safety policy in place. The National Minimum Standards for Care (Number 11.2) states that:

'The agency delivering the care has a comprehensive health and safety policy written procedures for health and safety management defining:

● individual and organisational responsibility for health and safety;

● responsibilities and arrangements or risk assessments under the requirements of the Health and Safety at Work Regulations (1999) (management regulation).'

Source: DOH, 2000

The CQC and the HSE have different roles and responsibilities in the regulation of health and social care but agree that both organisations share appropriate information so that people who use services are properly protected. In 2013 the CQC/HSE Liaison Agreement was drawn up, with the roles and responsibilities for both groups being firmly agreed. The HSE is responsible for enforcing the Health and Safety at Work Act 1974 (HASAWA), with specific aims to reduce death, injury and ill health by securing the health, safety and welfare of workers and protecting others, such as contractors or patients, who may be affected by work activities. It also has a role in patient safety. The CQC is the independent regulator of health and social care and protects the interests of vulnerable people. It monitors compliance with the HSC Act and associated regulations, and has powers to conduct investigations into serious failures of care. In serious breaches of the HSA and when work-related death, unexpected deaths of service users and serious safety incidents resulting in an injury to a service user occur, both the HSE and the CQC have regulatory responsibilities.

The HSE is responsible for control and monitoring of the risks within the workplace to ensure that workers remain safe. The belief that 'prevention is better than cure' informs its mission statement: 'to protect people's health and safety by ensuring that risks in the workplace are properly controlled' (www.hse.gov.uk).

Failure to comply with the legislation and guidelines for health and safety as laid down by the HSE can result in prosecution of the employer. This makes it imperative to ensure that staff comply with all your policies and procedures and demonstrate a responsible attitude towards health and safety.

LO2 Be able to implement and monitor compliance with health, safety and risk management requirements

AC 2.1, 2.2 Demonstrate compliance with health, safety and risk management procedures and support others to comply with legislative and organisational health, safety and risk management policies, procedures and practices relevant to their work

Demonstrate compliance

One of your duties as an employer is to ensure policies are in place and, more to the point, being used. You will also need to carry out risk assessments for the premises and then put risk management measures in place.

Compliance with the Safety Representative and Safety Committee Regulations (1977) and the Health and Safety Consultations with Employees Regulations (1996) (www.hse.gov.uk) is part of the employer's role and, as a manager, you need to ensure that everyone in your team understands that they are responsible for their own safety and also of anybody with whom they interact in the workplace, and that staff are aware of their responsibility when it comes to compliance with the legal aspects of health and safety.

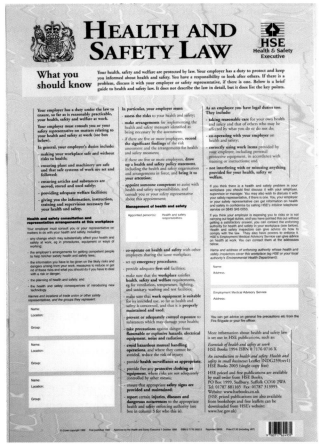

Figure 4.1 A health and safety poster should be displayed in your setting.

- **Make health and safety part of the agenda**: It is likely that you have made health and safety a regular agenda item for your team meeting. In this way, staff can be updated as to training opportunities, risk assessments and their outcomes, and general safety in the workplace issues. A poster giving details of the staff who are designated safety officers and first aiders is useful since it displays relevant information for staff and visitors to the area (see Figure 4.1).
- **Be a good role model**: By demonstrating good practice in a consistent manner, you will inspire others to follow your lead. For example, by ensuring that you take part in regular training updates for health and safety and manual handling with the staff you will be sending positive messages with respect to good practice.
- **Be aware of your responsibility to staff and others**: You need to ensure that visitors to the site are aware of the system in place for fire safety, infection control and COSHH. You might

also want to include information about how challenging behaviour will be dealt with should this occur.

As a manager, it is important that you monitor that staff are complying with the policies and procedures the setting has in place with respect to health, safety and risk management. Care setting failures have shown that although these policies may have been in place, lack of staff compliance led to poor performance and quality of care suffered. See case study on page 74 for more information on this.

Support others

Key term

Others in the care setting includes other workers/practitioners, cares, significant others, visitors to the work setting, inspectors and regulators and they all need to be made aware of how they will be expected to comply with legislative, organisational health, safety and risk management policies, procedure and practices relevant to their work. It is important to display notices and ensure that all visitors on-site are identified and are aware of their role in health, safety and risk whilst in the setting.

Reflect on it

2.1, 2.2 Demonstrating compliance and ensuring others follow protocol

Write a reflective account to show how you comply with the health and safety policies and how you ensure others are also following protocol.

AC 2.3 Explain the actions to take when health, safety and risk management procedures and practices are not being complied with

Your staff need to be aware of the responsibility they have to update their knowledge and to attend health and safety training on a regular basis. It is your responsibility to ensure that the opportunity to do this is available and that staff are encouraged to take time to attend training courses so that there is no reason for not complying with health, safety and risk management policies and procedures. Failure to comply could mean the staff member would be put at risk of losing their job and there will also be consequences for the organisation.

Inspectors from the HSE and from the local authority as well as the CQC enforce health and safety law and have the right to enter any workplace without giving notice. More often than not, notice is given, however, and on a normal inspection visit an inspector would expect to look at the workplace, the work activities, your management of health and safety, and your compliance with health and safety law. Often valuable guidance or advice is given, and occasionally improvement notices may be served and action taken if there is a risk to health and safety that needs to be dealt with immediately.

On finding a problem and a breach of health and safety law, action is taken to determine whether it is a fault of the person, or the systems in place, or the organisation. It may be that more training needs to be undertaken or more serious disciplinary action may be required. Managing risk in this way means that issues are identified before more formal inspections. The guidance from the HSE is as follows:

- **Informal**: if the matter is relatively minor, the employer will be advised as to what to do to comply with the law and the inspector will confirm and outline what constitutes a legal requirement from best practice advice.
- **Improvement notice**: an improvement notice is served when there is a more serious breach. In this case, the following process is generally followed:
  - The inspector discusses and clarifies understanding.
  - The notice will identify what needs to be done, why, and by when.
  - At least 21 days is given in which to take the remedial action. This allows the employer time to appeal to an industrial tribunal if they so wish.
- **Prohibition notice**: a prohibition notice is served when a risk of serious personal injury occurs or if there is potential for it. This means the activity will be prohibited immediately or after a specified time period, and will not be allowed to resume until remedial action (something that is done to remedy or improve

the situation) has been taken. If, for example, your form of transport for your service users or residents is unsafe, then this sort of action may be taken.

- **Prosecution**: this occurs when the inspector considers that it is necessary to initiate a prosecution and the decision to do so is informed by the principles in the HSE's Enforcement Policy Statement, which sets out the general principles and approach which the health and safety enforcing authorities (mainly the HSE and local authorities) are expected to follow. We have recently seen prosecutions of care homes for the neglect and cruelty meted out to residents; these were extreme cases. However, failure to comply with an improvement or prohibition notice carries a fine of up to £20,000, or six months' imprisonment, or both.
- **Appeals:** of course, the employer has the option to take legal action if they feel they have been treated unfairly and they have a right to appeal to an industrial tribunal when an improvement or prohibition notice is served.

It is clear, then, that health and safety in the workplace should not be taken lightly. Not only must you take care of yourself, your staff, service users and visitors to your workplace, you also have a responsibility to ensure that healthy and safety policies are up to date, current and being used.

In practice

2.1, 2.2, 2.3 Implement and monitor compliance with health, safety and risk management requirements

Imagine that you have an inspection happening and are required to provide information. What evidence do you have that you, staff and others in the setting comply with health, safety and risk management procedures? (2.1)

Show how you support others to comply with legislative and organisational health, safety and risk management policies in your setting. Give one or two examples (2.2).

Explain the actions you would take when health, safety and risk management procedures and practices are not being complied with in your own setting (2.3).

AC 2.4 Complete records and reports on health, safety and risk management issues according to legislative and organisational requirements

Importance of good record keeping

You already know the importance of good record keeping (Figure 4.2) and this is highly important in dealing with issues of health and safety. Should an accident happen at work, for example, you may be required to attend court if there has been a claim for compensation. Similarly, records can be used in court as evidence to show compliance with policies and procedures. Unfortunately, we live in a highly litigious society and in order to protect ourselves when we are being held accountable for the care we give, we need to be aware of the place records have. If a complaint is made against us, we would be hard pushed to answer if we had inadequately prepared records. If negligence or a breach of health and safety is suspected in any care setting, any records and statements pertaining to the case will be taken and scrutinised.

If your records are less than accurate, you may find yourself in a difficult situation. Any records maintained need to be:

● accurate
● ordered
● up to date
● stored safely and securely.

Data Protection Act 1998

The last point in the bullet list above is perhaps the most important point since it is a legal requirement

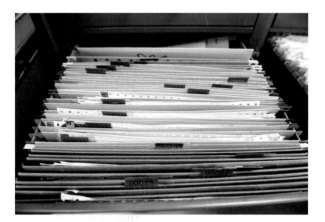

Figure 4.2 Good record keeping is vital in a health and social care setting.

to protect any data we may have on our service users or staff and to maintain it in a confidential way. Any use of such information in an unsuitable way or any breach of confidentiality needs to be dealt with promptly and must be reported to the manager. The security of information is a safeguard for vulnerable service users and any breach of that security can be detrimental to service users.

Compliance with the Data Protection Act (1998) is an imperative. This act gives individuals the right to access their records whether they are stored as paper files or electronically on computers. It is worth revisiting the eight principles concerning data the act refers to:

● Data must be secure.
● Data must not be kept for longer than necessary – you will need to check the requirements in your own organisation for the length of time. (For example, antenatal records are kept for 25 years.)
● Data must be accurate.
● Data must be fairly processed.
● Data must not be transferred without protection.
● Data must protect individuals' rights.
● Data must be processed for limited purposes only.
● Data must be adequate, relevant and not excessive.

Standards and accident and incident reports

The National Minimum Standards for care require that all organisation records relating to health and safety matters are accurate and kept up to date.

The CQCs Essential standard number 20 states that people's personal records must be accurate, fit for purpose, held securely and remain confidential. The same applies to other records that are needed to protect their safety and well-being.

You will be familiar with accident records and may have had to complete these from time to time. We can become blasé or relaxed about these, but we rely on these records, and if years later the case becomes part of a legal process, we need to be able to return to the records to remind us of what actually was done at the time.

Records, then, do the following:

● provide an account of the care given
● give a record of continuous care (in the case of nursing and medical records)
● provide a source of reference for care

2.4 Reporting and recording

You have been made aware of a case of neglect within your setting. One of the relatives of an elderly patient complained that she had found evidence that her elderly mother was not being cared for with dignity. She reported finding adult incontinence wear in the wardrobe in her mother's room and her mother had said she was told not to ring the bell to request being taken to the bathroom at night but to just wet the bed.

Staff then came in and removed the pads from the bed. The relative also said she had found wet nightclothes in the linen bag for her to take home to wash.

What systems have been breached here and as a manager how would you ensure that this does not occur again? How would you record and report on this particular health, safety and risk management issue according to legislative and organisational requirements?

- provide an audit and quality assurance trail
- are a legal requirement
- give evidence of compliance with health and safety guidelines and law.

Additionally, anything that is of a serious nature, such as a reportable disease, serious injury or death, must be reported under RIDDOR (1995).

Dimond (1997) highlighted the major areas of concern in such care reports. She revealed that in many records there were major omissions.

Our responsibility with respect to record keeping is clear. We need to make records on service users, but the way in which we use and store that information is paramount. We must handle all information effectively and be aware of the need to maintain confidentiality of that information. The following checklist may be useful to ensure that you and your staff are aware of good record keeping. It also addresses major omissions that Dimond highlighted.

- Have I written legibly?
- Have I put information in time order, as it happened (i.e. dates and times recorded accurately)?
- Have I got dates and times in the record, and are they accurately recorded?
- Have I put in signs and symptoms? I might even have written how the patient/client is feeling, i.e. client details are recorded accurately.
- Did I carry out a risk assessment?
- Have I included names of other people involved, e.g. of callers and visitors, and recorded information about them accurately?
- Have I written in a professional manner?
- Have I recorded it clearly, are abbreviations clarified?

- Have I signed the forms/records?
- Have I completed records in time, without delay?

2.4 Complete records and reports

Write a short account of how you maintain records in your own setting and how you comply with the eight principles of the Data Protection Act listed on page 83.

LO3 Be able to lead the implementation of policies, procedures and practices to manage risk to individuals and others

AC 3.1, 3.2, 3.3 Contribute to development of policies, procedures and practices to identify, assess and manage risk to individuals and others; work with individuals and others to assess potential risks and hazards and work with individuals and others to manage potential risks and hazards

Risk management

Under the Management of Health and Safety at Work Regulations, you have a responsibility to carry out risk assessment in the workplace in order to eliminate and reduce hazards and risks.

A health and safety risk can be anything that is hazardous. We often work in close contact with

In practice

3.1 Developing policies, procedures and practices

Evaluate your health and safety policy and determine its relevance in identifying, assessing and managing risk to individuals and others.

chemicals, medication and equipment, all of which may cause harm in some way. Risks may also be to do with activities staff are expected to carry out, such as moving and handling or dealing with service users who sometimes display difficult behaviour. The environment, with its stairs, lifts, hallways, beds, and even the people in it, may be potentially risky. As a manager, you need to be able to identify potential risk and eliminate it as far as you are able to. In some instances, you will not be able to eliminate the risk entirely, but you need to make sure you have identified it and put into place actions to minimise the possibility of harm occurring.

Contributing to policies, procedures and practices

In writing policies and procedures you will need to be aware of how detailed and prescriptive these documents can be. They describe the who, what, when, where and how of activities in a strict and rigid manner and can be very time consuming to write. However, once written they merely need to be updated every 12 months, so it is a useful exercise to undertake the task well in the first place so that no major changes need to be made each year. This could be based on the HSE's five steps to risk assessment, as outlined next.

The HSE has produced a free leaflet called 'An introduction to health and safety: health and safety in small businesses'. You are advised to look at this now – you can access it online by typing the title into your search engine. This document gives you a statement of general policy based on your responsibilities with respect to the Health and Safety at Work Act 1974. You are also able to record

your organisational responsibilities and your arrangements to ensure the health and safety of your employees within the sections supplied. There are notes and references for further information and, if you haven't got a policy in place, a template for you to develop your own policy.

Your policy should contain details such as responsibilities of staff, health and safety risks, health and safety staff representatives, staff responsible for maintenance, procedures with regard to handling and use of substances, details of who supervises and trains new recruits with regard to health and safety, where the H&S law poster is displayed, the provision of induction training, job-specific training and keeping training records, details of staff who keep records and those who are responsible for keeping records and reporting under RIDDOR, details about first aiders and where the first-aid kit is stored, details about safe working practices and about staff responsible for carrying out fire risk assessments, and how often checks are made on escape routes, fire extinguishers and alarms, and evacuation procedures.

Working with individuals and others to assess and manage potential risks and hazards

We may view the risk assessment and management as a somewhat onerous task, but we need to carry out such assessment prior to any activity being undertaken. The key stages within the process seek to address the following areas.

HSE's five steps to risk management

Step One: Looking for hazards. An investigation of the premises, activity or procedure needs to be undertaken. The hazards you identify will depend very much on the type of work being carried out. The risk assessment in a school is unlikely to be the same as that in a restaurant or a saw mill, for example.

Step Two: Identifying who could be harmed and how. This seeks to show special arrangements for the types of hazards that people may come into contact with, either through their daily work in an area or even as service users. We are all familiar with hard hats being worn by anybody entering a building site. In your own organisation your risk may be more to do with moving and handling service users or could be to do with issues around infection control. Care homes may need to risk assess their policy on security and entrances to the home, for example.

Step Three: Evaluation of the risk. In this part of the assessment you are making a judgement as to the arrangements already in place for dealing with a potential problem area. An example might be simply changing storage arrangements to free up the fire exit or identifying safer ways to transport service users to outpatient appointments.

Step Four: Record the findings. A record needs to include checklists identifying the hazards, the people likely to be at risk, and arrangements to reduce the hazard.

Step Five: Assess the effectiveness of the precautions in place. Following any dangerous occurrence, staff are expected to complete accident forms and sometimes to inform the HSE. If this occurrence shows up several times then clearly the risk assessment needs to be revisited and safer actions put into place.

The HSE provides an online risk assessment for office workers but with some changes you can use it for your work area also. Go to the HSE website for further help with this activity and find out more about risk assessment/management tools used in health and social care.

We need to be mindful of people such as others practitioners, carers, significant others, family, visitors, inspectors and regulators who come to the setting and ensure that they are also aware of the potential risks and hazards that they meet.

Research it

3.1 Policies, procedures and practices

Research the HSE leaflet 'An Introduction to Health and Safety: Health and Safety in Small Businesses.'

You can access it online by typing the title into your search engine. Make short notes on it, then show how it could contribute to development of policies, procedures and practices in your own setting. Does your policy need to be updated to ensure it identifies, assesses and manages risk to individuals and others?

In practice

3.2, 3.3 Assessing and managing potential risks and hazards

Complete a risk assessment with a member of your staff for an activity in the workplace and document the process.

Provide some evidence to show how you work with individuals and others to manage potential risks, and hazards.

LO4 Be able to promote a culture where needs and risks are balanced with health and safety practice

AC 4.1 Work with individuals to balance the management of risk with individual rights and the views of others

Care settings vary in type and as such the risks associated with them will differ. The rights of individuals in our care can occasionally be in conflict with health and safety issues and we need to be prepared to address such occasions. For example, a new client in a care home may wish to go out shopping by themselves or may wish to go along to the local pub in the evening. The client is clearly not imprisoned in the home and there should be no reason to deny them that right, but at the same time the staff may well have some concerns as to the client's safety when they are not in their care. The CSCI (Commission for Social Care Inspection) document *Rights, Risks and Restraints:*

Reflect on it

3.2 Potential risks and hazards

Think about one of the risks you have identified in your setting and say what you have learned about engaging with risk assessment. How do you think others view this practice in your setting?

Positive risk taking means identifying the potential risks and then developing plans and actions that reflect the potential benefits and harm of exercising one course of action over another. It is a way of seeing the risk in a positive way that enhances the quality of life for an individual.

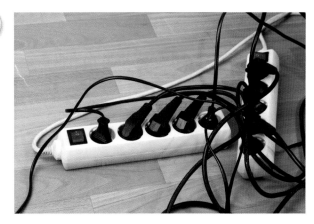

Figure 4.3 It is important to assess the environment for risks to individuals.

An exploration into the use of restraint in the care of older people (2007), although concerned mainly with how some older people have been restrained in some care settings, makes some useful points:

'Respecting people's basic human rights to dignity, freedom and respect underpins good quality social care. People may need support in managing their care and making decisions but they have the right, whether in their own home or in a care home, to make choices about their lives and to take risks.

'Social care services have responsibilities to keep people safe from harm and to ensure their safety. It is this need to balance people's rights to freedom and to make choices with ensuring people are safe that is at the heart of this exploration into the use of restraint in the care of older people.'

It is a case, then, of balancing your duty of care and the client's safety while also respecting their rights. The individual is at the forefront of any decision made and the risk assessment should enable rather than hinder. While workers might be afraid that they are neglecting their responsibilities when it comes to risk assessment, by putting measures in place and enabling risk, care can be transformed. One way in which this has been addressed is through the setting up of 'risk enablement panels'. The emphasis for the panel is on supporting **positive risk taking** while maintaining duty of care.

AC 4.2 Work with individuals and others to develop a balanced approach to risk management that takes into account the benefits for individuals of risk taking

Think about the risks you take on a daily basis. Did you perhaps pull out rather quickly into a busy road in the path of an oncoming car? Perhaps you had to run to catch the bus and didn't look too carefully at the road? Maybe it was simply

a case of standing on a chair in order to retrieve something from a high cupboard?

Our attitude to risk is likely to be different when it comes to risking our personal safety. As care professionals, though, we are bound by law and have a duty of care to our service users and this is likely to change our attitude to risk management. We may be more careful when dealing with service users and take the view that as 'vulnerable adults' they need to be protected in some way. But is this a fair assessment of the people we care for or merely a stereotypical view? Titterton (2005), in his work *Risk and Risk Taking in Health and Social Care*, takes the view that care workers tend to focus on what the service users cannot do and therefore take what he calls a 'safety first approach' to risk (Figure 4.3).

This type of approach focuses on the person's physical problems and disability and tends to ignore other needs. This type of treatment then leads to loss of self-esteem and denies the right to choice and an increase in independence. In this way, there is a danger that the care worker becomes more controlling of the client and person-centred approaches become less of a reality.

Risk in this instance then is thought of in terms of danger, loss, threat, damage or injury and the positive benefits of risk taking are lost. Therefore a more balanced approach needs to be adopted.

The Department of Health agrees with this. Its 2007 paper, 'Independence, choice and risk: a guide to best practice in supported decision making', makes the point that a 'safety first approach' may 'not be necessarily the best option for the person and may be detrimental to quality of life and a risk to maintaining independence'.

A more intelligent option is that proposed by Titterton in his Positive Risk approach. In this approach, risk is seen as positive and enhancing, and recognises the needs of individuals. It demonstrates that choice and autonomy are important and promotes the rights of vulnerable people. Steve Morgan (2004) summarises the approach:

'Positive risk-taking is: weighing up the potential benefits and harms of exercising one choice of action over another. Identifying the potential risks involved, and developing plans and actions that reflect the positive potentials and stated priorities of the service user. It involves using available resources and support to achieve the desired outcomes, and to minimise the potential harmful outcomes. It is not negligent ignorance of the potential risks … it is usually a very carefully thought-out strategy for managing a specific situation or set of circumstances.'

If we are to provide real choice and control for our service users we need to enable individuals to take the risks they choose, with support from the staff. This means allowing the individuals using our service to define their own risks and to plan and monitor any activity they wish to undertake that may entail some form of risk.

AC 4.3, 4.4 Evaluate own practice in promoting a balanced approach to risk management and analyse how helping others to understand the balance between risk and rights improves practice

Do you promote a balanced approach to risk management? Risk assessment and risk management are an essential part of adult social care, but it is often difficult to balance empowerment with the duty of care we owe our service users. For individuals to be able to lead independent lives and to take the risks they choose

to take, this needs to be constantly weighed against the likelihood of significant harm arising from that choice and the situation in question.

In assessing the seriousness of risk you may like to address the following aspects in your workplace:

● the sorts of factors that increase exposure to risk, e.g. environmental, social, financial, communication and recognition of abuse
● the existence of support to minimise risk
● the nature, extent and length of time of the risk
● the impact the risk may have on the individual and on others.

In addition to the above, you are bound by law as stated in Section 3(1) of the Health and Safety at Work Act 1974, which clearly states:

'It shall be the duty of every employer to conduct his undertaking in such a way as to ensure, so far as is reasonably practicable, that persons not in his employment who may be affected thereby are not thereby exposed to risks to their health or safety.'

Unfortunately, this can make us risk averse and you may have staff who err constantly on the side of caution and fail to allow service users to undertake certain activities that they consider to be a risk to safety. This sort of professional risk aversion will undoubtedly lead to a lack of choice for the service users, together with a loss of control and independent living. This will, of course, have an adverse effect on care and is potentially bad practice. Staff, then, need to be supported in carrying out risk assessment that they feel confident about. Balancing the risk against the benefits and the rights of an individual can significantly improve a person's quality of life.

In practice

4.3, 4.4 A balanced approach

Provide an account of your own practice to show how you promote a balanced approach to risk taking for your own setting.

Write a short account of how you have helped staff in your area to carry out risk assessments that support a positive risk-taking approach. How did you help them to understand the balance between risk and rights? Say how this practice has improved the care in your area.

Determine how you might help an employee to understand the balance between risk and rights.

LO5 Be able to improve health, safety and risk management policies, procedures and practices

AC 5.1 Obtain feedback on health, safety and risk management policies, procedures and practices from individuals and others

It is essential to evaluate the quality of your service with respect to health and safety on a continual basis and there are a number of ways in which this may be done.

The CQC is responsible for registering, inspecting and reporting on social care services in England and its main role is to improve social care and stamp out bad practice. Such inspections provide

In practice

5.1 Feedback

The health, safety and risk management policies, procedures and practices in place in your setting are all there to improve care for service users and others. How do you obtain feedback on these areas? How do you evaluate the quality of service in your workplace? List the various measures you use.

You may have identified these according to organisational, team and individual measures of performance.

invaluable feedback about the setting and its achievements. In order to be able to make a judgement, the CQC requires all registered adult social care services to submit an Annual Quality Assurance Assessment (AQAA). This is a legal requirement and in the assessment, care providers describe what they are doing well, what they could improve and how they are going to improve.

From an **organisational** point of view, there are a number of ways in which we are able to measure our performance on any aspect of health care. Feedback is one way to measure performance. This can be obtained in different ways:

- **Complaints and compliments:** complaints and compliments procedures can also provide a good indication of the areas of practice that are working well or badly. In a climate in which people feel able to complain without fear of recrimination, this is a useful way to check practice and to act upon the areas that require some work.

  You need to be aware that a low number of complaints does not necessarily mean that there are no issues. It may be that individuals feel unable to comment for fear of being victimised and this in itself needs investigation. We often get commended for the way in which staff have carried out their work and this needs to be rewarded in some way. A compliments system where service users and visitors can leave a small note to compliment a member of staff may be a useful way in which staff can be recognised for their work. Some organisations have a 'staff member of the month' scheme and this is a nice way to recongnise good work.

- **Focus groups:** service-user and focus groups may also be a part of your quality assurance strategy. The former are structured to gain the views of the people who actually use the service and additionally may provide an avenue of support by peers. If it is possible it should be a service user who runs the group and in this way the service users in the group feel more empowered. Focus groups can be set up to look at areas of practice and to give feedback on procedures or systems. These may be made up of staff, service users and even visitors or family, and are a way of gathering opinions in an open environment. These sorts of meetings are useful for gathering information that is crucial for the running of your setting and as such should be well conducted, with members of the group being clear about what they are being asked to do in a climate that is positive and welcoming. It is important to keep the members informed of the outcomes of the meeting.

- **Team meetings:** at a team level, your regular team meeting will provide much-needed information on health and safety issues. As mentioned earlier, it would be most useful if you had this as an agenda item for every meeting. In that way you can ensure that at least once a week there is a discussion about issues that may require attention and staff can be informed of any changes that require their consideration. The minutes of the meeting can be a part of the AQAA evidence, which must be made available to inspectors when they visit.
- **Appraisals:** Staff appraisals and supervision sessions provide feedback at an individual level and give staff the chance to evaluate their performance over time and to set goals for the future. This is covered in more detail in Unit SHC 52.

Other ways in which you can gain feedback about how your setting is performing with respect to health and safety might be to audit the accident records, the COSHH (Control of Substances Hazardous to Health) file, feedback from the HSE and other professionals, questionnaires, and staff training records to ensure that all are up to date and any problems are dealt with.

AC 5.2 Evaluate the health, safety and risk management policies, procedures and practices within the work setting

Auditing your workplace ensures that practices are in keeping with standards and protocols. For example, you might evaluate the organisation's performance for things such as COSHH assessment, health and safety, and first aid training and equipment; check for things like fire safety or anything in the environment that may be a hazard; cleaning and hygiene checks and data regarding accidents and incidents. These are just a few examples and you should check with your setting for a comprehensive list of health, safety and risk management policies, procedures and practices you will need to check and evaluate.

In practice

5.2 Evaluating health, safety and risk management

Undertake an evaluation of the health and safety activities within your work setting and compile a folder of evidence for your next AQAA.

AC 5.3, 5.4 Identify areas of policies, procedures and practices that need improvement to ensure safety and protection in the work setting and recommend changes to policies, procedures and practices that ensure safety and protection in the work setting

When identifying areas for improvement and recommending change, you need to consider the following:

- What has changed in legislation (regulations) or what recent innovations in care practice require the construction of new policies or procedures?
- Are all staff fully aware of the health and safety procedures within the workplace or is more training needed to ensure they have up-to-date knowledge?
- How will you go about recommending the changes needed and what will you need to do to ensure the changes are accepted?

By undertaking a review of your processes and your behaviour with respect to health and safety on a regular basis, you are in a good position to identify weak points and potential areas for improvement. In this way you can ensure that the policies you have in place are effectively protecting the individuals who come into contact with your setting.

In practice

5.3, 5.4 Identifying areas for improvement and recommending changes

Identify an area of practice that needs improvement to ensure safety and make a recommendation for change to a particular policy.

Document the process you undertake to do this and keep in your portfolio for assessment.

Legislation

See ACs 1.1 and 2.4.

Assessment methods

Learning outcome	Assessment criteria and accompanying activities	Assessment methods *To evidence coverage of the ACs, you could:*
LO1	1.1 Case study (p. 74)	Use the case study story as part of your next team meeting to discuss the consequences of breach of policy. Write up the minutes for your portfolio.
	1.1 Research it (p. 75)	Access the link and make short notes about the regulations.
	1.1 In practice (p. 76)	Prepare a Powerpoint or complete the table in the text listing the laws you are familiar with and explaining the purpose of them. Write a short piece stating what your responsibilities are with respect to implementing them.
	1.1 Research it (p. 79)	Place your written account into your portfolio for marking.
	1.2 Research it (p. 80)	Write short notes about how each regulation is met in your own setting.
	1.2 In practice (p. 80)	Present the analysis of the activity in a poster. Or write a reflective account to show your understanding of the policy and how it meets health, safety and risk management requirements.
	1.2 Reflect on it (p. 80)	Write a reflective account. Discuss your understanding about the activity with your assessor.
LO2	2.1, 2.2 Research it (p. 80)	Provide a written account. You could provide a written journal piece to show how you comply with the policies and how you ensure others are also following protocol.
	2.1, 2.2 Reflect on it (p. 81)	Write a reflective account to show how you comply with the health and safety policies and how you ensure others are also following protocol.
	2.1, 2.2, 2.3 In practice (p. 82)	Prepare a folder containing the evidence and alert staff to its use. Or provide a written account of a real incident from the workplace which shows the actions to take when health, safety and risk management, procedures and practices are not being complied with.
	2.4 Case study (p. 84)	Use this scenario for teaching staff. Prepare a short training session on the systems that have been breached and record and report such breaches.
	2.4 In practice (p. 84)	Write a short account of how you maintain records in your own setting and how you comply with the eight principles of the Data Protection Act listed on page 83.
LO3	3.1 In practice (p. 85)	Write a short piece which evaluates your own Health and Safety policy. Ensure that you include a comment about its relevance in identifying, assessing and managing risk to individuals and others. Provide a report for your assessor.
	3.2 Reflect on it (p. 86)	With your assessor undertake an observation of the area of risk and discuss how you risk assessed this.
	3.1 Research it (p. 86)	Discuss with your assessor the policies implemented as a result of this.

Learning outcome	Assessment criteria and accompanying activities	Assessment methods *To evidence coverage of the ACs, you could:*
	3.2, 3.3 In practice (p. 86)	Place a copy of the completed risk assessment in your portfolio and discuss with your assessor how you work with individuals and other to manage potential risk, and hazards. Or supply the documentation of a risk assessment you and a member of staff have carried out together.
LO4	4.1, 4.2 In practice (p. 88)	Produce a case study which shows how you promote a culture where needs and risks are balanced and how you help your staff to develop such a culture. Or access policies which show this or staff training records which identify how the culture has been developed
	4.2 Research it (p. 88)	Write up the findings from the interviews.
	4.3 Reflect on it (p. 88)	Prepare a short presentation to management about how you manage risk assessment in your setting.
	4.3, 4.4 In practice (p. 89)	Discuss the questions with your assessor and provide a written account.
LO5	5.1 In practice (p. 89)	Provide a list and discuss it with your assessor.
	5.2 In practice (p. 90)	Undertake an evaluation of the health and safety activities within your work setting and compile a folder of evidence for your next AQAA.
	5.3, 5.4 In practice (p. 90)	Document the process you undertake to do this and keep in your portfolio for assessment.

References

Care Quality Commission (2015) Enforcement Policy

CSCI (2007) *Rights, Risks and Restraints: An exploration into the use of restraint in the care of older people*. CSCI.

Department of Health (2000a) *Domiciliary Care – National Minimum Standards*. London: HMSO.

Department of Health (2007) *Independence, Choice and Risk: A guide to best practice in supported decision making*. London: HMSO.

Dimond, B. (1997) *Legal Aspects of Care in the Community*. Basingstoke: Macmillan.

HSE (2010) *An Introduction to Health and Safety: Health and safety in small businesses*. Sudbury, Suffolk: HSE.

Morgan, S. (2004) 'Positive risk-taking: an idea whose time has come,' *Health Care Risk Report*, 10(10), 18–19.

Nightingale, F. (1969) (first published 1858) *Notes on Nursing: What It Is, and What It Is Not*. Dover Publications.

Titterton, M. (2010) *Positive Risk Taking*. Edinburgh: Hale.

www.gov.uk/health-and-safety-executive

www.hse.gov.uk/pubns/indg449.pdf

www.hse.gov.uk/legislation/trace.htm

www.hse.gov.uk/pubns/indg232.pdf

www.telegraph.co.uk/news/health/news/10252991/Record-numbers-of-care-homes-warned-over-illegally-poor-standards.html.

Further reading and useful resources

Care Quality Commission (CQC) (2008) *Essential Standards of Quality and Safety*.

Health and Safety Executive: www.hse.gov.uk/news/subscribe/index.htm

Skills for Care (2011) 'Learning to Live with Risk': www.skillsforcare.org.uk

Unit M2c

Work in partnership in health and social care

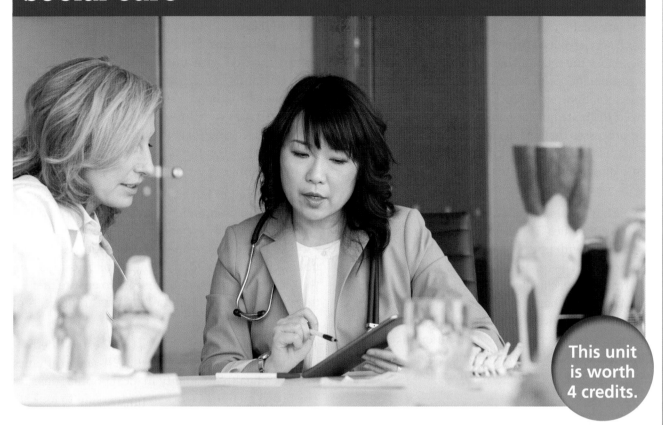

This unit is worth 4 credits.

Working in partnership defines a joint working arrangement where the partners from different services all agree to achieve a common goal for the service user despite being independent bodies. In a health and social care setting, and in your leadership role, this means sharing relevant information and creating a culture of shared ownership and common working arrangements across organisational and professional boundaries.

One of the aims of government in recent years has been to ensure that health and social care services work together to provide care that is integrated and personalised. This requires services from a variety of settings working as partners to ensure the service user receives the best possible care.

Joint health and social care managed networks have been put forward as best practice for ensuring service users with complex health needs benefit from services that share information and work towards common goals. In this unit we will look at how we can promote effective partnership working by establishing good working relationships with all care services we deal with on a daily basis, our colleagues, and the families of the people we care for.

Learning outcomes

By the end of this unit you will:

1 Understand partnership working.
2 Be able to establish and maintain working relationships with colleagues.
3 Be able to establish and maintain working relationships with other professionals.
4 Be able to work in partnership with others.

LO1 Understand partnership working

AC 1.1 Identify the features of effective partnership working

The idea of partnership working developed as a result of acknowledging that it was impossible for one health care provider to provide all care for a service user. Partnership working, then, describes the relationships between services with a responsibility for supplying a variety of care services. In order to work as partners, services need to create new organisational structures or processes that are separate from their own organisation and in which they plan and implement a jointly agreed programme, sometimes with joint staff or resources.

Working in this way is now integral to the way local authorities have developed community strategies with partners. The sharing of information has enabled councils and their partners to reach a better understanding of local problems and has helped to improve the efficiency of support services. With such a huge number of people all delivering services at different areas and locations, joint working with other health professionals is paramount if the service user is to receive the best service.

To work effectively as a partnership there are certain features that need to be in place:

- joint agreement that the service user is the central figure in the process and must be empowered through the process
- good communication
- strong leadership
- adequate resources
- trust between partners.

Working in Partnership – the NHS and the Health and Social Care Act 2012

It is important to remind ourselves of the wider organisation in which we work. We will deal with the National Health Service (NHS) as the main service although some of you may also work in partnership with the education system and local authorities.

With more than 1.3 million staff, the NHS is the biggest health service provider in Europe. Within such a large organisation there will be many different types of groups and teams working together in an effort to ensure that the best service is achieved.

The Health and Social Care Act 2012 brought new structures and working arrangements for the NHS in England. Primary care trusts (PCTs) and strategic health authorities (SHAs) were dispensed with and new bodies such as NHS England (known previously as the NHS Commissioning Board) and clinical commissioning groups (CCGs) were brought in with responsibility for commissioning NHS services. Local authorities took on the task of new public health commissioning.

All these changes have been a result of the need to focus on cooperation between services to provide 'joined up' health care and to streamline the services to reduce cost and use of resources. Other policy changes included the need to focus more on well-being and personalising care to ensure that the individual receiving the care was at the heart of their own care.

The Health and Social Care Act 2012 established health and well-being boards (HWBs) in an attempt to reduce health inequality in local populations. The board members work in partnership to look at local community needs, and work together to provide a seamless system of care.

As an effective way to deliver integrated care, the HWBs are the one forum that brings together elected members, clinicians and other members of the local community to discuss the integration of care and budgets. For more information, see www.local.gov.uk/health/-/journal_content/56/10180/3510973/ARTICLE#sthash.zYt1lodx.dpuf

Working in partnership with other professionals has significantly changed the experience of the service user, putting them firmly at the centre of the care given with greater access to shared resources, improved communication between teams and a more streamlined care service.

Research it

1.1 The Health and Social Care Act 2012

The Health and Social Care Act 2012 brought new structures and working arrangements for the NHS. As discussed, one such change was the development of more integrated care work through partnerships and HWBs.

Look at the following websites and find out more information about the various ways in which health care has been structured in other parts of the United Kingdom.

● The King's Fund's alternative guide to the new NHS in England – www.kingsfund.org.uk/projects/nhs-65/alternative-guide-new-nhs-england

● NHS Wales Shared Partnership Services – www.wales.nhs.uk/sitesplus/955/home

● Overview of Health and Care Structures in The Health and Social Care Act 2012 – http://www.local.gov.uk/health/-/journal_content/56/10180/3510973/ARTICLE

● NHS Scotland – www.show.scot.nhs.uk/

● Belfast Health and Social Care Trust – www.belfasttrust.hscni.net/about/Understanding-Health-Service-Structure.htm

Case study

1.1 Working in partnership

The following case studies from *The Guardian* in February 2015 show how the HWBs are working in partnership.

● One HWB worked together with key local players to share knowledge and ideas that link up local services.

There was acknowledgement, however, that HWBs lack formal powers to commission, which can be a hindrance to the process.

● In Newcastle the HWB is linked to the Change for Life programme, which is in place to meet

public health goals such as tackling obesity and smoking in the community.

Go to www.theguardian.com/healthcare-network/2015/feb/13/health-and-wellbeing-boards-bigger-role for the full stories.

As a manager comment on how your own local HWB works and how they ensure that all services link up.

What are your views on the approach put forward by Newcastle HWB? How does your HWB meet such objectives?

In practice

1.1 Features of effective partnership working

In your setting, report on the partners you work with on a regular basis and reflect on the effectiveness of the arrangements. What features are effective in these partnerships?

AC 1.2 Explain the importance of partnership working with colleagues, other professionals and others

The importance of partnership working with colleagues, other professionals and others should not be underestimated.

Partnership working has been set up to improve the experience and outcomes of people who use the service and this can be achieved by minimising barriers between different services.

As far back as 2002 the National Service Framework recommended 'more formalised structures and systems for achieving joint aims'. Through the use of Health Improvement and Modernisation Plans (HIMPs), partnership working between the NHS, local agencies and communities became the main focus. More recently, the Health and Social Care Act 2012 has developed the need for a more integrated way of working through partnerships and HWBs.

Colleagues are people you work with in providing care services. They may be in similar job roles as yourself or may have a different status. To work in partnership with colleagues there needs to be collaboration and commitment to the service user to ensure best practice.

Other professionals include people who are from different agencies and disciplines but still part of the wider health care team. They may be advocates for the service user or from social care agencies or other health disciplines such as physiotherapists and mental health workers, etc.

Others refers to those people who may not come under the umbrella of health professionals. They could be family, carers and friends, or children and young people.

Colleagues and others professionals

For our colleagues and health professionals, partnership working has improved the quality of the service offered and has proved to be more cost effective, thus securing jobs. By recognising common goals, a 'whole person' approach to care can be taken, there has been a growth in the understanding of other care professionals' roles and mutual respect is therefore built. The personalisation agenda has put service users firmly in charge of ensuring that the care and support they require has been designed with their involvement to meet their unique needs.

Others

This way of working has benefits for all involved in the care process. For service users it has meant a more 'joined up' approach to the care they receive. Having a single assessment process instead of multiple assessments by different agencies has been well received by clients and extends their choice.

The service users are ultimately our customers and they are at the centre of designing and delivering health and social care services. The Department of Health has actively promoted the involvement of service users and the public in decisions about the planning, design, development and delivery of local services and service users see themselves as

In practice

1.2 The importance of effective partnership working
Identify the features and importance of effective partnership working for your organisation.

having a particular role to play, not least because they are 'experts in their own experience'.

Family carers also play a huge role in caring for their family members and are a major part of the partnership in care. It is important for health professionals to recognise and respect the role of lay carers and to support the role. Over the last 20 years or so there has been greater recognition of the benefits of family members providing care, particularly if it helps to keep the family member in their own home. With detailed knowledge of their loved ones' preferences, illness, culture and value systems, these 'lay carers' (those with no care qualifications) are better equipped to provide the loving support the service user needs. In the past, however, lay carers were rather neglected and felt isolated and unsupported. Health professionals therefore need to ensure that the relatives of service users are involved in care planning processes and assessments.

Also see Unit LM1c (on leading a team) and AC 3.3 for more information on working with others.

AC 1.3 Analyse how partnership working delivers better outcomes

In the government White Paper 'Improving health and care: the role of the outcomes frameworks', published in 2012, a pledge to enable people to live better for longer was made and a number of outcomes for enabling this were put forward. With three outcomes frameworks, for Public Health, Adult Social Care and the NHS, published since 2010 the intention was to focus on improving all aspects of health care across the system, one focus of which was the strengthening of joint or partnership working.

Reporting on the outcomes in 2012, the NHS Future Forum found that patients were still experiencing gaps in service provision, communication breakdown and poor transitions between services. The Future Forum concluded

1.3 Analyse how partnership working delivers better outcomes

Using an example from your own practice, show how partnership working has delivered better outcomes.

the need for integration of services as a 'vitally important aspect' to improving care.

Integration of care is seen as the assimilation of organisations and/or services into single entities, allowing for greater transparency between partners as well as enhanced benefits for service users (Tilmouth *et al*., 2011).

Better outcomes

Partnership working enables the strategic goals and vision of the organisation in which we work to be jointly discussed and understood. It enables agreement to be reached on how the care for a service user can be implemented in the best interests of that service user and their families, as well as staff.

The Social Partnership Forum's website highlights the benefits of good partnership working as being:

- trust and mutual respect
- openness, honesty and transparency
- top-level commitment
- a positive and constructive approach
- commitment to work with and learn from each other
- early discussion – no surprises
- confidentiality when needed.

Source: http://www.socialpartnershipforum.org/1111

Working in partnership therefore provides safe, quality care from a range of providers who have the client/patient at the centre of the whole process.

AC 1.4 Explain how to overcome barriers to partnership working

Health and social care professionals work together at three levels (Department of Health, 1998):

- Strategic – planning and sharing information.
- Operational management – policies that demonstrate partnership.
- Individual care – joint training and a single point of access to health care.

However, all these working arrangements involve individuals from different professional backgrounds, and locations, with different funding and resources and philosophies of care and as such are potentially prone to challenges.

Armistead and Pettigrew (2004) argued that:

'It is important to recognise that the very term "partnership" might increasingly be perceived pejoratively, synonymous with lengthy, fruitless meetings, forced upon unwilling organisations by … government policy.'

Barriers to partnership working

Lack of role clarity

The various roles that come together in partnerships can make joint-working difficult, particularly where there are perceived differences in status between occupational groups. Some practitioners may feel that their professional status is threatened and this can lead to problems in coming to joint decisions.

Joint employment

Conditions between different organisations can also be a barrier to joint-working, particularly where new patterns of working are being requested at the same time. This can lead to resistance to change, resulting in poor morale among staff and other partners, particularly service users and other professionals and colleagues.

Financial barriers

When professionals have different pay scales according to their professional group and their role within it, this can cause conflict. Additionally, there may be resentment if staff notice that money is used to employ staff from one group to provide a service normally provided by their own staff. Staff shortages can also damage interaction and the groups will start to withdraw from partnership working in an attempt to limit demands that are being made. Where money is in short supply for some partners, this can become a huge issue when establishing budgets and costs for various initiatives. There are costs involved when it comes to partnership working and this can be frustrating and may also become a barrier.

Information

Information poses constraints and these revolve around not only reluctance to share data but also linking incompatible IT systems and the way in which records are kept in each organisation.

Time

Time is another area where barriers are widespread. With increasing numbers of partnerships developing, the time spent on meetings and travelling can be an issue and may lead to the outcomes achieved being far less than originally perceived.

Different priorities and cultures

Staff working in different disciplines prioritise the care they give in a variety of ways. If we lack understanding about how a service works and constantly question the way staff carry out care, this can lead to barriers forming. In addition, our whole ethos of working may be vastly different to that of the partner and this can lead to questioning the care they give. An underlying lack of understanding about how care can be delivered in different ways could damage the partnership.

Overcoming barriers

Working together: There have been a number of initiatives to try to break down barriers and we can learn a lesson from education here. It has long been a tradition to segregate students in universities based on their chosen professional pathway, but it has been shown that this way of teaching can lead to 'professional arrogance' (Leathard, 1994) and the notion that some groups and degrees are 'better than others'.

Postgraduate education has addressed this and now offers a significant number of Master of Science (MSc) and Master of Arts (MA) level programmes which encompass multi-professional participation, for example. This active development to include a varied studentship has led to a greater understanding of other disciplines with which we might not usually come into contact. The same could be true of multi-disciplinary working. By working in close contact with someone from another professional area, we are able to enhance our knowledge of their role and can better understand how they approach care from a different perspective.

Improved communication systems: A further way in which barriers can be broken down is to address the communication systems between professional groups. Successful collaboration depends on open and transparent discussion. Traditionally, communication has relied on written formats – referral forms, feedback forms, case notes, care plans, letters and faxes. However, while quality record keeping and evidence-based policies and procedures are necessary, there does need to be more one-to-one collaboration and **active participation** in meeting with partners on a regular basis.

Engage family and put interests of service user first: By engaging the family in all decision making and supporting them in their aims to help their loved ones, barriers to the partnership can become a thing of the past. The Care Act 2014 encourages 'person-centred care' and this requires complete recognition of the needs and choices of the person receiving care. By ensuring that support is available to families and the service user, and by listening to those on the receiving end of care, a better quality of life can be expected.

The increasing pressure put on health and care services has resulted in barriers to working and the policy goal of 'putting people first' has been slow to achieve. To help overcome this, the charity coalition National Voices wants the health and care systems to set an ambition to achieve genuinely person-centred care by 2020. This would improve the quality of life, health and well-being of people, and make care systems more sustainable.

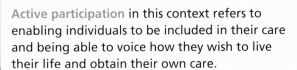

Key term

Active participation in this context refers to enabling individuals to be included in their care and being able to voice how they wish to live their life and obtain their own care.

In practice

1.4 Overcoming barriers

Write a report to explain how you have managed to overcome barriers to partnership working within your work area.

Reflect on it

1.4 Features of effective of partnerships and barriers

Think about a partnership you have set up in your setting and reflect on the effective features within it. What did you find particularly difficult? How have you worked to improve the barriers you experienced, if any?

LO2, LO3, LO4 Be able to establish and maintain working relationships with colleagues, other professionals, and be able to work in partnership with others

AC 2.1, 3.1 Explain own role and responsibilities in working with colleagues and other professionals

As we read in LO1, working in partnership means you will be working alongside different people from a variety of disciplines, as well as colleagues within your own team and members of the service user's family. One of the responsibilities you have is to maintain an open mind about the way in which other services work and to respect the roles of others in the care they give. For your colleagues you also need to create a working environment which promotes national policies with respect to partnership working.

Emphasis upon collaborative working will ensure that the service users in your care are provided with the support they require to live the lives they want with dignity, something that the Care Act 2014 stresses and was also highlighted in the White Paper 'Equity and Excellence: Liberating the NHS' (2010).

Effective working in health and social care requires collaboration. Additionally, effective team work enhances patient care and safety as members of the team coordinate and communicate their activities and have the patient at the centre of the care. One of your main roles will be to act as a link person in the partnership, whether it is with families or other professionals, and also to develop a climate of **trust** between all partners.

Build trust
Trust is such an important issue in management and leadership and is at a premium in today's working climate. If partnerships are to work, you need to ensure that you have created trust in your organisation by being open and reliable in your decision making and by articulating a commitment to the way in which the partnership is to work. Jobs are being lost on a daily basis, there is a

Key term
Trust is having the belief that something or somebody is reliable and honest.

climate of downsizing and outsourcing of work, and this will have had an effect on your workforce and the partners with whom you work.

When there is a lack of trust, the result is fear, suspicion and insecurity and this all leads to lowering of morale in general, with resultant resistance to change and reduced productivity.

The Authentic Leadership approach developed by George (2003) focused on characteristics of good leaders. He found that authentic leaders have a strong desire to serve others and demonstrate five basic characteristics:

1 They have a purpose.
2 They have strong values and are clear about the right thing to do.
3 They establish trusting relationships.
4 They demonstrate self-discipline.
5 They are passionate about their mission.

George (2003) further noted that individuals wanted their leaders to be open with them and to become more transparent, thus softening the boundary between roles. A trusting relationship with the leader leads to greater commitment to the mission and also loyalty.

As a manager, your role in this will be to create a high-trust culture which ensures that your staff and the people in the partnership feel safe and valued. The document *Partnerships: A literature review* (2007) published by the Institute of Public Health in Ireland also highlighted that 'building trust between partners is the most important ingredient in success'.

Open communication
Communication is important and in an atmosphere where trust is central to the workings of the team, individuals will feel free to be able to contribute fully. Staff should feel able to be part of negotiations within an organisation.

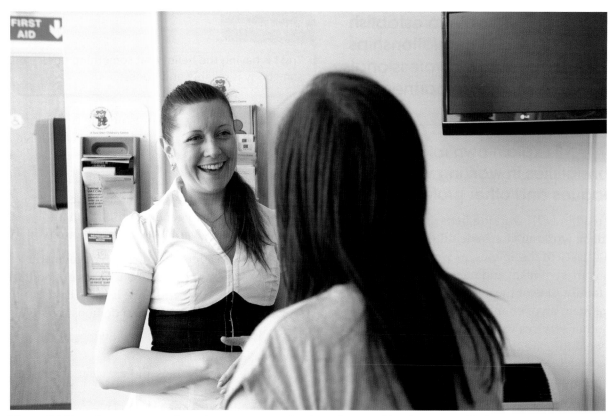

Figure 5.1 How do you ensure there is open communication when working in partnership?

Identifying and challenging discrimination/ difficult situations and managing conflict

This is also an area where staff must feel able to voice any concerns they may have. The transparency within the way you lead will also make dealing with conflict more palatable.

Unit LM1c LO1 on team working covers factors that enable good team working, such as negotiating. It also covers dealing with difficult situations and avoiding and managing conflict, momentum, respecting differences, recognising everyone's role, and positive relationships. It would be useful to the reading of this unit.

Reporting concerns and recording when working with colleagues

Should you have any concerns about a colleague and the way they are working, there needs to be a way in which you can report and record incidents. The policies in your workplace will show how you must address concerns and as a manager you should encourage staff to use the protocols in place. Should a member of staff report a concern to you, then there must be a record of the incident made and details about how the issue has been dealt with.

In practice

2.1, 3.1 Your role and responsibilities when working with colleagues and other professionals

Reflect upon your role and responsibilities (AC 2.1) in working with colleagues and other professionals (AC 3.1).

Provide evidence of partnership working you have been involved in and comment on its success. What might you change in the future?

AC 2.2, 3.3 and 4.3 Develop and agree common objectives when working with colleagues, with other professionals within the boundaries of your own role and responsibilities and with others

Objectives about policy and procedures, the way in which leadership is handled, and training and development all need to be agreed upon. There must also be some discussion about boundaries, and who is accountable for each part of the system of care. Communication and good personal relationships between specialist and more

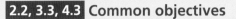
generalist workers will improve the trust among the wider partnership and thus enable a more effective way of working.

Colleagues

You will be familiar with the notion of setting objectives in order to achieve aims. Part of your role as a manager and leader will be to educate your staff and as such you set objectives as to what you hope the learners attending your session will gain as a result of being there. So, too, with partnership working – there needs to be a good balance between developing the partnership and its objectives in order for it to be successful.

It is all too easy to get carried away with the actual work that needs to be done within the partnership without recognising the differences that might exist between all concerned. For example, we may make assumptions about the way in which other organisations or individuals work and lose sight of what we are actually there for.

Other professionals

Partnership objectives need to be consistent with those of the partner organisations and other representatives and we also need to be fully aware of where the boundaries lie between the partnership's work and their own organisation's activities.

Others

The families, carers, advocates and friends of the individual are an important part of the care team surrounding the service user and so must be included in setting the objectives for care. These people are at the heart of the service user's life and as such can often see things like imbalances in the care being planned. They should be aware of the way in which each part of the team communicates and the relationship between the specialists and other workers involved in the care. They are then better placed to see where the boundaries between partners lie and who is accountable for the care in the setting.

 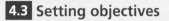
In practice

2.2, 3.3, 4.3 Common objectives

In making a more effective partnership, it is essential to invest in building good objectives from the outset. The following set of objectives may be useful. Think about your setting and the teams that you work with, including your colleagues, other professionals and others.

- Define the partnership role and purpose: What are we here for? What is the partnership actually supposed to do?
- Agree who is to be involved: Who should be invited onto the partnership and how will we select them?
- Establish protocols and procedures: What structures underpin the partnership?
- Ground rules and behaviour: Set your standards for behaviour and language to build trust and respect.
- Who is in charge? Share power and engage minority interests – ensure that equal parity is given to all groups, i.e. they are all treated equally.
- How will we ensure our activity is widely known? Communication and accountability – letting those outside the partnership know what's going on.

Using the objectives above, complete an action plan to show how you and your colleagues have set up a way of working with partners.

Part of your role as a manager is to encourage others to work effectively and one way to achieve this is to work towards the same goals and to cooperate with the decisions made. When properly managed and developed, such teamwork improves processes and produces results quickly and economically through the free exchange of ideas and information (Tilmouth *et al.*, 2011).

AC 2.3, 3.4 and 4.4 Evaluate own working relationship with colleagues, procedures for working with other professionals, and others

It is important to be able to measure how effective the work partnership is and to do so requires appraisal systems and outcomes measures.

Work performance appraisal systems can be used to assess how effective the partnership has been as well as the quality of the work produced. The evaluation methods used can take various forms and largely depend on the type of career professional being appraised. For example, doctors are required to undertake an annual medical appraisal to demonstrate to the GMC that they are up to date and fit to practise, and a specific process is followed. In health and social care work, evaluation of work performance may well rest on several basic techniques such as supervision and performance appraisals.

In evaluating your working relationship with your staff it might be useful to use a self-assessment tool in which staff are able to provide anonymous feedback about various aspects of the working relationship.

In evaluating procedures outside assessment, other professionals and teams may be asked to observe the workplace on a formal and informal basis, providing independent feedback. This can then be measured against the in-house evaluations by staff and service users.

Evaluation can also be gained through the use of written comment forms, telephone surveys or online questionnaires. Families and friends and others who may be supporting the service user may be included in evaluation and be asked to comment upon the service provision. We may also ask advocates to evaluate the service and comment on whether and how they have been included in discussions and planning regarding the service user.

Undertaking such measures can identify the successes of team working as well as the failures and can provide evidence for change. By making an evaluation of the way in which partnerships are working it is possible to assess the effectiveness of the care provided and make changes accordingly.

In practice

2.3, 3.4 Evaluating working relationships with colleagues and procedures for working with other professionals

Look at the way in which you work with people in your team and with professionals and others and identify your strengths and weaknesses in these arrangements.

Ask colleagues and other professionals to comment upon your assessment. Write a reflection of what you might do to improve your working arrangements. Include evidence from the outcome measures you use to audit the systems and procedures.

In practice

4.4 Evaluate procedures for working with others

Use the GROW model as shown in Unit 6 LM1c (Figure 6.5) or undertake a SWOT analysis to show how you might make changes to the whole process of partnership working and providing an integrated care system as a result of your evaluation.

Government guidance published in 2014 by Monitor, the sector regulator for health services in England, summarises the importance of working in partnerships and integrating care for service users.

With service users' care being provided by several different health and social care professionals, across different providers, it is possible that care may be fragmented or difficult to access if the partnership is failing. However, good integrated care can reduce this, improving outcomes for service users.

You may have received useful feedback from staff and other professionals. However, you may also have found some concerns with respect to the ways in which working relationships change as a result of partnership development.

In any environment where there is a range of groups working together from a variety of locations, problems can occur. Pearson and Spencer (1997) commented on this issue and said that the complexity of partnership working was

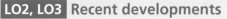

not always good for building inter-professional relationships. This way of working means that the team has too many members to be an effective size and planning meetings can be problematic, trying to get all professionals together at the same time.

With your own staff you may have had a more positive response. Being in close proximity to your team makes it so much easier to communicate and work together, making this type of working more stable and predictable.

AC 2.4, 3.5, 4.5 Deal constructively with any conflict that may arise with colleagues; with other professionals and with others

See Unit LM1c AC 1.7 on methods on addressing conflict within a team and Unit LM2c on professional supervision practice.

Conflict may arise at any time in any partnership and should not always be viewed as a negative occurrence. It may highlight an important issue and lead to a better outcome for all concerned. For example, in health care settings conflict between partners may arise if resources are threatened due to the introduction of another service. If staff feel that their role is undermined in any way by another service, this can lead to conflict. The main aims in any conflict resolution are to communicate, listen and keep an open mind about the situation.

The Research Briefing 41, commissioned by SCIE (2012), 'Factors that promote and hinder joint and integrated working between health and social care services' is a useful read and comments upon the findings from a large study about integrated (partnership) working.

The factors that cause conflict include some of the following:

- lack of understanding about joint aims and objectives or failure to establish a shared purpose

- lack of clarity about the roles and responsibilities
- confusion about policies and procedures underpinning the new service or way of working
- organisational difference or competing 'organisational visions' and lack of agreement about which organisation should lead
- absence of a pooled or shared budget and differences in resources and spending
- communicating across professional or agency boundaries, particularly when they are not located on the same site
- information sharing – difficulty sharing information, lack of access to information and incompatible IT systems
- lack of strong and appropriate managerial support (was thought to undermine attempts to work across agencies and professional boundaries)
- different professional philosophies

- lack of trust, respect and control
- difficulties in role boundaries
- constant reorganisation
- financial uncertainty
- difficulty in recruiting staff.

Dealing constructively with conflict

Occasionally others involved in care, family members or members of the wider disciplinary team may disagree about something in the setting and this needs to be dealt with in a sensitive and professional manner. There may be disagreements amongst other professionals or the family about the way in which care is given and this may be due to a lack of understanding about certain features of the care role. For example, the family or others involved in care may not understand the risk involved in certain lifestyle choices such as eating unhealthily or ensuring that medication is given on time. This can lead to the service user being compromised and may lead to conflict. The way in which this is handled needs to be specific to the person you are dealing with and will require a different approach to those who are health professionals.

AC 3.2 and 4.2 Develop procedures for effective working relationships with other professionals and others

The most important thing you can do to develop effective working relationships is to build your reputation as being a professional who is trustworthy and inspires confidence and respect in your team as well as between all team members. In this way you can show that you provide other professionals with information, advice and support within the boundaries of your role and expertise and as such can develop procedures for partnership working that are fair to all parties involved.

By being honest and open with staff you can develop a more cooperative way of working. Actively listening to the issues your staff and others have, and attempting to come to a mutual resolution when conflict arises, will go a long way

to ensuring that the workforce remains positive. Your policy on communication for example, can help effective working relationships by being robust and up to date.

In working with families and carers, service users and their advocates there are a number of ways that health and social care organisations develop their procedures to ensure they meet the needs of carers. Some of these may be:

- identify a mentor within the organisation who will be the first point of contact for carers and will take primary responsibility for making sure that carers' needs are considered
- provide 'carer awareness' training for all staff to ensure they understand what role the care will be taking
- develop links to local carers' organisations to explore ways of working together
- develop a carers' charter to ensure that best practice guidelines for working with carers and staff are identified and that staff are aware of these
- start up a staff carers' network
- make sure information for carers is available and well publicised
- involve carers in service planning and development
- provide training for carers in areas such as lifting and handling, intimate care, use of equipment, stress management and maximising their own health and well-being.

The HSE and other voluntary agencies supported by the HSE, such as Caring for Carers and The Carers Association, provide a national certified training course, 'Care in the Home', for carers and people working in the caring profession. This course covers practical caring skills such as feeding, washing and dressing and personal skills such as communication stress management and coping skills. (For more information on this, see ww.hse.ie/eng/services/list/4/olderpeople/carersrelatives/Support_for_Carers.html).

Key term

Others in this instance refers to individuals, children and young people, families and carers.

In practice

3.2, 4.2 Effective working relationships with other professionals and others
Write a case study of a service user or group of people you work with showing the procedures you have put in place to ensure effective work relationships.

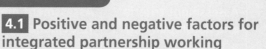

LO4 Be able to work in partnership with others

AC 4.1 Analyse the importance of working in partnership with others

We have seen from the previous ACs that the primary purpose of partnership working is to improve the experience and outcomes of people who use services, and this is achieved by minimising organisational barriers between different services. In addition, partnerships work by:

- delivering coordinated packages of services to individuals
- reducing the impact of organisational fragmentation
- bidding for, or gaining access to, new resources
- meeting a statutory requirement.

Partnership working is central to the care of service users and brings together a variety of other services such as those in the voluntary sector. The DOH launched the Voluntary Sector Strategic Partner Programme in April 2009 to improve communication between the department and voluntary health and social care organisations. It enabled voluntary sector organisations to work in equal partnership with the Department of Health, NHS and social care for the benefit of the sector and has improved health and well-being outcomes. You may also be working with other agencies within the wider multi-disciplinary team such as advocacy agencies or other health care teams. Advantages of working closely with other organisations are that they may be able to offer advice on specific issues, for example. Disadvantages of purely relying on other organisations are that some may be affected by

Research it

4.1 Positive and negative factors for integrated partnership working

Access the Research Briefing 41, commissioned by SCIE (2012), 'Factors that promote and hinder joint and integrated working between health and social care services' and make a list of the positive and negative factors for integrated partnership working.

In practice

4.1 Analysing the importance of working in partnership with others

Compile a case study which shows how you have set up a partnership with either a service user and their carer or another organisation and show the whole process of that venture. In analysing you should make sure you examine the partnership in detail and provide an in-depth explanation about its advantages and disadvantages.

lack of funding which may make it difficult for the sector to fund its work.

Legislation

- The Health and Social Care Act 2012 brings together the White Papers which led to its development.
- Health and Social Care (Safety and Quality) Act 2015.
- Government White Paper *Our Health, Our Care, Our Say: A New Direction for Community Services* (2006).
- The White Paper *Equity and Excellence: Liberating the NHS* (2010).

Assessment methods

LO	Assessment criteria and accompanying activities	Assessment methods *To evidence coverage of the ACs, you could:*
LO1	Research it (p. 95)	Make some notes on the way healthcare has been structured in other parts of the United Kingdom and discuss with your assessor the HWBs and integrated care work and their impact upon your setting.
	1.1 Case study (p. 95)	Provide a written account answering the questions.
	1.1 In practice (p. 95)	Report on the partners you work with on a regular basis and reflect on the effectiveness of the arrangements. Comment upon the ways in which roles differ. Write a short piece to show your understanding.
	1.2 In practice (p. 96)	Discuss with your assessor your thoughts on this activity.
	1.7 In practice (p. 97)	Provide evidence from your own practice which shows positive outcomes from partnership working. Prepare mind map which shows this.
	1.4 In practice (p. 98)	Write a report to explain how you have managed to overcome barriers to partnership working within your work area.
	1.4 Reflect on it (p. 98)	Prepare a report or a table which answers the activity.
LO2 LO3 LO4	2.1, 3.1 In practice (p. 100)	Collect information about partnership working in your setting and compile an information sheet which shows roles and responsibilities when working with colleagues and others and factors which demonstrate the success of the venture.
	2.2, 3.3, 4.3 Reflect on it (p. 101)	Supply some evidence from supervision reports (be sure to anonymise them) which shows when you have used smart targets for staff.
	4.3 Reflect on it (p. 101)	Discuss the process with your assessor and document it.
	2.2, 3.3, 4.3 In practice (p. 101)	Prepare a table which shows the above information and share the action plan with staff at a team meeting. Or you could develop an action plan to show how you agree objectives with own colleagues, partners and others.
	2.3, 3.4 In practice (p. 102)	Collect evidence from audits and systems in the setting which show how your setting works with colleagues and other partners. Prepare a short report from the findings to share with management.
	4.4 In practice (p. 102)	Place a copy of the GROW model in your portfolio together with a copy of your SWOT analysis.
	LO2, LO3 Research it (p. 103)	Place the findings from the research into your portfolio and write a short piece which evaluates what you found.
	2.4, 3.5 Reflect on it (p. 103)	Discuss with your assessor. Write a reflective account.
	4.5 Reflect on it (p. 103)	Give one example of the conflict experienced and comment upon how you have changed as a result of your learning here.
	2.4, 3.5, 4.5 In practice (p. 103)	Prepare a Powerpoint presentation which shows how staff can deal with conflict.
	3.2, 4.2 In practice (p. 104)	Write a case study of a service user or group of people you work with showing the procedures you have put in place to ensure effective work relationships.
	4.1 Research it (p. 105)	Prepare the list and discuss it with your assessor.
	4.1 In practice (p. 105)	Compile a report of the whole process which identifies how the partnership was planned, developed and evaluated.

References

Armistead, C. G. and Pettigrew, P. (2004) 'Effective partnerships: building a sub-regional network of reflective practitioners,' *The International Journal of Public Sector Management*, 17(7), 571–85.

Audit Commission (1998) *A fruitful partnership – Effective partnership working*.

Boydell, L. (2007) *Partnerships: A literature review*. Dublin: Institute of Public Health in Ireland.

Cameron, A., Lart, R., Bostock, L. and Coomber, C. (2012) 'Factors that promote and hinder joint and integrated working between health and social care services,' Research Briefing 41, SCIE.

Department of Health (2002) *National Service Framework: A practical aid to implementation in primary care*. London: HMSO.

Department of Health (2010) *Equity and Excellence: Liberating the NHS*. London: HMSO.

Department of Health (2011) *The Department of Health Voluntary Sector Strategic Partner Programme*. Crown.

DfE (2004) *Removing Barriers to Achievement: The Government's strategy for meeting special educational needs*. London: HMSO.

DOH (1998) *Information for Health: An information strategy for the modern NHS 1998–2005 – executive summary*. Crown Copyright.

DOH (2012) *Improving Health and Care: The role of the outcomes framework*. Government publications.

George, B. (2003) *Authentic Leadership: Rediscovering the secrets to creating lasting value*. San Francisco: Jossey-Bass.

Leathard, A. (1994) *Going Inter-professional: Working together for health and welfare*. London and New York: Routledge.

Monitor (2014) 'Delivering better integrated care,' Crown Copyright.

Office of Health Economics (2009) https://www.ohe.org/

http://changesuk.net/themes/partnership-working/

Pearson, P. and Spencer, J. (1997) *Promoting Teamwork in Primary Care: A research-based approach*. London: Arnold.

The World Health Organization (WHO) (1978) www.who.int/publications/almaata_declaration_en.pdf

Tilmouth, T., Davies-Ward, E. and Williams, B. (2011) *Foundation Degree in Health and Social Care*. London: Hodder Education.

Whitmore, J. (2003) *Coaching for Performance: GROWing people, performance and purpose* (3e). London: Nicolas Brealey.

www.bristol-inquiry.org.uk/final_report/report/Summary.htm

Useful resources and further reading

Department of Health (2006) *Our Health, Our Care, Our Say: A new direction for community services*. London: HMSO.

Health and Wellbeing Boards Leadership Offer. www.local.gov.uk/health/-/journal_content/56/10180/3510973/ARTICLE#sthash.zYt1lodx.dpuf

National Voices (2014) Person-centred Care 2020: Calls and Contributions from Health and Social Care Charities.

Unit LM1c

Lead and manage a team within a health and social care setting

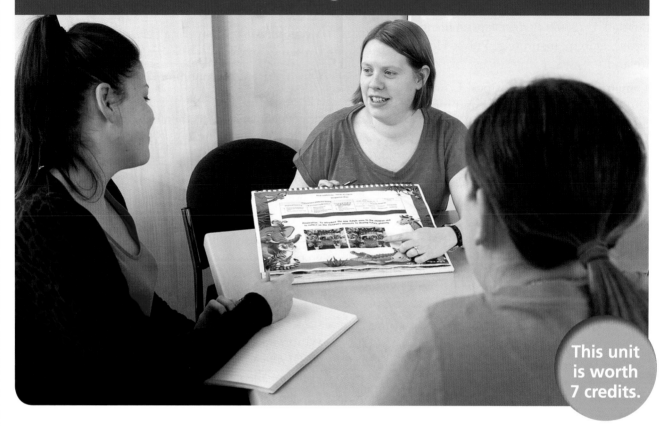

This unit is worth 7 credits.

A team is a group of people who work together and a group is a collection of two or more people who communicate together because they have interests in common. From the beginning of time, people have used work groups to get things done and to generate new ideas.

(Wheelan, 2005)

Team working means taking responsibility for your own work, as well as respecting the contributions of all your colleagues, and good communication is essential to effective team working.

Effective team performance requires the development of a positive and supportive culture in an organisation. Only in this way can we expect staff to be supportive of a shared vision to meet the agreed objectives for a health and social care setting. The most important person in your team will be the service user or client and they need to be central to any team working.

In this unit you will learn how to lead and manage a team and enhance their performance in a health and social care setting. The unit will introduce you to team function and the roles that are adopted in teams and will examine models of leadership relevant to the health and care sector. The features and activities in the unit will encourage you to examine strategies of team working and leadership in order to identify your own strengths, responsibilities and learning needs, and to reflect on best practice within the care context.

Learning outcomes

By the end of this unit you will:

1 Understand the features of effective team performance.
2 Be able to support a positive culture within the team.
3 Be able to support a shared vision within the team.
4 Be able to develop a plan with team members to meet agreed objectives.
5 Be able to support individual team members to work towards agreed objectives.
6 Be able to manage team performance.

LO1 Understand the features of effective team performance

AC 1.1 Explain the features of effective team performance

Imagine a group of footballers who have little idea about the rules of the game, what the objectives of the game are and how the position they play works with the rest of the team. Picture the first match and guess the outcome. Of course, it is likely to be a mess, isn't it? With nobody working together and without any direction, the game will be lost.

What is it that makes a group of people a team?

Just like in the example above, effective teams in your setting work together towards common goals and objectives and it is important you know what the features of effective team performance are.

Pearson and Spencer (1997) suggest that teams are formed because of a belief that having people work on shared goals interdependently will lead to synergy (or cooperation and interaction) the aggregate or total of individuals' performances will be exceeded by the work group's performance (Tilmouth *et al.*, 2011). In other words, individuals who work together can achieve more than individuals who work on their own.

Effective teams display certain features and the following are eight characteristics identified by Larson and LaFasto (1989) in their book *Teamwork:*

What Must Go Right/What Can Go Wrong. According to Larson and LaFasto, the team must have:

1 a clear goal
2 a results-driven structure
3 competent team members
4 unified commitment
5 a collaborative climate
6 high standards that are understood by all
7 external support and encouragement
8 principled leadership.

To sum up, goals, roles, procedure, relationships and leadership are the essential pre-requisites to effective team working (McKibbon *et al.*, 2008). The members in a team need to be able to communicate and collaborate effectively to function effectively. If we coordinate the work of a group of people and develop shared goals, working towards a common aim, then we are almost there. See page 110 for reflect activity.

AC 1.2 Identify the challenges experienced by developing teams

New teams coming together need to establish themselves and this in itself can prove to be a challenge. Your ability as a manager and leader of a diverse group of staff to develop positive relationships is very important here and requires the ability to communicate effectively with people at all levels within the organisation.

Tuckman's (1965) theory of the phases of team development and how groups develop over time demonstrates the process of forming a team. His mnemonic or cue for common stages of team development is outlined in the box on page 110. The challenges experienced by developing teams are highlighted in each stage.

It is therefore important that the setting manages this situation sensitively. A period of debriefing may be required when roles are redefined and clarified and a plan for the way forward for a new team is put in place. Any change within a team or a setting is likely to present a challenge and meet with resistance since it pulls a team out of its comfort zone. A manager who can lead in a flexible way to enable the team to reform and re-establish themselves, and to put policies and procedures in place, will maintain a cooperative workforce.

Tuckman's Stages of Team Development

Forming

The members of the team are new to each other and the group and as such are unsure and wary of each other and the purpose of the team. Individual roles are unclear and there is a heavy reliance on the team leader for direction and support. Your approach at this time is very important. Being too directive may result in people not joining together as a team and this will slow down the process of team cohesion.

Storming

As team members become more familiar with each other, it is here that challenging the team leader occurs. The clashes of personality and differences in opinions often lead to the need for a scapegoat and at times this will be the team leader. It is far easier to blame the manager for all of the problems within the team because you are the one who is perceived to be different from the rest of the team. The stormy stage occurs when the group atmosphere becomes uncomfortable and blame is apportioned to the manager, who is seen as the problem.

Norming

Ideas that emerged during the storming stage are now given clarity and a mutual direction and consensus is reached. Harmony brings with it positivity among the group.

Performing

The team members start to apply themselves to the job in hand and simply get on with the work that needs to be done.

Mourning/Adjourning

The team reviews the past work achieved and looks forward to new challenges. This often needs to happen when you or team members leave or a group is disbanded. At this stage it is natural to experience negative feelings for the team as a way of coping and feeling better about leaving them.

Reflect on it

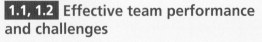

1.1, 1.2 Effective team performance and challenges

What makes for effective teamwork and what are the challenges your own team experiences?

Reflect on why this is the case and how it might affect the team's performance.

Write a journal piece to use as part of the evidence you require for assessment criteria. You may wish to use Tuckman's stages of development.

AC 1.3 Identify the challenges experienced by established teams

In the reflective activity you completed for AC 1.1 and AC 1.2, it is possible that you came to the conclusion that effective teamwork relates to relationships and communication. It is important that you understand what challenges established teams may encounter and how you can overcome these.

Momentum

Once the team is established, the major challenge is to ensure that it continues to work towards the objectives of the setting as outlined in your strategic plan. For this to happen everyone in the team needs to be working to keep operations running smoothly. For you as the manager, this requires keeping the team together and the communication lines open.

Respect differences and avoid conflict and clashes

Effective teamwork requires that all team members relate well to each other and as a manager you need to recognise the similarities as well as the differences in the individuals who make up your team. Your biggest challenge is to respect those differences in personality and to work with these to ensure the team members do not clash or that the team does not become dysfunctional.

Recognise everyone's role

Teamwork also requires a good knowledge of the individuals who make up your team and the roles they play. Teamwork is not about getting people together and dictating your orders to them but rather about developing a commitment to the goals by establishing **trust** and cohesion, and recognising everyone's efforts and work.

Belbin's research (1981) on the various roles needed in an effective team is worthy of note here. The study looked at determining how problems in teams could be predicted and avoided by controlling the dynamics of the group.

The results revealed that the difference between success and failure for a team was dependent not on factors such as intellect but more on behaviour. The research team began to identify separate clusters of behaviour, each of which formed distinct team contributions or team roles (www.belbin.com). Belbin identified nine team roles. Briefly summarised, these are:

- **Shaper**: task focused and generates action in a team.
- **Implementer** (company worker): the person who carries forward the strategies and gets the task done.
- **Completer-finisher**: the perfectionist of the team.
- **Coordinator** (chairman): the delegator who clarifies what needs to be done.
- **Team worker**: they carry out the work and turn ideas into action.
- **Resource investigator**: they explore what is happening locally and nationally and develop contacts.
- **Plant**: creative, lateral thinker/problem solver.

- **Monitor evaluator**: focused, logical, dispassionate and able to see all options.
- **Specialist**: they focus on their own subject area, rather than being team focused.

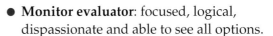

Research it

1.3 Belbin's team roles

Go to http://www.belbin.com/about/belbin-team-roles/ and find out more about the roles listed above and the strengths and weaknesses of each.

Think about your setting. How do these relate to the members of your team? How do these present a challenge?

In practice

1.1, 1.2, 1.3 Effective team performance and challenges

1 Study the team you work with over the next couple of days and try to get to know the members in a little more detail. How do the features of effective team performance present themselves in your team? How do these apply to a developing team you have worked with and an established team?
2 Using Tuckman's stages of development, identify and reflect upon the challenges experienced by your team.
3 Following on from the 1.3 research activity, at the next team meeting try to identify the roles that Belbin established. How do the different roles present as challenges in your team?

Key terms

Conflict is a disagreement or an argument.

Trust is having confidence in something or someone.

Reflective exemplar

You may wish to use this to write your own reflective account and use it as an example of how to evidence this assessment criterion.

I am a perfectionist. There is no other way to put it. I like to see the job done well; more than that, I *need* to see the job done. I like to make sure every 't' is crossed and 'i' is dotted and that the detail is attended to. It goes without saying then that errors and gaps always leave me feeling a little out of control and occasionally cross. With respect to Belbin's categories I guess that makes me a completer-finisher: 'conscientious, anxious' and 'inclined to worry'.

At the team meeting last week I asked the staff to work on the rota for the client's activities for July. We

had anticipated that there would be some visits out of the care environment and I had asked two of the staff to arrange these and the others to arrange for external speakers to attend on other days. At the team meeting this week I got quite irritated when A said he had not quite finished the task. I felt at first that he was irresponsible and lazy since he knows very well that I like to get the job done on time and I felt he had been unreasonable in asking for more time. J had completed the task and presented her work to the team but I became aware of an atmosphere developing and I feel she may have irritated some of the staff. I noticed the other team members were looking a little cross at some of the suggestions being put forward.

I had to think about what this all meant and reflected on the task, the team and the individuals I had specifically asked to do the job.

J is the most creative member of the team and comes up with some really good ideas, which is why I had chosen her to lead on the activity rota. In Belbin's category I guess she is what is called 'the plant'. She solves difficult problems and comes up with some real 'out of the box' thinking, which I like. But her communication skills leave a lot to be desired at times and I feel this might have been the issue here. I think she may have got carried away with all these wonderful activities and was not communicating this well to the rest of the team. The team were therefore unable to state their case and to put forward some of the down sides of her suggestions.

With A I simply did not read the situation well. I think A takes on the role of the coordinator and as such was able to clarify the task to others and set the goals but then tried hard to get the team to do the work for him!

When they did not come up with the goods he realised he had run out of time.

So I learned a lesson this week about my team and went away to reread Tuckman's theory.

Tuckman's stages of team development helped me to understand and manage the team in a more meaningful way. We are a relatively new team and as such we need to 'form', with each member of staff finding their niche and recognising how they 'belong' in the group. As the team leader I really should be developing the staff to ensure they have the opportunity to become clearer about their roles. Therefore, next week, I want to push forward with an activity that will help the forming stage. Instead of delegating to a couple of staff members, I think we need to make it a whole team effort and maybe then we can see how each of us will work effectively together. Perhaps this will help us all to really become part of a collective rather than individuals in a new group. I think this week's efforts show that we might already be in the storming stage, so we need to take a step back and ensure we rectify this.

Case study

1.3 Belbin and Tuckman

Reflect on the examplar above and think about what you would do if you were in the same scenario.

1 What do you understand by the term 'completer-finisher?'
2 How might you have dealt with the situation this team leader found herself in?
3 How might Tuckman's stages of team development help the leader manage the team?
4 What might she find happens at each stage?

AC 1.4 Explain how challenges to effective team performance can be overcome

From completing the above activity you may have identified areas within the workplace that require some thought. For example, you might be at a stage with the team where performance is being affected in some way and needs to be addressed.

The reality of modern health and social services is that the care we get depends as much on how health and social care employees work with each other as on their individual competence within their field of expertise (Tilmouth *et al.*, 2011).

Newly formed teams need to go through a development process and well-established teams have to be motivated to perform in roles in which they fit comfortably. Effective teams are those which comprise groups of people who complement each other in the roles they undertake within the team and who are managed and led in an efficient way. This can help to overcome challenges to effective team practice. As we discussed in ACs 1.2 and 1.3, the challenges to team working are many and varied. We discuss how to overcome some of these below.

Retaining momentum

In order to retain momentum, it is important to ensure that everyone knows where the project is heading and what they need to do to get there. As a manager you need to be aware that team members who fall behind schedule or fail to complete a task will have a negative effect on the team's momentum as a whole. Task sharing is one way this can be reduced. Time allocation is also important in maintaining momentum: too little and team members can get stressed, too much and the momentum can flag.

Overcoming conflict

Consider the divide between social care staff working alongside medical staff who may be separated by geographical boundaries, working in external settings, and with communication boundaries and status inequalities. These sorts of boundaries can be a source of conflict and as such may undermine team working. They can be frustrating and make the completion of tasks difficult. In addition, the mismatch of cultures, behaviours and understanding of services as well as a lack of understanding of each other's roles in the setting can be challenging and may affect the work we do. In order to overcome this challenge, joint working between professionals is critical and meetings need to be set up on a regular basis with members of the multi-disciplinary team to jointly plan and deliver services.

Positive relationships

A key factor in developing good team working and overcoming challenges is the manager's ability to develop positive relationships with the wide range of staff from different disciplines. This requires the ability to communicate effectively with people at all levels within the organisation. In the next AC we look at how leadership and management styles can help to overcome such challenges.

Communication

Poor communication is an area which is consistently upheld as a reason for underperformance and can also lead to conflict (Yoder-Wise, 2003). Therefore, as a manager and leader of a team, you need to hone these skills and improve any deficit or shortfall where you can. It is also important to communicate a clear vision to staff, and what teams are expected to achieve in their timeframes, a point that West (1994) emphasises. One aspect of communication is that of negotiation.

Negotiating

Much of the manager's day is spent in **negotiation** with other people and it can become an almost unconscious thing. We may simply be setting up a meeting or planning care with a member of staff, but the way in which this is carried out can mean the difference between an effective outcome or a failed one. Successful negotiation is linked to assertiveness and we aim to negotiate in an open and flexible manner in order to achieve a positive outcome.

Key term

Negotiation is taking part in a discussion which aims to reach an agreement.

We might consider the following points when addressing any challenge to the team's effectiveness.

- Are we empathetic? Have we really considered what it feels like to be in the shoes of the particular team worker with a problem?
- Can we seek clarification to make sure that we fully understand the other person's position and their needs?
- Are we calm or taking things personally?
- Are we prepared to support our case?
- Can we keep to the point and not allow ourselves to be side-tracked?
- Can we offer a compromise?

In practice

1.4 Reflecting on challenges

Reflect on the challenges you experience within your team and that you detailed in Activity 1.2 and determine how you could have improved your approach to them.

Apply the above checklist and say how you used those areas and what you might have improved upon.

Explain how the challenges you have encountered in your own team have been overcome.

Write up as a reflective account for your journal.

Figure 6.1 shows an example from the reflective exemplar.

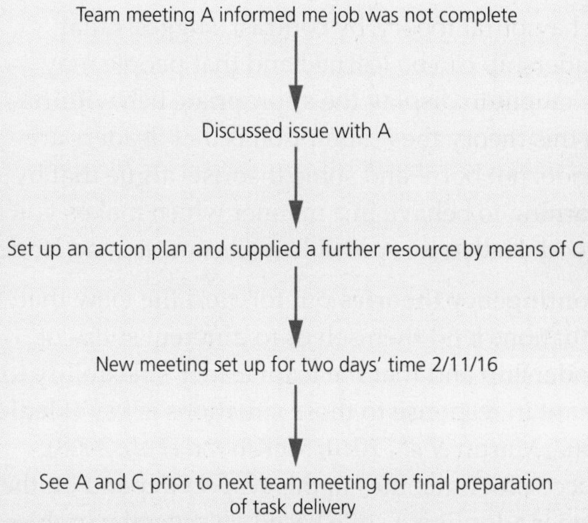

Team meeting A informed me job was not complete

↓

Discussed issue with A

↓

Set up an action plan and supplied a further resource by means of C

↓

New meeting set up for two days' time 2/11/16

↓

See A and C prior to next team meeting for final preparation of task delivery

Figure 6.1 Example from reflective exemplar

AC 1.5 Analyse how different management styles may influence outcomes of team performance

Theories

Leadership and management are terms often used simultaneously, but they are different. Management is concerned with process and developing systems that relate to organisational aims and objectives. It is about communicating those systems across the organisations. Leadership, meanwhile, is about the behaviour and personal style of the person leading.

Stewart (1997) stated:

> *'Management is essentially about people with responsibility for the work of others and what they actually do operationally, whereas leadership is concerned with the ability to influence others towards a goal.'*

At team-level management, it is unlikely that you are in a position to change very much in the wider organisation (Kouzes and Posner, in Tilmouth *et al.*, 2003) and therefore you may function more as a manager rather than as a leader. Nevertheless, the way you manage can influence others and in this respect it is worth looking at leadership traits.

Gordon Allport's (Allport and Odbert, 1936) trait theory suggests that certain characteristics that people possess make them good leaders. The idea that 'leaders are born rather than made' asserts that by identifying those characteristics in a person, we could identify who might be an effective leader. Behavioural theory, by contrast, suggests that leadership can be learned and that people may be taught to display the appropriate behaviours. In this theory the assumption is that 'leaders are made, not born' and some theorists argue that by learning to behave in a manner which makes you a 'good' leader, it is possible to become a good leader.

Contingency theories put forward the view that situations lend themselves to different styles of leadership and that the team leader's flexibility to adapt in response to those situations is key (Fiedler, 1967; Martin *et al.*, 2010; McKibbon *et al.*, 2008). Successful outcomes in this respect depend on the leader adopting a style based on several variables: the job in hand, the qualities of those in the team and the context in which the team is working.

Key term

Contingency theories state that there is no one best style of leadership. In this case the leader's effectiveness is based on the situation.

Research it

1.5 Characteristics of a good leader

What do you think are the characteristics of a good leader/manager?

Conduct some primary research and ask your peers and colleagues for their views. Figure 6.2 outlines some of these. All these are, of course, correct and there are many more you may have included.

The following may be helpful for secondary research and will help you to gain a greater understanding of the traits of good leadership and management:

Adair, J. (1983) *Effective Leadership*. New York: Pan Books.

www.businessballs.com/dtiresources/TQM_development_people_teams.pdf

Tilmouth, T., Davies-Ward, E. and Williams, B. (2011) *Foundation Degree in Health and Social Care*. London: Hodder Education.

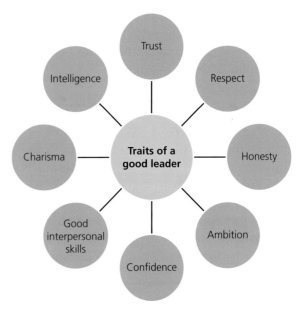

Figure 6.2 Some traits of a good leader

Adair (1983), a most influential writer on leadership and management, identified three key roles for leaders:

1 Achieving the task.
2 Developing team members.
3 Maintaining the team.

These may sound obvious but how often do we become so task orientated that we forget the needs of the team?

Team members need to understand the task and be given the resources to achieve that task if the outcome is to be successful. In this respect, team and individual development is critical to ensure that individuals can perform in the team (Martin *et al.,* 2010).

Traits of a good leader

Figure 6.2 highlights some of the traits of a good leader including confidence, good interpersonal skills and charisma.

Kouzes and Posner's (2003) Leadership Challenge model identifies the following character traits that are generally associated with good leaders:

- Honest
- Inspiring
- Forward-looking
- Competent
- Intelligent
- Dominant
- Conscientious
- Enthusiastic
- Sense of humour
- Integrity
- Courage
- Visionary

The bottom line is that good leaders and managers are able to generate enthusiasm and commitment in others. They lead by example, with consistent values, and break down barriers that stand in the way of achievement. Kouzes and Posner (2003, cited in Tilmouth *et al.,* 2011) argue:

- A good leader will also inspire a shared vision and enlist the commitment of others.
- A good leader will promote collaborative working, which builds trust and empowers others.

- A good leader recognises others' achievements and celebrates accomplishments.

Different leadership styles
Adjusting styles

The social skills needed in different leadership roles vary and leaders need to adjust their styles at different times to help group process (Wheelan, 2005).

At times we may need to be more directive and assertive to address and reduce any anxiety in team members, but this needs to be accomplished in a positive and open way. Supplying the resources needed to get the job done helps the team to accomplish their tasks and feel supported. When the team members start to work well and demand to participate more, a good leader will recognise this and step back rather than risk resentment due to undue influence from the leader. At times the leader's competence may be questioned and it is important not to take the attacks personally. Ultimately you want the team to take the leadership role on themselves in order to become more autonomous and responsible.

Whatever qualities we possess or need to develop, we will use these in various ways and adopt certain styles with respect to how we lead and manage.

Lewin *et al.* (1939) described leadership styles and although somewhat dated they remain relevant to team leadership and management today. He identified three very different leadership styles. The traits of these styles and their advantages and disadvantages are as follows:

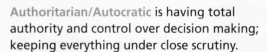

Key terms

Authoritarian/Autocratic is having total authority and control over decision making; keeping everything under close scrutiny.

Democratic/Participative is a sharing type of leadership in which employees' participation in the decision making is favoured.

Laissez-faire is the leadership style that favours leaving things to take their own course, without interference.

Autocratic/Authoritarian or 'I want you to …'

- The leader/manager makes decisions on their own without consulting the team.
- They expect the team to follow the decision exactly.
- The task is to be accomplished in the least amount of time possible.
- Instructions have to be clear and concise.
- Team members may become dissatisfied when they have ideas but are unable to voice these.
- Team members are not consulted on decisions being made.
- This can make them feel less involved and their commitment to the task is likely to be lukewarm.
- This type of leadership is good in situations requiring immediate or emergency action – for example, in emergency departments or in a crisis situation decisions have to be made quickly.

Democratic/Participative or 'Let's work together to solve this'

- Involving the team in the decision-making process leads to the team members feeling they have ownership of the task.
- This style is democratic and is the most popular style of leadership.
- The drawback is that teams are made up of individuals with vastly different opinions and decision making can therefore be a lengthy process.

Laissez-faire or 'You two take care of the problem while I go'

- The team are allowed to make their own decisions and get on with the tasks.
- This works well when people are capable and motivated in making their own decisions.
- The problem with this style is the tendency to go off task, with the result that the outcome

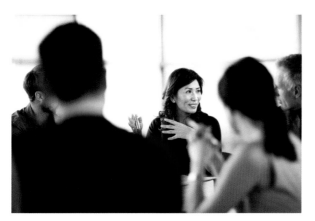

Figure 6.3 A collaborative leader values participation from employees

---

In practice

1.5 Management styles

a Interview your manager and ask about their particular style of management. Perhaps arrange to shadow them for a day.

b Comment on your own style and how it is similar to or different from that of your manager.

c Analyse how different management styles may influence outcomes of team performance.

Write this up as a reflective account for your journal.

---

is never achieved. It may lead to the team becoming impatient with the amount of time it takes to make a decision.

Part of a manager's role is to encourage others to work effectively and whichever style you adopt, you need to be able to rationalise why you chose that way to work. The outcomes will be affected if you fail to recognise the effect your style of leadership is having on the team. An effective team is committed to working towards the same goals and the team members will cooperate with the decisions made. In well-managed teams, results are produced quickly and economically where there is a free exchange of ideas and information (Tilmouth *et al.*, 2011).

AC 1.6 Analyse methods of developing and maintaining trust and accountability

Think about the managers you worked for in your first few roles. Picture them in your mind and then reflect on what it is that you either liked or disliked about them. Was it purely their friendly nature or were you a little in awe of them? Did they inspire you with confidence or were you just a little bit scared of them? Did they show an interest in you as a person or were they more task-focused?

Trust and accountability

One thing is certain: the managers and leaders we work for all have the same goal in mind and that is to get the job done and to get results. What differentiates a good and a poor working relationship between the manager/leader and the workforce is how that relationship is achieved and a lot of it is to do with **accountability** and trust. (See AC 1.3 for a definition of trust).

Your role as a team leader and a manager is a most important one, particularly in today's climate, which demands the delivery of quality care with fewer staff and resources. You are responsible for ensuring that staff morale remains high in a care service that changes constantly. So how do you accomplish this?

The American Management Association in 2011 collected data on the managerial effectiveness of 622 leaders across hundreds of organisations and highlighted three competencies that spanned all industries. This is reflected in work by Terry (1993) and George (2003) on authentic leadership.

The three competencies are as follows:

1 **Building trust and demonstrating personal accountability:** A leader who keeps their promises and honours commitments to the staff will be regarded by the staff as somebody who can be trusted. Far from being weak, the leader/manager who accepts responsibility for their actions and communicates honestly is seen as accountable and trustworthy.

2 **Action orientation:** Staff want somebody to act decisively and to suggest a solution in a crisis, so **action orientation** is about maintaining the momentum and sense of urgency about a project or a piece of work.

3 **Flexibility and agility:** Working for somebody who has fixed ideas can be demoralising, so if you are able to adjust to the situation and change your behaviour according to the change in circumstances, you demonstrate that you are open to new ways of doing things.

By being authentic in this way you develop a sense of trust with the staff and they can then be held accountable for their actions.

Trust, accountability and employees

Good management demands that we hold people accountable for what they do or don't do and the way in which you do this can make or break the relationship.

When goals were not met due to something the employee has failed to do, then it is appropriate for them to be held accountable for this failure. But if we are trying to hold employees accountable for things that are out of their control, that is unreasonable and we will lose the trust we have with the staff.

- **Be consistent:** the key ingredient is consistency and your staff will expect to be called to account if goals are not met or jobs are not done. The way in which you do this is also important – dealing with someone about a performance error in a firm but kind way in private is much better than berating or criticising them in public. Additionally, it is important that all staff are dealt with in the same way, otherwise the sense of injustice is great and trust is lost.
- **Build relationships:** as a manager there is a distance between you and your staff. But those leaders and managers who take the time to build relationships will gain the trust of their staff. It is a wise manager who takes time to find out a little about their staff and to share a little about themselves. You are likely to remember a manager who takes an interest and asks about your family or is happy to share a few words, for example.
- **Be honest:** trust builds respect and it is this that gets results. We can cultivate trust by being transparent and honest in what we are thinking and doing. We show ourselves to be trustworthy managers by being consistent and the sort of person who can be relied upon.

It is important to remember service users require staff who are confident and happy in their work and this can be achieved only if managers are able to encourage this in their team.

Key terms

Accountability is taking responsibility and being liable or answerable for something.

Action orientation is a type of leadership in which practical action is taken to deal with a problem or situation.

Reflect on it

1.6 Maintaining trust

Write a reflective account of the methods you use to ensure that you maintain the trust of your staff. Include a **critical incident** that demonstrates the way in which you maintain accountability and trust in your work.

AC 1.7 Compare methods of addressing conflict within a team

Conflict within teams is not uncommon but can be unpleasant and lead to disruption in performance. However, when resolved effectively, conflict can lead to personal and professional growth since it can be creative and productive.

There are two types of conflicts:

1 Those that revolve around the disagreements in relation to approaches to work.
2 Those that may arise between individual members of the team stemming from differences in personal values and beliefs.

Badly managed conflict leads to ineffective team work and people start to avoid each other and rifts develop. This inevitably leads to ineffectual or weak care of service users, clients and patients.

Larson and LaFasto (1989) suggest an effective way of solving this sort of conflict. In unit LM2c we look at their CONECT model (2001) for resolving conflict and it would be useful for you to look at this to achieve this outcome.

Thompson's (2006) RED approach to managing conflict is for situations with a high degree of tension associated with them. He suggests:

R – Recognise the conflict; do not sweep it under the carpet.

E – Evaluate the conflict to see how detrimental it would be if it was allowed to develop.

D – Deal with the conflict; keep open communication.

The two destructive extremes, either pretending the conflict does not exist or overreacting to the situation, are best avoided, according to Thompson.

In LO2 a number of practical ways of managing conflict and promoting a positive team environment are suggested.

LO2 Be able to support a positive culture within the team

AC 2.1 Identify the components of a positive culture within own team

An effective team works towards the same goals and the team members will cooperate with the decisions made. When properly managed and developed, team work improves processes and produces results quickly and economically through the free exchange of ideas and information.

Components of a positive culture

Your team is a unique one in that it is made up of individuals who all come with their own values, beliefs and attitudes. The term 'culture' is a complex one but refers to the rules, norms, values or beliefs that are shared by a group. In the work setting, then, **team culture** is about the professional values and beliefs shared by that team.

In health and social care there is a shared belief in anti-discriminatory practice, client autonomy and creating a tolerant and caring environment for the service user. A positive culture in this respect will be one in which team members all work towards the same goals and vision of the organisation. To do this requires each team

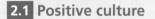

Research it

2.1 Positive culture

Wheelan (2005) provides a useful list of characteristics of high-performing teams. Research Wheelan's work. How far does this reflect your own team?

See the following website for more information: www.businessballs.com/dtiresources/TQM_development_people_teams.pdf

Write a short piece in your journal to show how you understand what is meant by a positive culture in team work.

In practice

2.1 Induction into a team

a Conduct some primary research. Interview a new member of staff and find out how they learned the team culture.
b How were they inducted into the way in which the team works and how aware are they of the overall goals of the organisation?
c How have you helped them to fit into the team?
d Reflect upon the positive nature of your team and give an example of how practice supports positive culture.
e What team structures are in place that directly influence a positive team culture?

member to have a clear understanding of their responsibility within the workplace and to be able to reflect upon the practice in order to monitor their performance.

The organisation that promotes openness and creativity, encouraging the team members to share information, to innovate and take calculated risks, will provide a positive climate in which to work.

AC 2.2 and 2.3 Demonstrate how own practice supports a positive culture and use systems and processes to support a positive culture in the team

The norms, beliefs and values you have brought into the workplace can be a valuable asset to the team in which you work and the way in which you work will reflect the professional values the

Reflect on it

2.2 Personal practice

Think about and reflect on how your own way of practising supports a positive team culture.

organisation expects. In working with individuals in health care we value such things as choice, individuality and independence. When working with service users it is essential that you have a good understanding about your role and responsibility in the workplace and are able to reflect on your practice, identifying your strengths and limitations. Moreover, your personality (general friendliness and a positive outlook) can support a positive culture. In a positive team culture you will feel valued by your team and there will be structures in place to help you work in an effective manner. Structures that can support a positive culture include information systems and systems of appraisal and training that enable staff to improve their performance.

AC 2.4 Encourage creative and innovative ways of working within the team

Transformational leadership and encouraging creativity and innovation

Effective teams are cohesive – they share goals and vision and operate in an atmosphere of openness and cooperation. The manager and leader who wants to encourage the team to be innovative and creative needs to adopt a management style that can transform the team further. The transformational leadership approach is one in which the leader sets out to create change by empowering the team to try new things, to be creative and innovative.

James MacGregor Burns developed the concept of transformational leadership in 1978. He believed that positive change could be created in teams by fostering a culture of interest in each other and in the interests of the group as a whole. Group motivation, morale and performance were enhanced by a leader who was 'energetic, enthusiastic and passionate'. If you have ever been in the presence of somebody who is enthusiastic and passionate about what they do, you will recognise just how powerful an influence this can be.

As Burns suggested, it is through the strength of their vision and personality that such leaders are able to inspire team members to change their expectations and motivations to work towards common goals.

Transformational leadership then goes beyond more traditional methods of leadership. Such leaders have a clear collective vision which they manage to communicate effectively to all the team. As effective role models, they inspire their team members to put the good of the whole organisation above self-interest and are not afraid to use unconventional methods to achieve the collective vision (adapted from Epitropaki, 2001).

Creativity and innovation address ways of doing things better and differently and in health and social care settings change will always require new perspectives. One such creative change to health and social care in recent years was the introduction of the personalisation agenda in 2007, which empowers people to be active citizens in control of their care. This required creativity and innovation with respect to the provision of person-centred care and support and changes to funding arrangements.

In practice

2.2, 2.3, 2.4 Problem solving

Problems that are unusual or out of the norm require an innovative or creative response.

1 What practices, systems and processes support a positive culture in your team?
2 How do you encourage the staff in your setting to adopt creative and innovative ways of working? Give an example. Or you might like to use the exemplar reflection on pages 111–112 to demonstrate how you would have solved the issue there.

Key term

Reflection is giving serious thought or consideration to something.

LO3 Be able to support a shared vision within the team

AC 3.1 Identify the factors that influence the vision and strategic direction of the team

The factors that influence the vision and direction for care work are those imposed by legal and professional groups and changes that come about as the result of research and new development.

Skills for Care in its Adult Social Care Management Induction Standards (launched in 2008 but a 'refreshed' 2012 web edition is also available) identifies eight common principles to support self-care and highlight the need for leaders and managers to have a clear vision and be committed to making a positive difference. You can find out more about these at www.skillsforcare.org.uk/ Document-library/Standards/Manager-Induction-Standards/Manager-Induction-Standards.pdf

The Care Act 2014 is a new law concerning the care and support people receive. It sets out the key responsibilities of local authorities, including the need to promote individual well-being, the integration of care and support, and co-operation with other local authorities and their relevant partners such as the NHS and the police. You can find out more about this at www.legislation.gov.uk/ukpga/2014/23/ contents/enacted/data.htm

The Department of Health provides guidance for health care in the UK and shapes the delivery of adult social care services through leadership and policy. In addition, local councils with social services have a responsibility to commission public, private and voluntary sector providers to deliver services that meet the needs of their local population. This whole process shapes the shared vision for the delivery of care services and your work is directly influenced by this.

Effective working in health and social care settings requires that we collaborate in order to achieve the national outcomes and to influence the achievement of a shared vision, both nationally and locally. As a team this means you will work towards your organisation's strategic plan, which has been set to reflect the government initiatives. It is likely that these will have been translated into targets, which clearly identify what level of service is to be provided, for example, and reflect the needs of the service user in your setting. You will also be looking to meet the standards set out at a national level.

AC 3.2 and 3.3 Communicate the vision and strategic direction to team members and work with others to promote a shared vision within the team

We may not always agree with what we are expected to do in health and social care and occasionally there are decisions made at national level which impact on local delivery of care. For example, recent cutbacks in budgets in the public sector have left many organisations with fewer resources at their disposal and little option but to reduce the number of staff to save money. These sorts of decisions are less than conducive or helpful to good team relationships, but as a manager you are likely to be involved in promoting a shared vision, making such changes, and you need to be able to ensure the staff are also fully aware of the need for change.

Communicating vision and change

Managing change in this situation is crucial to keeping the team focused on the vision and the **strategic direction**.

In health care, change happens for various reasons:

● New research in practice becomes available.
● New policies and regulations appear.
● There is overspending on budgets.
● Occasionally the need to update buildings or premises leads to disruption in the working day.
● The turnover of staff constitutes a change to team working and can be a challenge.

Any change is a challenge and can cause anxiety for some, so managers need to be aware of how to minimise this and keep the team focused.

Key term

Strategic direction is a course of action that leads to the achievement of goals in an organisation's strategy.

Managing change requires a planned and systematic approach to ensure that the team's motivation is maintained.

John P. Kotter (1995) devised 'eight steps to successful change', which provide a useful starting point. Each stage recognises how individuals respond to and approach change, and Kotter identifies this through how we see, feel and then act towards change.

Kotter's model shows well how managers can motivate people to buy into the change by 'owning' the change and this is the important element of any successful change.

We can reduce the eight steps model down to four major factors:

● **The urgency factor**: the pressure to change is on the organisation and you need to get the team behind you to ensure successful outcomes.
● **The vision factor**: a clear shared vision is an imperative and as managers, it is necessary to ensure that team members are with you and not against you. Motivation is the key here and you need to be aware of what motivates your team.
● **The resource factor**: the resources you need to implement change have to be identified before you proceed and you need to ensure these are provided. Without the necessary tools, your team cannot be expected to do the job.
● **The action factor**: when all else is in place, the next part of any change is to act. Having planned for change and implemented it, you then need to check that it is working and act if it is not.

If the change is working, then maintaining the effectiveness and appropriateness of the change is good practice. By monitoring and analysing data produced you are in a position to evaluate the success or otherwise and to keep the team informed of progress.

The fear of the consequences of change can have a damaging effect on the team's morale. Ensuring that staff feel secure in their roles is a management task to maintain motivation. Honest and open communication is essential and it should be provided on a continuous basis.

Change raises the level of stress and takes us out of our comfort zone. We start to fear not only for our jobs but also for the upset in our routine and the status quo. As a manager, the need to communicate to the team that the change will bring about a new 'comfort zone', once implemented, will be most welcome.

Money as a motivator must also be considered, but is surprisingly way down on the list for most people. Any change that requires low-paid staff to do more for little recompense is likely to be viewed negatively and staff will feel undervalued. If more pay cannot be part of the agreed changes, then other motivators and perhaps other packages can be implemented to improve motivation.

How to communicate strategy and vision

When staff are being requested to buy into something new, communication and ensuring the team understands the vision and strategic direction are crucial to success. Team meetings with agendas giving team members opportunities to offer their ideas should be set up and other forms of communication, such as email may also be useful, but you should consider the advantages and disadvantages of these. Communicating through discussions and appraisals are also good ways to ensure that all are aware of the changes and how they might be affected. Suggestions from staff should be encouraged and considered. See LO4 for information on meetings.

Working with others to promote a shared vision

Your team will also work with a range of people, including the individuals/service users, their loved ones/significant others and families, carers

Research it

3.2, 3.3 Kotter's eight-step change model

Go to www.businessballs.com/changemanagement.htm and research Kotter's eight-step change model. How does this help to promote a shared vision within a team?

and members of wider groups of professionals, including staff and practitioners. For example, you may find yourself liaising with and calling on the services of those who work in social work, community nursing staff, infection control teams, the justice system and education staff.

In working with others we need to promote a shared vision in the team by ensuring that everyone is involved in decision making and is aware of any change and the need for the change.

In the past, groups of staff from the same discipline rarely communicated with other specialists around patient issues and this led to a number of problems in service provision. The push towards multi-disciplinary team working has been encouraged over the last 20 years or so and the Laming Report (2003) highlighted the importance of working closely with people from other professional groups and agencies.

AC 3.4 Evaluate how the vision and strategic direction of the team influences team practice

To check how well the team has performed, targets must be reviewed regularly and feedback given to the team on performance. This should be an on-going process and not a one-off event.

The evaluation phase of any project involves a sequence of stages that includes:

- **forming** objectives, aims and goals and hypotheses of the project
- **conceptualising** the major parts of the project, the participants involved, the setting and how you will measure the outcomes
- **designing** the evaluation of the project and giving details of how these components will be managed and coordinated
- **analysing** the information, in qualitative and quantitative ways
- **using what is learned** through the evaluation process.

Adapted from www.socialresearchmethods.net/kb/pecycle.php

You might also use a model of reflection in your evaluative process which you and the team are likely to be aware of. Kolb's (1984) cycle of experiential learning can be adapted well here. Kolb recommends that we need to recall our observation of an event, or the change in this case, reflect on those observations, develop and research some theories about what we saw and then decide on some action as a result of the process (Jasper, 2003).

The purpose of sharing your strategic direction is to enable the team to focus its energy on the organisation's wider objectives and vision and to help the team to formulate a picture of what is needed to move forward. In addition, any changes that may be needed can be clarified and the rationale behind these changes can be articulated. By outlining strategic priorities, you can enable the team to appreciate how these connect to the wider needs of the organisation.

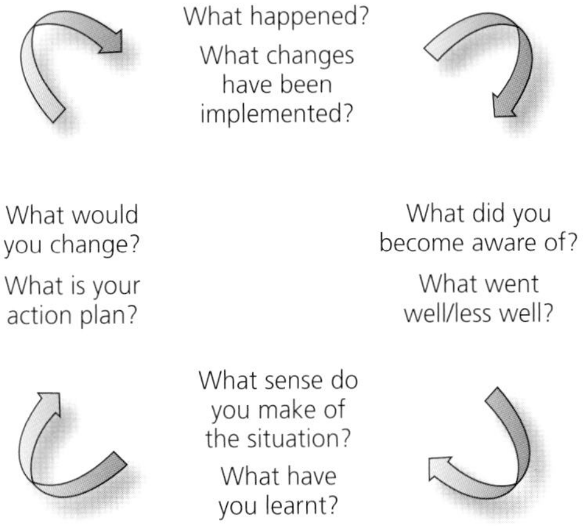

What happened?
What changes have been implemented?

What would you change?
What is your action plan?

What did you become aware of?
What went well/less well?

What sense do you make of the situation?
What have you learnt?

Figure 6.4 A reflective cycle based on the work of Kolb (1984)

Source: Tilmouth *et al.*, 2011

Reflect on it

3.4 Effects of change

Write a reflective account of a recent change you made, looking specifically at the response of staff. Say what you have learned about the management of the team as a result of this.

What might you do differently next time?

What were the major motivating factors for your team members?

In practice

3.1, 3.2, 3.3 A shared vision

a Reflect on your organisation's vision or mission statement and identify the points that are necessary for your team to understand.

b Set an agenda item for the next team meeting, ensure this is communicated to staff and check their understanding of the goals for the organisation.

c Introduce something you wish to change in the way in which the team works and show how you will go about managing change within the team.

d Find out what the chief motivators are for your staff.

e Construct a spider diagram which shows the other people you work with to promote a shared vision within the team.

f How does the vision and strategic direction of the team influence practice? Discuss the positive and negative impacts of this.

LO4 Be able to develop a plan with team members to meet agreed objectives

AC 4.1, 4.3 and 4.4 Identify team objectives, facilitate team members to actively participate in the planning process and encourage sharing of skills and knowledge between team members

Identifying aims and objectives

To enable the achievement of a shared vision, the team will need to work to a set of objectives. Aims are the goals you hope to achieve or, in this case, may be the overall shared vision. Objectives are the activities you undertake in order to reach those goals.

Any objective your organisation has is likely to be linked to national strategies. For example, NHS England's 'business plan for 2013/14 – 2015/16', called 'Putting Patients First', describes an 11-point scorecard to measure performance of key priorities, designed to ensure 'high quality care for all, now and for future generations' (www.england.nhs.uk/pp-1314-1516/).

One of the outcomes (6) aims to ensure that people have a positive experience of care. In your own setting, this wider agenda will be a part of your strategic plan in order to meet this government-set initiative.

In practice

4.1, 4.3, 4.4 Objectives, planning process and sharing of skills and knowledge

1 Look at the following example of an overall aim and specific aims and then see if you can identify the objectives to meet those aims.
2 Encourage members of the team to participate in the planning process and show how you managed this.
3 How did you enable the team members to share their skills and knowledge with others in the team?

The overall aim of the project:

To improve the quality of **person-centred care** in your setting.

Specific aims:

● To increase an individual's quality of life.
● To increase an individual's comfort and well-being.
● To increase an individual's confidence and motivation.
● To empower an individual to engage in their own care to enhance well-being.

Perhaps you had something along these lines in your answer:

● To provide information and advice on care packages available.
● To provide an excellent living space and health care for all.
● To offer a variety of activities to enhance well-being and health and fitness.
● To support individuals in accessing clubs, jobs, external activities and training.
● To facilitate a support group for clients.
● To enable individuals to be represented at staff meetings.
● To encourage open communication between staff and clients to undertake problem solving.

Key term

Person-centred care is the process of life planning for individuals based around the principles of inclusion and individualised care.

Facilitating team members to actively participate in the planning process and encouraging sharing of skills

One of the best ways to get staff involved in planning is to allow time during the regular team meeting for them to express their views and to communicate their opinions or ideas. So often, our team meetings become mere information-giving sessions, without an adequate venue for the exchange of ideas. If this is the case, then valuable expertise, the skills and knowledge of the staff, will not be accessed. Through a mentoring process team members can learn a great deal from each other, and the expertise each one possesses as a result of their experience and training can be used as a valuable resource for planning.

Meetings

A meeting is an opportunity to communicate with the whole team present and can be a useful vehicle through which to encourage staff to discuss the overall aims of the team with the shared vision in mind.

Meetings afford the opportunity for the team members to get to know each other and to open discussion and make action points. Day (2006) suggests that the success of a meeting can depend on the way it is chaired and this is an important role for the manager to learn.

As the chair leading the meeting, you need to ensure that you encourage participation from the entire group using open questions and occasionally directing your attention to one person in particular. In this way you are giving everybody in the team the chance to express what they know and to demonstrate their skills, which may be useful for achieving the whole team's outcomes. It is very important to come away from the meeting with some action points or objectives, if appropriate.

When a planning activity is required the team meeting can be a useful vehicle for this. If all team members understand the background to the project and its relevance to the organisation they will be more focused on the changes needed and be motivated to ensure a successful outcome.

At the meeting there can be a collaborative approach to the collection of data such as service-user requirements, and timescales can be set which are clear and achievable. With the project broken down into manageable tasks and assigned to team members for completion, the planning process can reach a successful conclusion in a timely manner.

AC 4.2, 4.5 Analyse how the skills, interests, knowledge and expertise within the team can meet agreed objectives and agree roles and responsibilities with team members

Team objectives and skills, interests, knowledge and expertise

You will now be more familiar with the roles your staff take on in their work and have been encouraged to identify what motivates them through the previous activities in this unit. You are likely to have also noticed the types of skills that they have. For example, you may know a member of staff who is particularly good at dealing with conflict, whereas others are much more creative and tend to be able to engage with the clients in this way.

The success of the team will depend on bringing together people with diverse skills and knowledge and if they lack these, encouraging them to undertake training and education. For example, doctors, nurses, occupational therapists and physiotherapists working together in an orthopaedic ward to best meet the needs of the patients on the ward make up a multi-disciplinary team (MDT).

Agreeing roles and responsibilities

Each team member needs to have a clearly defined role within the team and this should be based upon their knowledge and skill. Team members feel valued when they are able to contribute to the work in roles they feel qualified and confident to perform. By recognising each individual's differences and training, you as a manager can ensure the team members have some say in the roles they undertake.

It is possible that you may have had to make some uncomfortable decisions and staff members may not have been fully on board with the responsibilities you agreed with them. An

assertive approach to dealing with difficult issues will go a long way to ensuring the team remains focused and motivated.

Working towards a win/win outcome shows that you respect the person and the differences they have. In this way they are likely to be more prepared and committed to work towards an outcome that is mutually acceptable.

Research it

4.1, 4.2, 4.3 Action research project

1 With your team, undertake an action research project which identifies the team's objectives and encourage the team members to participate in the planning process.
2 Analyse how the skills, interests, knowledge and expertise within the team can meet the agreed objectives.

Reflect on it

4.5 Roles, responsibilities and objectives

Think about the roles and responsibilities within your team. How does knowing this help with your planning objectives for your setting?

In practice

4.2, 4.5 Roles and responsibilities

Agenda an item for the next team meeting in which you discuss the roles and responsibilities of team members for a particular task.

Identify the task objectives with the team and demonstrate your understanding of their skills, interests and knowledge.

Reflect on how you have encouraged your team members with this task.

Place a copy of the minutes of the meeting in your portfolio and give a reflective account to show how you agreed the roles and responsibilities.

LO5 Be able to support individual team members to work towards agreed objectives

AC 5.1 and 5.2 Set personal work objectives with team members based on agreed objectives and work with team members to identify opportunities for development and growth

All care workers have to take part in performance reviews, supervision and appraisals and such meetings are a good time to set objectives and discuss changes to their workload or requests for training.

A good way to identify personal objectives is to use Smart targets. Staff must ensure that they remain 'fit for purpose' and are required to update their portfolio of evidence which shows the professional development activities and training they have undertaken.

By undertaking this course and carrying out the activities throughout this book you are engaging in **continuing professional development (CPD)** and providing evidence through the activities you complete. Your staff also require development. In supervision or appraisal sessions you need to work with them to identify their strategies for development.

Key terms

Smart targets are those objectives that are specific, measurable, achievable, realistic/relevant and time-related.

Continuing professional development (CPD) is training and education activity to ensure staff remain fit for practice.

In practice

5.1, 5.2 Setting objectives

1 Case study 5.1 shows one way in which we might set objectives. Set your personal work objectives for the coming year and discuss these with your manager.
2 Now work with a member of your team to identify opportunities for their development and growth.

Case study

5.1 Workload and training and development

Meeting with Susie
Workload

Susie feels that currently her workload level is fine and she is enjoying the work with the newer clients. She feels the change the team made to specifying a named staff member to a group of allocated clients is useful. Susie feels her confidence has grown and she is relishing the more independent way of working. I commented that as her team leader I had noticed she was making appropriate decisions for her clients and was working well in the team.

Training and development

So far this year Susie has attended the health and safety update and two further in-house training courses. She seems very keen to undertake a foundation degree in health and social care at her local sixth-form college. We discussed what this would entail and Susie mentioned that it was one day a week in college for two years, with additional days off to undertake further work placement activity. We devised the following action plan:

- Susie to advise of fees and days required out of work – date 17/10/16.
- Susie to approach the college and get an application form and start the process of applying by 20/11/16.
- TT (the team leader) will approach the area manager to obtain permission in principle for attendance and to inform Susie of the decision by 20/11/16.
- Further meeting to take place on 21/11/16 to discuss next steps.

AC 5.3 Provide advice and support to team members to make the most of identified development opportunities

Case study 5.1 looks at how we might approach the development of a member of staff, in this case Susie. She has requested to undergo further training to enhance her career, and CPD is required to ensure staff remain skilled and can evidence updated practice.

Sometimes, however, training on the job in new skills and techniques or simply to update the staff in new policies, practices and procedures is required. The use of coaching as a strategy to advise and support team members and to enhance team performance is now a well-respected factor in team development.

Parsloe and Wray (2000) define coaching as:

'A process that enables learning and development to occur and thus performance to improve. To be successful, a coach requires a knowledge and understanding of process as well as the variety of styles, skills and techniques that are appropriate to the context in which the coaching takes place.'

Clutterbuck and Megginson (2006) have further identified four main styles that coaches have defined themselves. These are:

● Assessor
● Tutor
● Demonstrator
● Stimulator

The assessor and tutor roles in this instance are more directive, whereby they give more instruction and are teacher led, whereas the roles of demonstrator and stimulator tend to be less so, taking on a more supportive role. As a manager providing coaching, you need to be able to move between styles and to use a high degree of reflection to recognise when and how to use the styles.

The GROW model developed by Whitmore (2002) and further adapted by Alexander and Renshaw (2005) is a useful framework to adopt – see figure 6.5.

● Goal (**G**)
● Current situation (**R** = Reality)
● Options (**O**)
● Obstacles (**W** = Wrap up)

Hawkins and Shohet (2009) suggest supervision is an important part of taking care of the team members. Supervision involves education, support, self-development and self-awareness but is sometimes seen in a negative way, with a certain amount of suspicion and a lack of trust. There may be a feeling that supervision is management's way of judging individuals and their performance and the team may feel defensive and uncomfortable.

The main advantage of supervision is that team members are able to continue to learn and move forwards at work and it can help people use their resources better. It therefore needs to be viewed as a positive tool for change in the team.

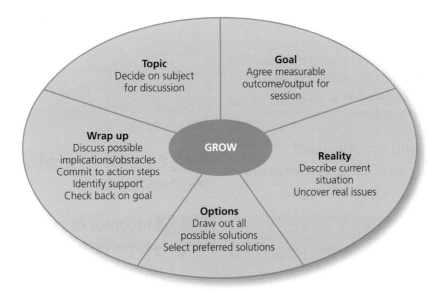

Figure 6.5 The GROW model (based on Whitmore 2002)

Key term

Personal development planning is the process of planning for future education or career development. In order to make the most of development opportunities staff need to be guided to various opportunities for improving their knowledge and skills. This will include opportunities for improving their knowledge and skills, for example.

Reflect on it

5.3 Training and development

Think for a moment how your team view training and development. How might you provide advice and support to team members to make the most of identified development opportunities?

In practice

5.3 The GROW model

Using the GROW model (as expressed in Figure 6.5), work with a team member to identify opportunities for their development and growth and set personal objectives towards which they can work.

In addition to supervision, mentoring can be a source of support for staff. By working with or 'shadowing' a colleague, a team member can learn a great deal and be guided in tasks and situations. Peer support is also useful as staff are able to access the experience of others in the team and gain emotional support or practical help if required. Developing staff members is part of CPD and **personal development planning** (PDP) is a process all staff must be prepared to undertake.

AC 5.4 Use a solution-focused approach to support team members to address identified challenges

The solution-focused approach to management started with a psychotherapy background. Insoo Kim Berg, a young American therapist in the 1960s, was dissatisfied with the traditional way of carrying out therapy and looked to develop a new means of looking at problems. He and Steve

Research it

5.4 Solution-focused approaches

Research solution-focused approaches and determine how you might use such approaches in developing your team.

In practice

5.4 The solution-focused model

Using the four points in the solution-focused model, identify a solution-focused approach to support the team to address a challenge.

de Shazer devised a new way of approaching problems in the 1980s and switched to studying 'solution behaviour'.

This led to further models being put forward and the Four-Step Method of Solution-Focused Management is now a favoured approach in management circles.

- **Step One: identify and acknowledge the problem** – how does it hinder and affect you? By asking these questions, you can address the issue in a constructive manner.
- **Step Two: describe the success – what do you want to achieve?** This ensures you can focus on the solution and know what defines 'success' in this situation and when you have achieved this.
- **Step Three: identify and analyse positive exceptions** – when did the same or a similar challenge occur in the past? What did you do differently that time to achieve that? Whatever you did positively before, repeating it could change the behaviour for the better.
- **Step Four: take a small step forward. Try it out!**

Adapted from © 2004 Coert Visser and Gwenda Schlundt Bodien

LO6 Be able to manage team performance

AC 6.1 Monitor and evaluate progress towards agreed objectives

In AC 3.4 we looked at ways in which the vision and strategic direction of the team influence team practice and you are advised to revisit this now.

There is little difference in the way you will monitor and evaluate progress and you may decide to use a reflective model to do this as suggested previously.

There will be a variety of evidence within your own workplace which measures quality of provision and performance, for example. You will have access to staff appraisals, service user evaluation data and a complaint process which may provide evidence. In addition, service user and patient forums give a good indication of how a team is functioning. You might also look at budgets/savings and time allocation for tasks to measure performance.

AC 6.2 and 6.3 Provide feedback on performance to the individual and the team and provide recognition when individual and team objectives have been achieved

Feedback

We all need to know how we are progressing in anything we do and feedback, whether positive or negative, is a necessary part of managing people well. Providing feedback means we acknowledge what the team members are doing and this in itself can be a huge motivator. It also helps the team to stay focused and on track.

Figure 6.6 is a useful model to adopt for both individuals and teams.

Recognition

A good starting point is to ask the member of staff to evaluate their own performance and in so doing you will be able to gain an understanding of how they perceive their level of performance. You may find they are critical of themselves, but this will give you the chance to praise them and give them some good news about their performance. Not only can this type of feedback be a huge motivator but giving them feedback from other staff, managers and clients complimenting them on their work can really boost morale.

BOOST feedback

Balanced: Focus not only on areas of development, but also on strengths.

Observed: Provide feedback based only upon behaviours that you have observed.

Objective: Avoid judgements and relate your feedback to the observed behaviours, not personally.

Specific: Back up your comments with specific examples of observed behaviour.

Timely: Give feedback soon after the activity to allow the learner the opportunity to reflect on the learning.

Figure 6.6 BOOST feedback

Source: Tilmouth *et al.*, 2011

Good practice demands we feed back to staff our views on how they are progressing and performing.

Rewarding staff and showing them how they are valued can be done in many ways, such as hosting events to celebrate achievement, making them 'employee of the month' or even mentioning them in staff newsletters.

If there is an issue with a staff member's performance, they may find it difficult to express this themselves and this might cause issues. In the next AC we look at how we might approach the more challenging issues associated with poor performance.

AC 6.4 Explain how team members are managed when performance does not meet requirements

Occasionally it is necessary to give negative feedback to staff in order to address issues with unsatisfactory performance. This can inevitably cause conflict and can be quite uncomfortable.

Individuals receive criticism in different ways and you need to ensure that you are sensitive to how they will be feeling at this time. A good approach is to provide a positive point initially and to say clearly what was good about it. You can stress how well they did and what you liked about their performance. When critiquing their performance, you could highlight this as an area for improvement. Again, you must specifically draw attention to what you expect the team member to do and give a clear indication of how they might achieve this. You can then constructively give advice on how they can change. Finally, by ending with a positive point you can do much to rebuild self-esteem in what can often be a rather uncomfortable situation.

The following points might help:

- Do not make it a personal issue. Keep a clear picture of the person and yourself separate from the issue. It is the behaviour, not the person, you have issues with.
- Do not blame and accuse, just point out what changes you feel need to be made.
- Be clear and specific about your perception of the issue to be addressed and your desired outcome.
- Look and listen to each other. (If this becomes a conflict issue then often we start to avoid looking directly at each other and stop listening. We need to look and listen to each other so that we can respond appropriately.)
- Ensure that you understand each other and if you are unclear or confused about the issue, ask open questions and paraphrase back what you think you hear.

In practice

6.4 Dealing with underperformance

Being mindful of confidentiality and anonymising your records, provide evidence of a meeting with a member of your staff who is underperforming. Describe how you prepared for the meeting before you met the member of staff and how you approached the subject.

Evaluate your performance by writing a reflective account of what you did, why you did it in that way and the outcome of the whole meeting.

- Choose your place and time carefully when you need to give negative feedback. Make sure both parties feel comfortable. Set a time limit.
- Following the feedback, acknowledge and show appreciation of one another.
- If necessary, outline the disciplinary process and the legal nature of the position. Be sure to deal with the member of staff in a fair and even manner.

Legislation

Exploring the Care Act 2014 would be useful to the understanding of AC 2.4 in this unit. While there is no direct reference in law to team working, if we are to achieve excellent quality and safety in care it is imperative that strong teams are built. Health care staff work in a multi-disciplinary way and often across professional boundaries. To ensure service users are given the best quality care, staff must coordinate the services and collaborate in ways that are helpful and cooperative.

Assessment methods

LO	Assessment criteria and accompanying activities	Assessment methods *To evidence these assessment criteria you could:*
LO1	1.1 1.2 Reflect on it (p. 110)	Write a journal piece to use as part of the evidence you require for assessment criteria. You may wish to use Tuckman's stages of development. Or Supply a personal statement or reflection about your experience of the factors that affect team development and the roles people take on in the team in your work setting.
	1.3 Research it (p. 111)	Write an account of what you understand by Belbin's roles and how they relate to your team members.
	1.1 1.2 1.3 In practice (p. 111)	You might like to undertake a small study of the team you work with. Perhaps interview the team members and provide a written account. Answer the questions in the activity and put them into your portfolio as evidence of work carried out.

LO	Assessment criteria and accompanying activities	Assessment methods *To evidence these assessment criteria you could:*
	1.3 Case study (p. 112)	Produce a written account answering the questions in the activity.
	1.4 In practice (p. 113)	Answer the questions in the activity. Produce a flow chart of how the outcome was finally reached.
	1.5 Research it (p. 114)	What do you think are the characteristics of a good leader/manager? Conduct some primary research and ask your peers and colleagues for their views. Provide a written account. Or directly observe your manager in your workplace and supply and analyse an account of the observation.
	1.5 In practice (p. 116)	You may answer the questions in the activity and write this up as a reflective account for your journal. Or Produce a piece of written work to show a comparison of different management styles and how they impact upon the workplace. Or directly observe your manager in your workplace and supply and analyse an account of the observation.
	1.6 Reflect on it (p. 117)	Write a reflective account of the methods you use to ensure that you maintain the trust of your staff. Include a critical incident that demonstrates the way in which you maintain accountability and trust in your work. Or provide a written account of a real incident from the workplace (please anonymise) and show how the team demonstrated trust and accountability.
	1.6, 1.7 In practice (p. 118)	Compare two models of conflict management. Or research another to show your understanding of the ways in which conflict may be handled. Make sure you provide the different reasons for conflict and think about your own work setting and say why conflict sometimes happens. Also think about the methods you use to develop and maintain trust and accountability. Answer the questions in the activity. Provide a written account.
LO2	2.1 Research it (p. 119)	Provide a written account and explain how your team promotes a positive culture, giving examples. Be sure to include a definition of the term 'culture' Complete the activity and then write a short piece in your journal to show how you understand what is meant by a positive culture in team work.
	2.1 In practice (p. 119)	Complete the activity and provide a written account.
	2.2 Reflect on it (p. 119)	Think about and reflect on how your own way of practising supports a positive team culture. Provide a written account.
	2.2, 2.3, 2.4 In practice (p. 120)	Supply a piece of primary research and a reflective account which shows how your own way of practising supports a positive team culture. Provide a personal statement that comments on problems that are unusual or out of the norm that require an innovative or creative response and how you use systems and processes to support a positive culture. Provide a reflection to show how you have solved staff issues in creative ways and answer the following questions in the activity.
LO3	3.2 3.3 Research it (p. 122)	You could supply an action plan for staff about an item of change for the team.
	3.4 Reflect on it (p. 123)	Supply evidence from your reflective account and journal for your assessor.

LO	Assessment criteria and accompanying activities	Assessment methods *To evidence these assessment criteria you could:*
	3.1, 3.2, 3.3 In practice (p. 123)	You can answer the questions in the activity. Show your understanding of the influences and strategic direction of your team and how you communicate this and promote a shared vision by providing evidence of oral/written questioning or team meeting minutes.
LO4	4.1, 4.3, 4.4 In practice (p. 124)	Complete the task in the activity and show it your assessor. You might include observation and reflection, a written piece to demonstrate or show your understanding of how you met the objectives, and an evaluation of the task.
	4.1, 4.2, 4.3 Research it (p. 125)	With your team, undertake an action research project and complete the activity.
	4.5 Reflect on it (p. 125)	Provide a written account answering the questions.
	4.2, 4.5 In practice (p. 125)	Complete the activity and provide a written account.
LO5	5.1, 5.2 In practice and 5.1 Case study (p. 126)	Complete the case study before taking it to a team meeting to work with individual staff members. Write an account of how this went and place a copy in your portfolio.
	5.3 Reflect on it (p. 128)	Provide a reflective account and then present an action plan to show your coverage of working with a member of staff.
	5.3 In practice (p. 128)	Complete the activity. Write up your meeting and let your assessor see it.
	5.4 Research it (p. 128)	Undertake the activity and discuss this with your assessor.
	5.4 In practice (p. 129)	Provide a written example of a stepped approach to the solution of a team problem or challenge.
LO6	6.1 Reflect on it (p. 129)	Provide a written account about how you supply evidence of the team's progress towards goals.
	6.2, 6.3 In practice (p. 129)	Collect the documents from the activity, carry and discuss them with your assessor. Present the report to your manager to show how far the team have progressed towards goals.
	6.4 In practice (p. 130)	Complete the activity and prepare a report to show how you went about covering the activity and evaluate its effectiveness.

References

Adair, J. (1983) *Effective Leadership*. New York: Pan Books.

Alexander, G. and Renshaw, B. (2005) *Supercoaching*. London: Random House Business Books.

Allport, G. W. and Odbert, H. S. (1936) 'Trait-names: A psycho-lexical study', *Psychological Monographs*, 47(211).

Belbin, M. (1981) *Management Teams: Why they succeed or fail*. London: Heinemann.

Burns, J. M. (1978) *Leadership*. New York: Harper & Row.

Clutterbuck, D. and Megginson, D. (2006) *Making Coaching Work*. London: CIPD.

Day, J. (2006) *Interprofessional Working*. Cheltenham: Nelson Thornes.

Epitropaki, O. (2001) *What is Transformational Leadership?* Sheffield: Institute of Work Psychology, University of Sheffield.

Fiedler, F. E. (1967) *A Theory of Leadership Effectiveness*. New York: McGraw-Hill.

George, B. (2003) *Authentic Leadership: Rediscovering the secrets to creating lasting value*. San Francisco: Jossey-Bass.

Hawkins, P. and Shohet, R. (2009) *Supervision in the Helping Professions* (3e). Berkshire: Open University Press.

Kolb, D. (1984) Cycle of Experiential Learning, in Tilmouth, T., Davies-Ward, E. and Williams, B. (2011) *Foundation Degree in Health and Social Care*. London: Hodder Education.

Kotter International, www.kotterinternational. com/the-8-step-process-for-leading-change/

Kouzes, J. M. and Posner, B. Z. (2003) *The Leadership Challenge* (3e). San Francisco: Jossey-Bass.

LaFasto, F. M. J. and Larson, C. (2001) *When Teams Work Best: 6,000 team members and leaders tell what it takes to succeed*. Thousand Oaks, CA: Sage Publications.

Larson, C. E. and LaFasto, F. M. J. (1989) *Teamwork: What must go right/what can go wrong*. London: Sage Publications.

Lewin, K., Lippit, R. and White, R. K. (1939) 'Patterns of Aggressive Behaviour in Experimentally Created Social Climates', *Journal of Social Psychology*, 10, 271–301.

Martin, V., Charlesworth, J. and Henderson, E. (2010) *Managing in Health and Social Care* (2e). London: Routledge.

McKibbon, J., Walter, A. with Mason, L. (2008) *Leadership and Management in Health and Social Care for NVQ/SVQ Level 4*. London: Heinemann.

Parsloe, E. and Wray, M. (2000) *Coaching and Mentoring: Practical methods to improve learning*. London: Kegan Paul.

Pearson, P. and Spencer, J. (1997) *Promoting Teamwork in Primary Care: A research-based approach*. London: Arnold.

Skills for Care (2008) *Adult Social Care Management Induction Standards*. Leeds: Skills for Care.

Stewart, R. (1997) *The Reality of Management* (3e). Oxford: Butterworth-Heinemann.

Terry, R. W. (1993) *Authentic Leadership: Courage in action*. New York: John Wiley.

Thompson, N. (2006) *People Problems*. Basingstoke: Palgrave Macmillan.

Tilmouth, T., Davies-Ward, E. and Williams, B. (2011) *Foundation Degree in Health and Social Care*. London: Hodder Education.

Tuckman, B. (1965) 'Developmental sequence in small groups', *Psychological Bulletin*, 63(6), 384–99.

Visser, C. and Schlundt Bodien, G. (2004). The four steps outlined on page 128 are adapted from a blog written by Visser and Schlundt Bodien. The blog is, however, no longer available on the website.

West, M. (1994) *Effective Teamwork*. London: Blackwell.

Wheelan, S. A. (2005) *Creating Effective Teams: A guide for members and leaders* (2e). London: Sage.

Whitmore, J. (2002) *Coaching for Performance: Growing people, performance and purpose*. Boston, MA: Nicholas Brealey Publishing.

Yoder-Wise, P. S. (2003) *Leading and Managing in Nursing* (3e). St Louis: Mosby.

Insoo Kim Berg and Steve de Shazer at www. solutionmind.com/approach/solution_focused_ origins.html. This website no longer exists but you can find some useful information on http://erica-oneil-miller.blogspot.co.uk/2013/03/postmodern-approaches.html.

Useful resources and further reading

Bass, B. M. (1990) 'From transactional to transformational leadership: learning to share the vision', *Organizational Dynamics*, Winter, 19–31.

DOH (1998) *Our Health, Our Care, Our Say: A New Direction for Community Services*. London: HMSO.

DOH (2010) *Equity and Excellence: Liberating the NHS*. London: HMSO.

DOH (2014) Care Act 2014, www.legislation.gov.uk/ ukpga/2014/23/contents/enacted; www.england. nhs.uk/pp-1314-1516/

Jasper, M. (2003) *Beginning Reflective Practice*. Cheltenham: Nelson Thornes.

www.businessballs.com/changemanagement.htm

www.businessballs.com/dtiresources/TQM_ development_people_teams.pdf

Unit LM2c

Develop professional supervision practice in health and social care settings

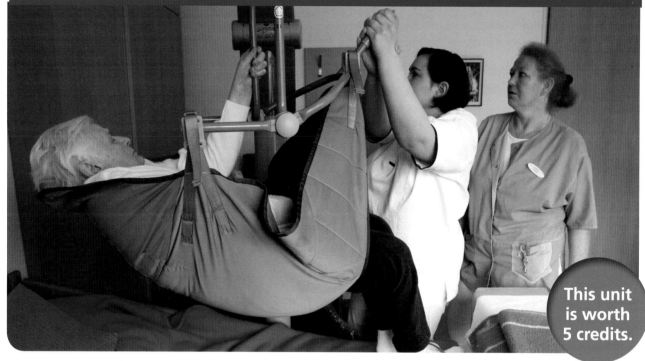

This unit is worth 5 credits.

Supervision has been introduced into practice to provide professional support and learning for staff, to enable them to develop knowledge, skills and competence in their work. This enhances the experience of the service user and in turn improves quality and safety in the care setting. As a manager, it is your responsibility to provide professional supervision for the staff to ensure they are supported in their roles and to enhance their skills and performance.

In this unit we will cover the purpose and processes of professional supervision together with performance management and dealing with conflict. It would also be useful for you to read the unit on understanding professional supervision practice (LM2a). There is some overlap but it will complement and aid your understanding of this unit. Cross references to the unit have been added to make navigation easier for you.

Learning outcomes

By the end of this unit you will:

1 Understand the purpose of professional supervision in health and social care settings.
2 Understand how the principles of professional supervision can be used to inform performance management in health and social care settings.
3 Be able to undertake the preparation for professional supervision with supervisees in health and social care settings.

4 Be able to provide professional supervision in health and social care settings.
5 Be able to manage conflict situations during professional supervision in health and social care settings.
6 Be able to evaluate own practice when conducting professional supervision in health and social care settings.

LO1 Understand the purpose of professional supervision

AC 1.1 Analyse the principles, scope and purpose of professional supervision

What is professional supervision?

Supervision is a process whereby a manager or supervisor oversees, supports and develops the knowledge and skills of a supervisee. It is the way in which a manager can enable a worker to carry out their role in an effective way.

Carroll (2007) in his article One More Time: What is Supervision? provides us with a fantastic potted history about the development of what we now know is supervision, from its inception during Freud's time to now:

'At its simplest, supervision is a forum where supervisees review and reflect on their work in order to do it better. Practitioners bring their actual work practice to another person (individual supervision), or to a group (small group or team supervision), and with their help review what happened in their practice in order to learn from that experience. Ultimately, supervision is for better quality service.'

As a care worker and manager, you will have your own ideas about how you see supervision. It is important, though, to focus on the purpose of the activity as well as the main principles.

The scope and purpose of supervision

All social care workers and managers in care settings are required to undergo supervision and meet particular standards and requirements.

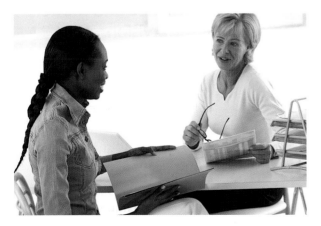

Figure 7.1 Professional supervision involves supporting care workers to carry out their roles effectively.

Meet standards of practice
You are expected to:

> *'Meet relevant standards of practice and work in a lawful safe and effective way.*
>
> *'Seek assistance from your employer or the appropriate authority if you do not feel able or adequately prepared to carry out any aspect of your work or you are not sure how to proceed in a work matter.'*

(The General Social Care Council 2010)

In order to do this, there should be policies and procedures to enable such working to take place, as well as a vehicle for you to discuss your practice and to support you in changing any deficiencies in practice.

Improve the quality of service
The whole purpose of this clear directive is to improve the quality of the work we do in order to achieve agreed objectives and outcomes. Our intention through supervision is to ensure that all people who use services in social care settings have the capacity to lead independent and fulfilling lives. It also ensures that staff themselves feel supported in their work and have recourse to a system of help should they require it.

The British Association of Social Workers and the College of Social Work (BASW/CoSW) England Code of Good Practice for Supervision in Social Work highlights the purpose as being:

> *'to support social workers to provide good quality services. Social work is a complex and demanding profession. Effective supervision of social workers enables social workers to maximise their effectiveness.'*

SCIE's 2013 research paper quotes Morrison's work and defines supervision as:

> *'a process by which one worker is given responsibility by the organisation to work with another worker in order to meet certain organisational, professional and personal objectives which together promote the best outcomes for service users.'*
>
> *Further features of this relationship are that:*
>
> ● *it occurs in a safe environment on a regular basis*
>
> ● *it is based on a respectful relationship*
>
> ● *the process is embedded in the organisation's culture and is understood and valued.'*

(Lambley, S. and Marrable, T., 2013)

Clinical supervision therefore allows the health professional access to professional supervision by a skilled supervisor.

People involved and principles of supervision

The relationship between supervisor and supervisee

The supervisor, who is likely to be you in your own area, is usually a skilled professional who assists staff to develop their skills and helps them to attain knowledge and professional values. You are also required to give advice in supervisory situations and to counsel staff on practice guidelines and policy. Supervisors require training in the process and should provide a good role model for the supervisee.

The person being supervised or the supervisee is a practitioner who receives professional advice, support and guidance from a supervisor who is engaged in observing and assisting staff in delivering good quality care and then giving feedback. In the case of an experienced person, the supervisor may impart support and guidance on reflective practice, for example. We occasionally manage people who have more experience than ourselves and in this case we may be used more as a source of support in their practice.

The principles of supervision

Supervision is a practice that should provide regular, ongoing support for staff and as such time should be set aside for it. Staff need to be clear about the need for supervision and what it is for and also given space to discuss issues in a confidential and safe environment.

The Nursing and Midwifery Council (NMC) has defined a set of principles, which it believes should underpin any system of clinical supervision that is used. So rather than specifying a framework for our use, it would ask us to look to the principles of supervision and use those to guide our practice. These principles are:

- Clinical supervision supports practice, enabling registered nurses to maintain and improve standards of care.
- Clinical supervision is a practice-focused professional relationship, involving a practitioner reflecting on practice guided by a skilled supervisor.

In practice

1.1 Principles, scope and purpose

Write a short account to answer the following questions:

a) What do you understand the purpose of supervision to be?
b) What policies and procedures are in place for your own supervision and how does it help you in practice?

- Registered nurses and managers should develop the process of clinical supervision according to local circumstances. Ground rules should be agreed so that the supervisor and the registered nurse approach clinical supervision openly and confidently and are aware of what is involved.
- Every registered nurse should have access to clinical supervision and each supervisor should supervise a realistic number of practitioners.
- Preparation for supervisors should be flexible and sensitive to local circumstances. The principles and relevance of clinical supervision should be included in pre-registration and post-registration education programmes.
- Evaluation of clinical supervision is needed to assess how it influences care and practice standards. Evaluation systems should be determined locally.

The NMC supports the establishment of clinical supervision as an important part of clinical governance and in the interests of maintaining and improving standards of care.

See unit LM2a AC 2.1 for more information on key principles of effective professional supervision.

AC 1.2 Outline theories and models of professional supervision

While there are a number of models for supervision, including one-to-one supervision, group supervision, and peer group supervision, the approach used will depend on a number of factors, including personal choice, access to supervision, length of experience, qualifications and availability of supervisory groups.

Professional supervision has in the past been likened to the apprentice system or the 'student learning at the feet of a master'. Clinical and professional supervision is now recognised as a complex exchange between supervisor and supervisee, with supervisory models/theories developed to provide a frame for it. It is an ethical requirement of professions where one-to-one contact with clients is an ongoing process and the models that have been developed lend themselves more to this type of process.

As a process for learning, three models are apparent. These are:

- developmental models
- integrative models
- orientation-specific models
- solution-focused models.

www.mentalhealthacademy.com.au is a useful website to visit for more information.

Developmental models

Developmental models of supervision simply define progressive stages of supervisee development from novice to expert (Bernard and Goodyear, 1998). This has been a dominant model for a number of years and focuses on stages within the process (Hogan, 1964; Holloway, 1987).

Stoltenberg and Delworth's (1987) developmental model has three levels for supervisees – beginning, intermediate and advanced – and the focus in each level is on the development of self-awareness, motivation and autonomy.

Supervisees at the beginning or novice stage have limited skills and are presumed to have a lack of confidence. At this stage the supervisee is likely to be highly dependent upon the supervisor and may feel quite insecure.

The supervisee starts working in a dependent manner, imitating the supervisor in their role and becoming more self-assured as they gain in confidence. Movement to the intermediate level happens when dependence on the supervisor is restricted to more difficult work cases and conflict may happen in this stage as the supervisee's self-concept is threatened when they start to question the supervisor's actions.

At the middle stage supervisees have built on their skills and confidence and there may be a tendency to question more and to move between feeling dependent and at the same time fairly autonomous. The supervisee is likely to demonstrate good problem-solving skills and reflection, is more confident and begins to integrate theory into their practice, and is able to reflect on why they are practising in the way they are.

Independence occurs at the advanced level and supervisees start to be accountable for the decisions they make.

The supervisor has to have an accurate picture of the current stage of the person being supervised and be able to facilitate progression to the next stage. The term 'scaffolding' has been used to describe this (Stoltenberg and Delworth, 1987; Zimmerman and Schunk, 2003).

Scaffolding

Scaffolding means the supervisee uses knowledge and skills they already have to produce new learning. As they gain skills at this stage they are encouraged to incorporate these skills and some from the next stage and in doing so, build up a more advanced repertoire. This continual growth is a two-way process in that the supervisor–supervisee relationship changes as they both progress in their learning.

Integrative models

These types of models utilise a number of theories and models and tend to integrate several types of approach. Many of these models refer to the supervision that exists for counsellors and the requirement they have to seek supervision in order to maintain their practice.

Some examples of integrative models are those developed by Bernard (1979) with the discrimination model, Holloway (1995) and the systems approach to supervision, and Ward and House's (1998) reflective learning model. We will look at two of these models.

Bernard (1979)

Bernard's discrimination model was published in 1979 and later developed in 1998. It identified three parts of supervision, namely intervention, conceptualisation and personalisation, and three possible supervisor roles, that of teacher, counsellor and consultant (Bernard and Goodyear, 2009). It focuses on the relationship a counsellor would have with their supervisor and promotes effective skill building through the three areas shown above.

> ### Key term
>
> Scaffolding is the process of moving students progressively towards better understanding and independence in their learning using various instructional techniques (adapted from http://edglossary.org/scaffolding/).

Within the roles taken on by the supervisor, the 'teaching' role occurs when the supervisor lectures or instructs the supervisee. Counselling happens when they assist supervisees in noticing how they may be responding to a client's issues and need to be more objective in their approach. They may have been caught up in a client's problem: they feel empathy but cannot move on. The consultant role occurs when co-therapy is required and the supervisee works with the supervisor and client.

In addition to the three roles taken on by the supervisor, there are within these three different types of supervision:

● **Intervention,** where the supervisee's intervention skills are the main focus.
● **Conceptualisation,** or how the supervisee understands what is going on in the session.
● **Personalisation,** or how the supervisee deals with the potential issues of counter-transference responses, the process whereby emotions are passed on from one person to another, and how they deal with their personal issues.

Holloway (1995)

In Holloway's systems approach model, the emphasis is on the relationship between the supervisor and the supervisee. Holloway describes seven aspects of supervision, which are represented as six wings all connected by the supervisory relationship which takes centre stage. These aspects or 'wings' are the functions of supervision, the tasks of supervision, the client, the trainee, the supervisor and the institution (Holloway, from Smith, 2009).

Orientation-specific models

These models are more useful in psychotherapeutic/counselling settings since there is a firm belief that the supervisor and supervisee should share the same theoretical orientation in order to optimise the relationship. For example, if the supervisor favours a particular approach to psychoanalysis/therapy, such as behavioural or client-centred therapy, for effective supervision to occur, the supervisee should understand the concepts of the theory. In this way orientation-specific models of supervision often mimic the therapy itself, with the terminology, focus and techniques from the counselling session becoming part of the supervision as well.

More fitting for social work is the model proposed by John Dawson (1926). Kadushin (1992) restates the functions of supervision and clarifies this earlier work as being:

● **Administrative** – the promotion and maintenance of good standards of work and coordination of practice. In this role the primary concern is to ensure adherence to policy and procedure and is therefore one of control and authority.
● **Educational** – the primary goal in this role is improve the skill of the worker and to encourage reflection.
● **Supportive** – the maintenance of harmonious working relationships, the cultivation of *esprit de corps* cited by Smith (1996, 2005).

Within this role the supervisor must attempt to improve morale and job satisfaction. With staff facing job-related stress, there is a need to help them and enable them to face the potential problem of 'burnout'.

Solution-focused models

'Solution focus' is about looking for solutions rather than merely focusing on the problems. These models give the supervisor a range of options with which to help the supervisees to move forward positively.

Components of clinical supervision

The Open University (1998) and Proctor (undated) outlined three components of clinical supervision:

● **Formative educative function**, which refers to the part of supervision that encourages the professional development of the practitioner through reflection on practice and self-awareness.
● **Restorative supportive function**, which is the supportive relationship between the supervisor and the supervisee, dealing with the emotional stress arising from practice.
● **Normative managerial function** – this aspect deals with the responsibility of the employer or manager to put in place the means for developing competence and supporting employees in the interest of clinical governance and risk management.

These types of models may fit much better in an organisation where the manager's supervisory role is determined by performance standards and quality. But which model can we use? Interestingly, the NMC, while supporting the principle of clinical supervision, does not

'advocate any particular model of clinical supervision and we do not provide detailed guidance about its nature and scope.'

See unit LM2a AC 1.1 for more information on all of these models as well as information on managerial, clinical and professional supervision.

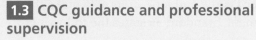

Research it

1.2 Models of supervision

There are a number of other models you may have used for supervision. Research a couple of the following to enhance your learning:

- Hawkins and Shohet (Double Matrix Model)
- Proctor Functional Model
- Waskett 4S Solution Focused Strategy Model
- Cutcliffe and Proctor (1998) Three function interactive model
- Intervention analysis framework
- Davys and Beddoe (2010).

Reflect on it

1.2 Which model of supervision do you use?

Which model of supervision do you use in your own practice? Highlight how you undertake the process and determine where it fits with the models shown. Write a reflective piece to show your understanding of the models and frameworks.

In practice

1.2 Theories and models

Compare and contrast the two types of models you have researched and say how they might relate to your own setting.

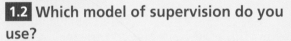

AC 1.3 Explain how the requirements of legislation, codes of practice and agreed ways of working influence professional supervision

Legislation, codes of practice and agreed ways of working

Key term

Agreed ways of working are your setting's policies and procedures as well as guidelines, for the care and support you provide for service users.

Research it

1.3 CQC guidance and professional supervision

Look at the actual document at

http://www.cqc.org.uk/sites/default/files/
documents/20130625_800734_v1_00_
supporting-information-effective_clinical_
supervision_for_publication.pdf

The document describes effective clinical supervision and applies to registered providers, registered managers and staff across all care sectors and settings.

How can you use the guidance within your own setting to influence the supervision practice you currently have in place?

It would also be useful for you to research recent stories to understand the importance of supervision.

The Health and Social Care Act 2012 is the legislation that the service regulator, the Care Quality Commission, inspects under. More recently, the Care Act 2014 highlighted further responsibilities of local authorities.

Although not specifically mentioned, Outcome 14 (supporting workers), which is required under Regulation 23, refers to appropriate training, professional development, supervision and appraisal.

In 2013 CQC published a paper entitled 'Supporting information and guidance: supporting effective clinical supervision' following the recommendations made from the Winterbourne View Serious Case Review. It sets out what effective clinical supervision should look like, and although it was developed primarily for people with a learning disability, it does provide a useful guide for all care sectors and settings. As a result of this case, codes of practice have changed and ways of working mean that staff are required to undertake realistic workloads and are entitled to training and regular skills updates.

From a legal point of view, supervision is a requirement for all staff. The Skills for Care Council in its document *Providing Effective Supervision* (2007) states that:

> 'High quality supervision is one of the most important drivers in ensuring positive outcomes for people who use social care and children's services. It also has a crucial role to play in the development, retention and motivation of the workforce.'

Not only is it good practice to supply supervision, the National Minimum Standards for Care Homes for Older People and for Adults also make this a requirement. Standard 36 states the following:

36.1 The registered person ensures that the employment policies and procedures adopted by the home and its induction, training and supervision arrangements are put into practice.

36.2 Care staff receive formal supervision at least six times a year.

36.3 Supervision covers:
- all aspects of practice
- philosophy of care in the home
- career development needs.

36.4 All other staff are supervised as part of the normal management process on a continuous basis.

36.5 Volunteers receive training, supervision and support appropriate to their role and do not replace paid staff.

While the standards outline the minimum requirements, it goes without saying that you may well need to see and supervise staff on other occasions. Effective management demands that you support your staff to develop areas of practice in which they are deficient or not coping well.

As a manager you are responsible for the effectiveness of the work the team undertakes and for the quality of that work. By focusing more on the outcomes for the organisation and not, for example, on the supervisee and their development, supervision becomes a tick-box exercise at best, checking compliance with policy and procedure. At worst it may not be done at all and may be left out of your role.

In support of supervision as a vital management tool for improving the practice in a team and questioning practice and custom, SCIE (2012) carried out research to evidence the worth of supervision. The findings suggested that:

- good supervision is associated with job satisfaction, commitment and retention
- supervision helps to reduce staff turnover and is significantly linked to employees' perceptions of the support
- for service users, anecdotal evidence suggests that supervision may promote empowerment, fewer complaints and more positive feedback.

In addition, the Skills for Care and the Children's Workforce Development Council (CWDC) have

promoted the widespread provision of high-quality supervision across adult and children's social care, by providing a supervision tool. This tool links to the Skills for Care and Children's Workforce Development Council social care leadership and management strategy suite of products and provides links to other frameworks, including the Championing Children Framework (2006).

As the document suggests:

'Professional supervision can make a major contribution to the way organisations ensure the achievement of high quality provision and consistent outcomes for people who use services (adults, children, young people, families, carers). High quality supervision is also vital in the support and motivation of workers undertaking demanding jobs and should therefore be a key component of retention strategies. Supervision should contribute to meeting performance standards and the expectations of people who use services, and of carers and families, in a changing environment.'

The codes of practice, legal requirements and the way in which we work and address the quality of the care in our settings influence the supervision we give our staff.

See unit LM2a AC 1.2 for more information on how requirements of legislation, codes of practice, policies and procedures impact on professional supervision.

Reflect on it

1.3 Guidance into practice

Read the Skills for Care Council's document *Providing Effective Supervision* (2007) or the Children's Workforce Development Council's guidance on supervision or the document from the 1.3 Research it activity and reflect on how the guidance has been worked into the practice in your own area.

In practice

1.3 Your codes of practice, policies and procedures

Determine how your code of practice or policies and procedures reflect current thinking about supervision.

As a result of legislation, do you need to change your policy on supervision to bring it up to date?

AC 1.4 Explain how findings from research, critical reviews and inquiries can be used within professional supervision

Evidence-based practice

Evidence-based practice is about incorporating evidence from research and making professional judgements as a result of the new knowledge, and applying it to formulate care decisions. In supervision, staff need to be informed of how they can research and review new information and should be made aware of how inquiries inform guidelines and standards.

As practitioners we are duty-bound to perform care in a safe way and in a way in which we are able to question our practice and be accountable for what we do. To 'do no harm' then is the essential premise of evidence-based practice and the need to be able to demonstrate that the care we provide is safe and effective is a reasonable expectation. It is no different in our practice with respect to supervision.

As an effective practitioner accountable for your own safe practice, you need to have access to and be up to date with the research related to your own area and be able to critically appraise such work. As a manager of staff in your setting, you are accountable when it comes to ensuring that the staff have embraced the notion of evidence-based practice.

In making a decision about how and what care is to be given, it is important to have an accurate picture of the research available and to construct sufficient evidence from it to support our actions. In supervising staff we need to ensure that their practice is based on good, sound evidence and that they are informed as to how they might be able to improve their practice consistent with new initiatives in care.

An ethical consideration

From an ethical viewpoint, practising in an informed way means we can be assured that staff are delivering enhanced care that is safe. Each member of staff should be aware of the need to

Key term

Evidence-based practice (EBP) refers to using information from high-quality research and applying it within practice to make informed decisions about a service user's care.

In practice

1.4 Findings, critical reviews and inquiries

Write a short report about how findings from research, critical reviews and inquiries can be used within professional supervision.

How might you help a member of staff during supervision to undertake a piece of work for a course?

---

contribute to their knowledge base by accessing continuing professional development (CPD) and knowledge updates to ensure safe practice. This will reduce the number of incidents surrounding patients and their care and risks in the workplace and thus the potential for litigation. It can also raise the profile of the organisation.

See unit LM2a AC 2.2 for more information on the importance of managing performance in relation to governance, safeguarding and key learning from critical reviews and inquires.

AC 1.5 Explain how professional supervision can protect individuals, supervisors and supervisees

The Royal College of Nursing, in its document *A Vision for the Future* (1993), defined supervision as:

> *'a formal process of professional support and learning which enables individual practitioners to develop knowledge and competence, assume responsibility for their own practice and enhance consumer protection and safety of care in complex clinical situations.'*

This definition clearly points out how the process of supervision protects the public and highlights how we are accountable for what we do. It follows that the supervisor will also benefit, not only from being supervised themselves but also through enabling the staff in the setting to be able to work in an efficient and safe way.

Personal supervision has a protective function for both supervisees and supervisors as well as for the individuals they are caring for. As a manager and leader in a health and social care setting, supervision at its very best can benefit all those working in the area. To enable you to monitor and review the work, supervision can prove to be one of the main ways in which your organisation can do this. It ensures that all staff are being properly supported and can develop their skills and you can be assured that the clients and patients in your care are being safely looked after by competent and knowledgeable staff.

Reflect on it

1.5 Protecting individuals, supervisors and supervisees

Write a reflective piece which shows how your professional supervision can protect the client, the supervisor and the supervisee.

In practice

1.5 How professional supervision can protect individuals, supervisors and supervisees

Working with a supervisee, discuss the protective function of supervision and determine their understanding of it.

LO2 Understand how the principles of professional supervision can be used to inform performance management

AC 2.1 Explain the performance management cycle

Performance management is the way in which managers and employees work together to set work objectives and to monitor and review how they contribute to the work of the organisation. It is the process of communication between a supervisor and a supervisee which is ongoing, occurring throughout the year and supports the accomplishment of the strategic goals of an organisation.

The Chartered Institute of Personnel Development (CIPD, 2006) describes the Performance Management Cycle as 'a systematic approach' which includes:

- setting objectives
- using relevant performance indicators and other measures for determining output
- regularly monitoring and appraising individuals and teams to identify achievements
- identifying training and development needs
- using the knowledge gained to modify plans.

This approach can be represented in a four-stage Performance Management Cycle (see Figure 7.2).

Stage One – Planning
At the planning stage of the Performance Management Cycle you will need to evaluate an employee's current role and performance in order to ascertain where areas of improvement may be needed and to set realistic goals and aims.

Stage Two – Develop
The focus is on improving expertise by allowing the employee to develop new skills and knowledge through CPD.

Stage Three – Perform
At this stage the staff are enabled to practise or 'perform' new skills and new roles that they have learned. Job satisfaction and improved staff morale comes with doing the job well. A good manager will ensure that staff are working to their strengths in order to achieve this.

Stage Four – Review
The final stage is the evaluation by both parties to consider what has been done and what has been achieved. It is here that we can ascertain whether the goals have been reached. By assessing the results of the planned changes, it is possible to determine what next needs to be done, hence the cyclical nature of the process.

See unit LM2a ACs 4.2 and 4.3 for more information on the cycle and methods that can be used to measure performance.

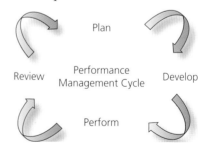

Figure 7.2 The four-stage Performance Management Cycle

In practice

2.1 Performance management cycle

With a member of staff, undertake to plan, develop, perform and review a set of measures, a task or a change in practice. Use the four-stage performance management cycle to help.

142

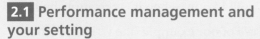

AC 2.2 Analyse how professional supervision supports performance

By using a Performance Management Cycle you impose structure and process to the management of staff and their training and development needs.

In any organisation the aim is to produce and deliver high-quality services and to ensure that all opportunities for improvement, change and innovation are clearly identified and worked towards. To achieve that end, the organisation must realise its potential against performance targets, and equally ensure that the performance management systems in place get the best out of people in the workplace, and deliver the best for people who use services. This can be monitored through the supervision process.

Standards and policies to support performance management

The essential standards of quality and safety consist of 28 regulations (and associated outcomes) that are set out in two pieces of legislation: the Health and Social Care Act 2008 (Regulated Activities) Regulations 2010 and the Care Quality Commission (Registration) Regulations 2009. Together with national occupational standards and codes of practice, they are all helping to change the performance management framework in the social care sector and this is something to celebrate. The inspection process and even the supervisory framework you adopt should be seen as an opportunity to improve performance and service delivery rather than be used as a punitive or disciplinary measure to be feared. Critics argue

that performance management is not a good thing for this very reason and there are also some people who do not value supervision. However, effective performance management and supervision can promote good quality service delivery and result in more highly motivated staff (SCIE, 2011).

As a supervisor there is a need to measure performance against results and not merely focus on behaviours and activity. Think for a moment about the member of staff who always seems to have a lot to do but rarely accomplishes what actually should be done. In this instance, the employee needs to be made aware of the organisational goals together with methods by which those goals may be achieved. This can be done through good supervision, continuing professional development and effective line management.

AC 2.3 Analyse how performance indicators can be used to measure practice

Your organisation's objectives are the starting point when it comes to setting targets for performance. You will also be aware of the staff's job descriptions and the competencies required to carry out certain roles.

Staff must understand what is expected of them and how what they do contributes to the continued success of the work setting. As the manager, you need to ensure that the first step you take in performance management is to define clearly what the staff are required to do, why they need to do it and to what standard.

A good way in which to do this is to have a set of performance criteria made up of measures and standards which clearly state the level of performance required in areas such as:

- deadlines or delivery
- cost or budgets

- colleagues' and service users' views of your performance
- the quality that is expected
- how much is expected or the quantity.

You also need to ensure that the objectives you set are:

- consistent with the member of staff's job description
- consistent with the organisational goals
- clearly expressed
- supported by measurable performance criteria
- challenging.

Setting objectives is not an easy task by any means, but objectives that are Specific, Measurable, Achievable and agreed, Realistic and Time-bound, or, SMART are a useful way to start (see Figure 7.3).

Specific – being specific means we have a much greater chance of success and the way to set such a goal is to plan with these questions in mind:

- Who: is involved?
- What: do I want to accomplish?
- Where: will this happen?
- When: in what timescale?
- Which: identify requirements and constraints.
- Why: do we need to do this?

Example: TT to rewrite the Safeguarding Policy by the end of (date).

Although we have not specified here the reason for doing this, it can be assumed that safeguarding being a huge area in care work is a firm enough reason.

Measurable – to ensure your target is measurable, you might ask questions such as:

- How much?
- How many?
- How will I know when it is accomplished?

In the case of our example (the writing of the safeguarding policy) we will know it is done when it is written. We might also add how much we would expect to be written; we could specify a word count, for example.

Achievable and agreed – an achievable target for a member of staff is one which they agree is needed and one they can actually do. In helping a member of staff in this part of target setting, you could identify small steps towards the larger goal and outline dates by which they should achieve these.

Realistic – to be realistic, the member of staff and you as the manager must believe that the person can actually accomplish the task. It is wise to check that the individual has done something similar in the past and is given the opportunity to identify what they might need in terms of support to accomplish the target.

Time-bound – without a timeframe, the target loses urgency and momentum. By setting a date for completion, there is a given point when the task is to be completed and delivered.

Having a large number of performance indicators will result in little progress being made and it is important to be wary of this. By measuring practice using Smart objectives, the information you obtain may then be used in staff appraisals, for example. The facts obtained provide firm evidence for performance and will show improvement or limitations. As a manager, it is crucial to focus your staff on essential areas for improvement.

Also see unit LM2a LO4 for more information on understanding how professional supervision supports performance.

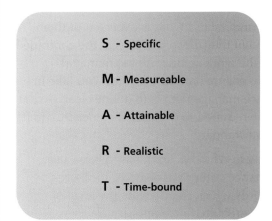

Figure 7.3 SMART objectives

In practice

2.3 How performance indicators can measure practice

Set a SMART target for yourself in which you show how you intend to complete the work for this particular unit.

Write the target in your evidence portfolio showing the steps you will take in order to reach a goal.

LO3 Be able to undertake the preparation for professional supervision with supervisees in health and social care settings

AC 3.1 Explain factors which result in a power imbalance in professional supervision

In most organisations, there will be people who have more power than others simply because they are in a higher position in a hierarchy. This power can be used in a positive way, but often the concept of power brings to mind negative connotations of abuse and harassment and this kind of thinking can lead us to distrust anybody who is in such a position of power. In this way, power can be perceived as influencing or controlling somebody in a negative way. This then can affect supervision.

If you are the manager in a work setting, you are already in a position of power. It is quite possible that you may even have recruited the people who you manage. You have influence and authority over those people. Furthermore, the concept of 'master–apprentice' in supervision evokes a hierarchy of power that favours the master and this is likely to affect the supervisory relationship.

Factors that result in power imbalance

Two main types of power, personal and organisational, are worthy of further investigation here.

When we refer to personal power, we are noting the knowledge, skills and competence associated with an individual that make them an expert. As an expert, the individual can exert a certain amount of power in various situations. Think about the teacher–learner relationship.

Organisational power can be of four types:

- **Reward power** – the manager's ability to give inducements such as pay, promotion or praise to move an organisation forward.
- **Coercive power** – the use of punishment such as disciplinary procedures.
- **Legitimate power** – that which comes with a rank in an organisation that gives authority.

> ### Reflect on it
>
> #### 3.1 Power imbalance
>
> Think about the sorts of power imbalances that you may have come across in the course of your work life. Write an account of how they affected you.

- **Information power** – based on access to information or data that is valued and not open to all (from Gopee and Galloway, 2009).

Being the manager means you invariably supervise the work of the team and this in itself may lead to power imbalance. Supervision in care has become one of the ways in which it is possible to monitor employees' work, ensuring that performance indicators are being met, and this in itself can lead to conflict. With this in mind, we need to look at ways to address the imbalance.

AC 3.2 Explain how to address power imbalance in own supervision practice

If you recognise that a power imbalance exists in the supervision relationship, then you can start to address it. What do we mean by this?

See unit LM2a AC 3.1 for information on anti-oppressive practice.

> ### In practice
>
> #### 3.1, 3.2 Factors leading to power imbalance and how to address this
>
> - What factors might you see resulting in a power imbalance in professional supervision in your setting?
> - How do you deal with power imbalance in your own setting?
> - What sorts of actions do you take, for example, when an important decision needs to be made which you know is likely to be unpopular?
> - Give an example from your workplace.

Case study

3.1, 3.2 Power imbalance

James was the manager in a large care organisation but found his role a difficult one. He always blamed the difficult, unpopular decisions he had to make on higher management with the line 'it's not my decision, it's what they have told me to do' and then took credit for the more palatable ones. In time, he lost credibility with staff who saw through his lack of integrity.

What do you think was the problem here and how might James gain the staff's trust again?

James was clearly trying to be popular with the staff while failing to accept that he would sometimes have to make unpopular decisions. It seems he was not comfortable with that and did not want to adopt an authoritarian approach or an approach in which he would be seen to be dictating and directing matters. Unfortunately, staff are likely to lose confidence in this type of manager and conflict arises.

As a manager with responsibility for the smooth running of a department or organisation, your staff will be looking to you to lead with respect for them and honesty. You will always have the power in the relationship by virtue of the fact that you are accountable for the actions of the staff, that is, the buck stops with you. However, you are responsible for addressing power imbalances and there is no need to take an authoritarian approach to how you lead. Having a conscious awareness of how being 'in charge' can make or break a relationship means you can take control of decisions and set the tone for the work group. While it is good to be 'one of the team' and adopt a friendly manner towards staff, there is a fine line between this and taking control of the situation when you need to. It is always best policy to act with honesty, integrity, fairness and respect for others – this will help to ensure a positive relationship between the supervisor and the supervisee.

AC 3.3 Agree with supervisee confidentiality, boundaries, roles and accountability within the professional supervision process

Effective supervision is about sharing experiences in a safe environment, and informality will enable both parties to feel comfortable and safe. But if no structure is imposed, there is a danger that supervision sessions will not be viewed as meaning much and learning may not occur at all.

The importance of a supervision policy

The best way to impose structure on the proceedings is to first of all ensure there is a supervision policy in place. If this is the case then you will be expected to undertake this aspect of staff development and there will be guidelines as to how you can do this.

The whole process of supervision needs to be 'owned' not only by the organisation but also by the supervisee. Everybody needs to feel part of the process if the merits of such an activity are to be achieved.

Thompson (2006) writes:

'Some people unfortunately adopt a narrow view of supervision and see it primarily... as a means of ensuring that sufficient quantity and quality of work is carried out... a broader view of supervision can play a significant role in promoting learning and developing a culture of continuous professional development.'

A possible framework

You may wish to adopt the following framework to manage your supervision sessions:

- Establish ground rules and boundaries, reminding the supervisee of these at the start of each session.
- Remind the supervisee of the need for confidentiality of information on both sides and agree the boundaries of such and areas that may have to be divulged.
- Agree that the session will not be interrupted unless an emergency occurs and agree what constitutes an emergency. This will really help to confirm the importance of the process.
- Agree the appropriate reason for cancelling the session.
- Identify the agenda for discussion at the start of each session and agree an action plan following each item discussed. Both you and the supervisee should agree on this. These should fit within the categories of:
  - clinical issues/reflections on role and accountability
  - what support is needed/professional issues
  - educational issues/workload discussions
  - management issues.

Research it

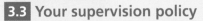

3.3 Your supervision policy

Obtain a copy of your supervision policy and write a short piece about how you might change it to fit what you have learned about supervision to date.

- Ensure appropriate allocation of time and agree that you the supervisor should act as timekeeper.
- A brief record of the contents of the session should be kept by the supervisor.
- Conduct the session in a non-judgemental/discriminatory manner.

AC 3.4 Agree with supervisee the frequency and location of professional supervision

With a policy in place, together with a supervision agreement, the frequency and location of the supervision can be agreed.

To ensure the supervisee is confident that the whole process will take place in a calm and confidential manner, the room must afford privacy and you will need to ensure that mobile phones are switched off or landlines re-routed to another line for the duration of the meeting.

How often you meet will depend upon the policy in your organisation, but you may agree to meet regularly on a fortnightly or monthly basis for 1–2 hours.

AC 3.5 and 3.6 Agree with supervisee sources of evidence that can be used to inform professional supervision and agree with supervisee actions to be taken in preparation for professional supervision

Evidence

The evidence you require a member of staff to bring to supervision will depend on the agreement you have made and the agenda set at the last meeting. The evidence will be linked to the supervisee's objectives and may include reflective accounts of critical incidents that have occurred, assessments undertaken, observations, and service user surveys.

Actions

An action plan which had previously been drawn up may require the supervisee to do something before the next meeting and to bring the finished piece. For example, the supervisee may be undertaking a course of study and will require some support in course work. In this instance, they may bring with them copies of work, course content and reflective accounts of their learning so far. You need to ensure that you do not fall into the trap of becoming a 'surrogate course tutor' for the staff member but allow them to reflect on their learning with respect to how it is affecting or changing their practice.

In preparing for the supervisory meeting, staff need to be aware of the agenda set at the previous meeting. If this required work to be completed, they should get into the habit of bringing with them evidence to support the work done.

Research it

3.6 Actions to be taken

Guidance provided by the Department of Health and the Department for Education and skills on supervision (2012) highlights the need for supervision meetings to be well prepared in terms of reviewing notes, readiness to share ideas and planning for future training and education events.

Access the CWDC and SfC (2012) *Providing Effective Supervision* paper, read and make notes on it.

In practice

3.3, 3.4, 3.5, 3.6 Agreeing details regarding the professional supervision process

Produce evidence of a supervision session you have carried out with a staff member. Include:

- How did you go about agreeing confidentiality, boundaries, roles and accountability with supervisee? (3.3)
- How did you agree the details of time and location? (3.4)
- What sources of evidence did you request the supervisee to bring? (3.5)
- What is the supervisee expected to do to prepare? (3.6)

LO4 Be able to provide professional supervision

AC 4.1 Support supervisees to reflect on their practice

This process of reflection is extremely important to you as a manager since it enables you to bring together practice and theory. Reflection on practice enables us to take a step back from what we are learning and assess what was good and what we might have done differently in any one situation.

In helping your staff to be more reflective about their work, there are a number of useful reflective tools, such as the one developed by Gibbs (1988):

Description – you may ask yourself where you were, who you were with, what happened and what the result was.

> ### Key term
>
> **Reflective practice** is the act of stopping and thinking about what we are doing in practice and analysing the decisions we make in the light of theory and the things we have learned. By doing this we are more able to relate theory to practice to help us to generate new knowledge and ideas.

Feelings – recollecting what you were thinking/feeling at the start and if the feelings changed during the event.

Evaluation – what was good and bad about the experience? How do you judge the event?

Analysis – what sense can you make of the situation? Break the situation down.

Conclusion – what else could have been done? How can you learn from the experience?

Action plan – if it arose again, would you do the same?

Source: Adapted from Jasper (2003)

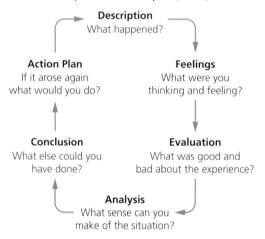

Figure 7.4 The process of reflection

Source: Gibbs, 1988

> ## In practice
>
> ### 4.1 Supporting supervisees to reflect on their practice
>
> Prepare a PowerPoint presentation detailing the process of reflection and showing the key elements of this for your staff.
>
> You may have highlighted the key elements of reflection as follows:
>
> - **Reflection** helps us to achieve a better understanding of ourselves and the roles we carry out. Reflection is where we actively analyse experience, attempting to 'make sense' or find the meaning in it.
> - **Stand back.** It can be hard to reflect when we are caught up in an activity. 'Standing back' gives a better view or perspective on an experience, issue or action.
> - **Undertake repetition.** Reflection involves 'going over' something, often several times, in order to get a broad view and check nothing is missed.
> - **Gain a sense of deeper honesty.** Reflection is associated with 'striving after truth'. Through reflection, we can acknowledge things that we find difficult to admit in the normal course of events.
> - **'Weigh up'.** Reflection involves being even-handed or balanced in judgement. This means taking everything into account, not just the most obvious.
> - **Achieve clarity.** Reflection can bring greater clarity, like seeing events reflected in a mirror. This can help at any stage of planning, carrying out and reviewing activities.
> - **Gain understanding.** Reflection is about learning and understanding on a deeper level. This includes gaining valuable insights that cannot be just 'taught'.
> - **Make judgements.** Reflection involves an element of drawing conclusions in order to move on, change or develop an approach, strategy or activity.

AC 4.2 Provide positive feedback about the achievements of the supervisee

> **Key term**
>
> **Feedback** is an open two-way communication between two or more parties.

Feedback needs to be provided on a regular basis and should be a daily part of your work as a manager. In a formal supervision session, the best way to approach this task is to ask the supervisee how they perceived their performance of a task before you launch in with your assessment. By linking the feedback to their professional development, the member of staff will be able to focus more on what they need to change. In this way you can see what they understand about how well they are doing their job and you are also encouraging them to be reflective about their performance.

Occasionally we are very critical about what we do and it is therefore nice to hear some positive praise for how we have completed a particular job. Positive feedback is often not forthcoming and yet it is motivator when it is genuinely felt. Thanking somebody at the end of the day for a job well done or acknowledging a person's work during a shift builds respect and ensures that the member of staff is secure in their work.

AC 4.3 Provide constructive feedback that can be used to improve performance

Think about the following.

Your manager wants to give you some constructive feedback and has called a meeting for that purpose. How are you feeling? You are probably approaching the meeting in a negative way, thinking that you are about to be criticised in some way. The term 'feedback' is often confused with criticism and how we might have done a job in a better way, and for that reason we view the whole concept less than positively.

So if that's how you feel about it, chances are your staff and supervisees share the same negative vibes. We cannot go through life without making any mistakes and without requiring some guidance on aspects of our work, and although the content of feedback may be negative, it can always be given in a constructive and encouraging manner. When done in such a way, you can help the member of staff to solve a problem, or even to address a part of their behaviour and work towards organisational goals. We give such feedback to ensure that the supervisee is helped to develop, grow and improve.

So how do you go about giving constructive feedback? You may have heard of the 'feedback sandwich' (Figure 7.5). This is a three-step procedure to help provide constructive feedback, consisting of praise, followed by the problem area or criticism, followed by more praise. In this way, the unpalatable news is sandwiched by good news and the blow of receiving it is softened.

Although it has come in for criticism (ironically) from some writers, it is a good way for new managers and supervisors to help to deliver news that may otherwise be seen as negative. Look at the case study on page 150 for an example of how it might work.

See unit LM2a AC 4.5 for more information on constructive feedback.

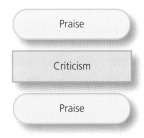

Figure 7.5 The praise 'sandwich'

> **In practice**
>
> ### 4.2, 4.3 Positive and constructive feedback
>
> Give an example of positive and constructive feedback you have used to help improve the performance of a member of staff. Record a real supervision session and anonymise it for your coursework.

Case study

4.2, 4.3 Positive and constructive feedback

Jenny is a member of staff who is undertaking a teaching qualification and has been asked to participate in some staff development. Her manager is aware that Jenny does not fully engage all the staff in the room when she teaches and has noticed some staff members not paying attention.

- **Praise:** 'Jenny, I really enjoyed your presentation to the staff this morning. I thought your PowerPoint presentation was very clear and you had some great handouts for the staff. This is such an important subject, isn't it? We need to ensure that all staff are clear about this.'
- **Criticism:** 'Did you notice that two of the staff were using their mobile phones while you were talking? And I think they got rather muddled about some of the points you were making. I think this might mean they have not fully understood how important safeguarding is. Can you be sure they are going to be able to cope

with the work you set them to do? Perhaps you could ask more questions of individuals to get them to voice their concerns.' Allow for discussion.

- **Praise:** 'I am pleased that your teaching seems to be going really well at the moment and the staff obviously enjoy it too. Well done.'

You will see here that the area for Jenny to work on has been highlighted but she has also been praised for the good points in her teaching. Hearing what someone likes about us or our performance is always encouraging and being specific about what is good is also a useful tool. We need to know what it is that is good or positive. By making reference to the issue you have a concern with and offering ways in which it can be addressed, the criticism is seen as more constructive and useful provided it is clear and specific. By focusing on the positives and then the areas for development, feedback can be usefully employed to improve performance.

AC 4.4 Support supervisees to identify their own development needs

Ongoing staff development is just one discussion you will have with your supervisees during the supervision session. These needs are likely to reflect their job role and the long-term goals of the organisation.

If the member of staff is seeking new responsibilities in the work setting, they may be helped to identify courses to enable them in a new role. It is important that you as a manager and supervisor are up to date with policy changes, national initiatives and legal requirements for the setting in order to specify the sort of training they need.

Professional development requirements attached to various roles and required by regulatory bodies such as the NMC or HCPC (Health and Care Professions Council) change over time and you need to have a good understanding of those required for your work setting. Supervisees should be encouraged to reflect on their practice with respect to these codes from time to time.

AC 4.5 Review and revise professional supervision targets to meet the identified objectives of the work setting

Using staff appraisals to review

Staff appraisals, performed at the end of an annual cycle for managing staff, are a vehicle for reviewing the goals set throughout the supervision process and planning for the year to come.

The targets set in the 'In practice' may well have been developed at a staff appraisal meeting, the purpose of which is described below:

- Review the job description and role.

In practice

4.4, 4.5 Identifying development needs and reviewing and revising targets

Using the supervision session carried out in 'In practice 4.2 and 4.3', record the developmental needs identified by the staff member and review them against the targets set.

How did you support the supervisee to identify their development needs?

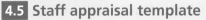
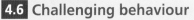

4.5 Staff appraisal template

The following website provides a useful template for staff appraisal: www.businessballs.com/performanceappraisalform.pdf

Read the information and reflect on its usefulness in your own work.

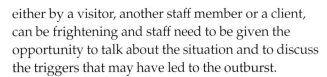

Reflect on it

4.6 Challenging behaviour

Remind yourself of your policies with respect to how you would help staff to deal with challenging behaviour.

- Look at individual performance and achievement and reward (performance-related pay or other incentives).
- Plan ongoing professional development.
- Give feedback.

The object of appraisal is to set goals for the coming year and to identify ways in which the staff member can improve their performance over the next year. It should be a positive process in which the member of staff can be given details about their performance and can start to plan for the forthcoming year. Staff who have been underperforming should have been made aware of this during supervision and at appraisal will be identifying ways in which they can meet the required standards in the year to come. They should not be surprised to learn of the problems with their performance at this stage in the proceedings since they will have received feedback in the previous supervision sessions.

The process of appraisal is similar to supervision. For example, you could check in with how they are going about their own CPD and whether the work they are doing is within their expertise or if they need to develop their skills further. You may also want to look at how the employee dealt with the workload and what they achieved with the service users.

See unit LM2a AC 4.6 for information on the use of performance management towards the achievement of objectives.

AC 4.6 Support supervisees to explore different methods of addressing challenging situations

In dealing with any challenging situation, your supervisees must be directed to the policies in the workplace and should be given the opportunity to undergo training. Any challenging behaviour,

either by a visitor, another staff member or a client, can be frightening and staff need to be given the opportunity to talk about the situation and to discuss the triggers that may have led to the outburst.

It is a good idea to discuss this with new staff and to remind experienced staff of the types of challenging behaviour your setting might come across and to ensure they are aware of how they are to deal with such incidents. By reflecting on these incidents, the staff can learn from challenging situations and can also start to be more aware of how they felt in such instances.

By evaluating the event in this way, staff can start to appreciate how they might have been affected by a situation and how others may also be affected. They will also see how circumstances at the time may have led to the event and this sort of examination can be useful in planning for a different reaction the next time it happens.

See unit LM2a ACs 3.2, 3.3 and 3.4 for information on methods, how conflict may arise within professional supervision and how it can be managed.

AC 4.7 Record agreed supervision decisions

All supervision meetings need to be properly recorded in order to identify and support agreed actions and their completion within agreed timescales. Without records we cannot be sure we have actually set tasks and actions and this can lead to confusion.

However you choose to record the meeting, the following are points to consider:

- Record decisions and actions which you agree on and ensure that these are signed and dated.
- Have clear timescales.
- Detail responsibilities.
- Ensure copies are filed in a safe place and supervisees know that other managers may have access to them.

LO5 Be able to manage conflict situations during professional supervision

AC 5.1 and 5.2 Give examples from own practice of managing conflict situations within professional supervision and reflect on own practice in managing conflict situations experienced during professional supervision process

What is a conflict situation and why does it occur?

In supervision the potential for conflict arises when there is a disagreement about a point of professional practice or the values and goals of the supervisor do not fit with those of the supervisee. For example, the supervisor may challenge the member of staff and this could cause some opposition. See also AC 3.4 in unit 17.

You may come across two types of conflict:

- **Task-based conflict** – disagreements related to approaches to work, processes and structural issues within the team and the organisation.
- **Relationship-based conflict** – conflicts between individual members of the team, usually caused by differences in personal values and beliefs.

Specific areas of conflict that you may come across during supervision may include:

- lack of clarity around team roles and responsibilities
- unfair distribution of work
- lack of clear vision on the part of the supervisee

- lack of understanding of the role of others
- poor communication.

Effects of conflict

Conflict can disrupt performance but within teams it is a common occurrence. When the resolution of the conflict is effective, it can have a positive effect, leading to personal growth and development.

If managed effectively it can be 'creative and productive and creative solutions to difficult problems can often be found through positive conflict resolution' (Tilmouth *et al.*, 2011).

How to deal with conflict situations

It is imperative to handle such conflict effectively since bad handling of these situations will lead to an ineffective team. Staff start to avoid each other and rifts occur, with staff taking sides. The ultimate downside of this happening is that this most certainly leads to poor and ineffectual care of service users. It is important to be assertive and provide fair feedback on problems or areas of conflict.

The most effective way of solving conflict in a team is for the people concerned to have a constructive conversation (Larson and LaFasto, 2001). By doing so, each person will be helped to see the other person's perspective and will gain some understanding about the way the other person feels about the situation. The conversation must result in each party committing to making improvements in the relationship (Tilmouth *et al.*, 2011). These conversations might be initiated by the staff members themselves or they may require the services of a neutral facilitator or another person to mediate in the situation. This can be set up in supervision.

Larson and LaFasto's (2001) CONECT model for resolving conflict by conversation is useful:

- **Commit** to the relationship by discussing the relationship and not the problem causing concern. Each person should say why they feel change should occur and what they hope to gain.

5.1, 5.2 Managing and reflecting on conflict situations

What sort of conflict have you managed in your own practice? Identify an area of conflict you have been involved in with a member of staff and write a short piece showing how you managed that situation.

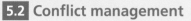

Research it

5.2 Conflict management

At your next team meeting, agenda an item on conflict management.

Collect information about how staff manage conflict in their roles with service users and with other staff members.

Collect the information to provide a record of types of conflict experienced and ways in which it is managed.

- **Optimise** safety, with both parties committing to maintain confidentiality and create an atmosphere of trust.
- **Neutralise** defensiveness, with each person explaining what they have observed, how it made them feel and the long-term effects of the other person's actions.
- **Explain** each perspective or each side of the argument.
- **Change** one behaviour and ask each person to change.
- **Track** the change and decide how improvements will be measured. Agree to meet to discuss whether changes have been successful (Tilmouth *et al.*, 2011).

In resolving conflict, when people's needs are discovered then a solution can be found. We may be tempted to compromise, but compromise means that people's needs are still not fully met and this can lead to resentment (West, 2004).

Ensuring that conflicts are addressed in the right manner means that relationships are maintained and can function smoothly.

Reflecting on practice

A conflict situation is never pleasant but by reflecting on the circumstances that led to the event and thinking about how it might have been handled

in a different way we can sometimes find more useful ways of managing conflict should it arise again.

LO6 Be able to evaluate own practice when conducting professional supervision

AC 6.1 Gather feedback from supervisee/s on own approach to supervision process

One way you can evaluate your work as a supervisor is to ask for feedback; however, this may be quite difficult to do. Nevertheless, if you are to improve your practice, you need evidence of what you can do to achieve this.

You might decide to ask staff to complete an anonymous questionnaire about your work. The following questions might be useful:

1 How did you find my approach to the session?
2 Was it positive?
3 How might I have improved it?
4 What was the best aspect of my approach?
5 And the worst?
6 What are the areas I need to improve?

Supervision requires that you are conforming to standards as set out in guidance supplied by governing bodies such as CQC which provide us with minimum standards. By working in line with such guidance we will be able to measure our performance against standards and we can highlight areas for improvement in our practice.

AC 6.2 Adapt approaches to own professional supervision in light of feedback from supervisees and others

Good supervision goes a long way to ensuring that staff and managers maintain a healthy working relationship. Gaining feedback from staff keeps the relationship healthy since we can learn and adapt our style and as a result change our practice to more efficient ways of working. Supervisors who are reflective will be able to change, develop and improve their practice for the good of their supervisees.

Legislation

While there is no specific law that demands supervision, in practice the various codes of conduct under which health care professionals work demand

In practice

6.1, 6.2 Gathering feedback and adapting approaches

Ask the member of staff you supervised to comment on your work. Collect the data and reflect on the comments.

How might you adapt or change your approach to your own professional supervision in light of feedback from supervisees and others.

Research it

6.1, 6.2 An evaluation sheet

Prepare an evaluation sheet for your supervisees and other staff members to enable you to gain feedback on your approach to the supervision process. Collate the information gained and say how you will adapt your approach in light of feedback from supervisees and others.

Reflect on it

6.2 Feedback and changes

Reflect on the comments and identify any changes you intend to make as a result of your feedback.

quality care and set standards for supervision. You might look at the list below for further information:

- The National Minimum Standards for Care Homes for Older People and for Adults.
- Skills for Care Council (2007); Providing Effective Supervision.
- CQC (2013) Supporting information and guidance: Supporting effective clinical supervision.

- SCIE (2011) Social Care Governance: A Workbook based on Practice in England. London: Social Care Institute for Excellence.

Assessment Methods

LO	Assessment criteria And accompanying activities	Assessment methods *To evidence these assessment criteria you could:*
LO1	1.1 In practice (p. 136)	You could discuss the role of supervision with your assessor or you might provide a written account answering the questions in the activity.
	1.2 Research it (p. 139)	Carry out some secondary research on two or three of the models of supervision in the activity. Discuss with your assessor the model you wish to use for your practice.
	1.2 Reflect on it (p. 139)	Complete the activity. Write a reflective piece to show your understanding of the models and frameworks you use and highlight how you undertake the process.
	1.2 In practice (p. 139)	Prepare a presentation for staff about the models and show how they say how they might relate to your own setting.
	1.3 Research it (p. 139)	Go to the webpage in the activity and make notes on the guidance which describes effective clinical supervision and applies to registered providers, registered managers and staff across all care sectors and settings. Undertake a professional discussion with your assessor to show how can you use the guidance within your own setting to influence the supervision practice you currently have in place?
	1.3 Reflect on it (p. 140)	Provide a written reflection for your assessor which shows how the guidance from the documents outlined in the activity have been worked into the practice in your own area.
	1.3 In practice (p. 140)	Provide details of how your code of practice or policies and procedures reflect current thinking about supervision. You might choose to add copies of the policies with areas highlighted. Discuss with your team at a team meeting whether the recent changes in legislation requires policy change to bring it up to date?

LO	Assessment criteria And accompanying activities	Assessment methods To evidence these assessment criteria you could:
	1.4 In practice (p. 141)	Either write a short report about how findings from research, critical reviews and inquiries can be used within professional supervision or ask your assessor to supply you with a witness testimony which demonstrates how you have used research, critical reviews and inquiries in your practice. Write an account of how you might help a member of staff during supervision to undertake a piece of work for a course?
	1.5 Reflect on it (p. 142)	Write a reflective piece which shows how your professional supervision can protect the client, the supervisor and the supervisee or give details of how you have helped a staff member during this process.
	1.5 In practice (p. 142)	Undertake an observation of a supervisee, and engage with them in a discussion about how they see the protective function of supervision. Write a short piece on their understanding of it.
LO2	2.1 In practice (p. 142)	Complete the activity. Prepare a hand-out to show the four-stage Performance Management Cycle and put a copy of it in your portfolio.
	2.1 Research it (p. 143)	With your assessor undertake a professional discussion to show the effectiveness of your performance management system. Show evidence of the structures you have in place to support the performance management process. Or you might complete a short piece of research in your own setting to determine the extent to which your organisation complies with the performance management process.
	2.2 In practice (p. 143)	Complete the activity and provide a written account.
	2.3 In practice (p. 144)	Complete the activity and provide a written account. Alternatively you may discuss this with your assessor and ask her to undertake to write a witness testimony of the discussion.
LO3	3.1 Reflect on it (p. 145)	Write a short reflective account for the activity.
	3.1, 3.2 In practice (p. 145)	Discuss the questions in the activity with your assessor and perhaps your manager.
	3.1, 3.2 Case study (p. 146)	You could use the case study and answer the questions or you could use a real life example which shows how power imbalance has played a part in your setting. Discuss this with your assessor.
	3.3 Research it (p. 147)	Complete the activity. Discuss your findings with a mentor or assessor.
	3.6 Research it (p. 147)	You might read and make notes on the guidance. Discuss with your assessor how you prepare for this in practice.
	3.3, 3.4, 3.5, 3.6 In practice (p. 147)	Provide a written account answering the questions in the activity. Refer to the Providing effective supervision document in the research activity.
LO4	4.1 In practice (p. 148)	Prepare a PowerPoint presentation as instructed in the activity.
	4.2, 4.3 In practice (p. 149)	Ask a member of staff if you may record a real supervision session and anonymise it for your coursework. Provide a report of positive and constructive feedback you have used to help improve the performance of a staff member.
	4.2, 4.3 Case study (p. 150)	You could use the case study and write a short response to how positive feedback is given here or you could use a real life example which shows how you give positive and constructive feedback in your own setting. Discuss this with the assessor.

LO	Assessment criteria And accompanying activities	Assessment methods *To evidence these assessment criteria you could:*
	4.4, 4.5 In practice (p. 150)	Provide a written account answering the questions.
	4.5 Research it (p. 151)	Complete the activity and write a short piece to show how you might use it.
	4.6 Reflect on it (p. 151)	Complete the activity. Or you may obtain copies of the policies and procedures in your workplace and highlight the areas which show how they might help staff to deal with challenging situations.
	4.6, 4.7 In practice (p. 152)	Complete the activity and discuss this with your assessor.
LO5	5.1, 5.2 Reflect on it (p. 152)	Provide a reflective account.
	5.1, 5.2 In practice (p. 153)	Provide a written account for your assessor.
	5.2 Research it (p. 153)	Complete the activity. Or invite your assessor to attend this.
LO6	6.1, 6.2 Research it (p. 154)	Complete the activity.
	6.2 Reflect on it (p. 154)	Provide a reflective account. Discuss with your assessor how you might adapt your approach in the light of the comments.
	6.1, 6.2 In practice (p. 154)	Complete the activity and provide a written account.

References

Bernard, J. M. (1979). 'Supervisor training: a discrimination model', *Counsellor Education and Supervision*, 19, 60–8.

Bernard, J. M. and Goodyear, R. K. (1998) *Fundamentals of Clinical Supervision* (2e). Needham Heights, MA: Allyn & Bacon.

Carpenter, J., Webb, C., Bostock, L. and Coomber, C. (2012) Research briefing 43: Effective supervision in social work and social care, SCIE.

Carroll, M. (2007) 'One more time: what is supervision?' *Psychotherapy in Australia*, 13(3), May. www.supervisioncentre.com/docs/kv/one%20 more%20time.pdf

CIPD (2006) *Coaching Supervision: Maximising the potential of coaching*. The Bath Consultancy Group.

CQC (2013) Supporting Information and Guidance: Supporting Effective Clinical Supervision.

CWDC and SfC (2012) *Providing Effective Supervision*. Leeds: Children's Workforce Development Council and Skills for Care.

Dawson, J. B. (1926) 'The casework supervisor in a family agency', *Family*, 6: 293–5.

Department of Health (2003) *National Minimum Standards: Care Homes for Older People*, DOH 2003b Standard 36. London: TSO.

DfES (2006) *Championing Children. A shared set of skills, knowledge and behaviours for those leading and managing integrated children's services*. London: DFES.

DfES (2007) *Providing Effective Supervision*. Skills for Care and the Children's Workforce Development Council (CWDC). London: TSO.

General Social Care Council (2010) *The General Social Care Council – Code of Practice*.

Gibbs, G. (1988) *Learning by Doing: A guide to teaching and learning methods*. Oxford: Further Education Unit, Oxford Brookes University.

Godden, J. (BASW/CoSW England) Code of Practice to Support Social Workers.

Gopee, N. and Galloway, J. (2009) *Leadership and Management in Health Care*. London: Sage.

Harkness, D. and Hensley, H. (1991) 'Changing the focus of social work supervision: effects on client satisfaction and generalised contentment', *Social Work*, 36(6), 506–12.

Hawkins, P. and Shohet, R. (2012) *Supervision in the Helping Professions (Supervision in Context)*. London: Oxford University Press.

Hogan, R. A. (1964) 'Issues and approaches in supervision', *Psychotherapy, Theory, Research & Practice*, 1, 139–41.

Holloway, E. L. (1987) 'Developmental models of supervision: is it development?' *Professional Psychology: Research and Practice*, 18(3), 209–16.

IDEA (2008) *Performance Management – The People Dimension*, www.idea.gov.uk/idk/aio/6237345/

Inskipp, F. and Proctor, B. (1995) *Art, Craft and Tasks of Counselling Supervision: Professional Development for Counsellors, Psychotherapists, Supervisor and Trainers Pt.1 and 2*. Twickenham: Cascade.

Jasper, M. (2003) *Beginning Reflective Practice*. Cheltenham: Nelson Thornes.

Kadushin, A. (1992) *Supervision in Social Work* (3e). New York: Columbia University Press.

LaFasto, F. M. J. and Larson, C. E. (2001) *When Teams Work Best: 6,000 team members and leaders tell what it takes to succeed*. London: Sage.

Lambley, S. and Marrable, T. (2013) 'Practice enquiry into supervision in a variety of adult care settings where there are health and social care practitioners working together,' London: SCIE.

Morrison, T. (2005) 'Staff supervision in social care', Brighton: Pavilion, in SCIE (2013) *Effective Supervision in a Variety of Settings*. London: SCIE.

Nursing & Midwifery Council (2008) *The Code: Standards of conduct, performance and ethics for nurses and midwives*.

The Open University, School of Health and Social Welfare (1998) *Clinical Supervision: A development pack for nurses*. Milton Keynes: Open University.

Proctor, B. (undated) 'Supervision: a co-operative exercise in accountability' in Marken, M. and Payne, M. (eds), *Enabling and Enduring*. Leicester: National Youth Bureau/Council for Education and Training in Youth and Community Work.

Royal College of Nursing (1993) 'A vision for the future', *Guidance for Occupational Health Nurses*.

Skills for Care and CWDC (2007) *Providing Effective Supervision: A workforce development tool, including a unit of competence and supporting guidance*. SCF01/0607.

Smith, K. L. (2009) *A Brief Summary of Supervision Models*, http://www.marquette.edu/education/grad/documents/Brief-Summary-of-Supervision.

Smith, M. K. (1996, 2005) 'The functions of supervision', *The Encyclopedia of Informal Education*.

Stoltenberg, C. D. and Delworth, U. (1987) *Supervising Counsellors and Therapists*. San Francisco: Jossey-Bass.

Stoltenberg, C. D., McNeill, B. and Delworth, U. (1998) *IDM Supervision: An integrated developmental model of supervising counselors and therapists*. San Francisco: Jossey-Bass.

Thompson, N. (2000) *Promoting Workplace Learning*. BASW Policy Press.

Ward, C. C. and House, R. M. (1998) 'Counseling supervision: a reflective model', *Counselor Education and Supervision*, 38, 23–33.

Waskett, C. (2010) 'Clinical supervision using the 4S model 1: considering the structure and setting it up,' *Nursing Times*, 106(15), early online publication accessed on 18/8/15.

West, M. (2004) *Effective Teamwork*. Oxford: Blackwell.

Zimmerman, B. J. and Schunk, D. S. (eds) (2003) *Educational Psychology: A century of contributions*. Mahwah, NJ: Lawrence Erlbaum Associates.

http://cdn.basw.co.uk/upload/basw_13603-1.pdf
www.mentalhealthacademy.com.au

www.scie.org.uk/workforce/peoplemanagement/staffmanagement/performance/index.asp

www.skillsforcare.org.uk

Useful resources and further reading

Buchner (2007) *Performance management theory: A look from the performer's perspective with implications for HRD*. Human Resource Development International.

https://www2.rcn.org.uk/development/learning/transcultural_health/clinicalsupervision

SCIE (2011) *Social Care Governance: A workbook based on practice in England*. London: Social Care Institute for Excellence

The British Association of Social Workers and the College of Social Work (BASW/CoSW) England Code of Good Practice for Supervision in Social Work.

Unit M3

Manage health and social care practice to ensure positive outcomes for individuals

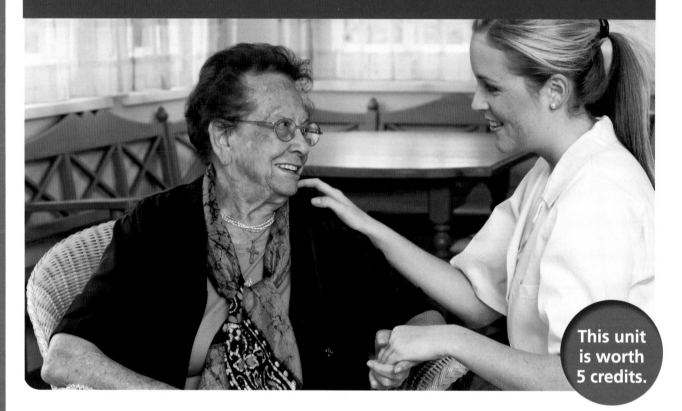

This unit is worth 5 credits.

Personalisation refers to the choice and control that people have over the support they receive, whether from statutory services or self-funded, and in recent years there has been growing importance placed on meeting outcomes that fulfil the needs of individuals.

The purpose of this unit is to assess the learner's knowledge, understanding and skills required in the process of planning and achieving positive outcomes that underpin the personalisation agenda. This unit also covers the key areas of practice that support the implementation of personalisation and is further covered in units M2c and HSCM1.

The unit also explores the role of the manager/senior worker in providing a supportive environment for individuals to achieve positive outcomes.

Learning outcomes

By the end of this unit you will:

1 Understand the theory and principles that underpin outcome-based practice.
2 Be able to lead practice that promotes social, emotional, cultural, spiritual and intellectual well-being.
3 Be able to lead practice that promotes individuals' health.
4 Be able to lead inclusive provision that gives individuals choice and control over the outcomes they want to achieve.
5 Be able to manage effective working partnerships with carers, families and significant others to achieve positive outcomes.

LO1 Understand the theory and principles that underpin outcome-based practice

AC 1.1 Explain 'outcome-based practice'

In an attempt to ensure that all individuals requiring care are dealt with holistically and with their needs being met, the 'personalisation 'agenda has been introduced into a lot of recent government documentation. A system of care and support tailored to meet the needs of the individual has replaced the 'one size fits all' approach previously in vogue. Seen as a user-centred approach to care, it involves the care worker acting as a facilitator in care pathways.

Based upon the social model of disability and empowerment, this approach has been hailed as a better option to the needs-led assessment, and research supports this (Harris *et al*., 2005).

Three dimensions of the model have been put forward as being:

● outcomes involving change, such as those that focus on developing self-confidence, or skills that enable self-care
● outcomes maintaining quality of life, occasionally referred to as maintenance outcomes
● outcomes associated with the process of receiving services, or those which involve being valued and listened to in the care process.

Harris *et al*. (2005) categorised the dimensions into a four-part framework, which might also be seen as showing how needs may be met. See Table 9.1.

Table 9.1 The outcomes framework

Autonomy outcomes include:	Personal comfort outcomes include:
● access to all areas of the home ● access to locality and wider environment ● communicative access ● financial security	● personal hygiene ● safety/security ● desired level of cleanliness in the home ● emotional well-being ● physical health
Economic participation outcomes include:	Social participation outcomes include:
● access to paid employment as desired ● access to training ● access to further/higher education/employment ● access to appropriate training for new skills (e.g. lip reading)	● access to mainstream leisure activities ● access to support in parenting role ● access to support for personal secure relationships ● access to advocacy/peer support ● citizenship

Source: From Maclean *et al*., 2002

Key terms

Personalisation refers to the way in which individuals are helped to become the drivers in developing systems of care and support designed to meet their unique needs.

Outcome-based practice, also referred to as outcomes management and outcomes-focused assessment, is one such approach to achieving desired patient care goals. It refers to activity that benefits patients and involves team work and quality assurance measures.

Outcomes management is a means to help patients, funding services and providers make care-related choices based on knowledge of the effects of these choices on the patient's life.

In practice

1.1 Outcome-based practice

Explain what you understand by 'outcome-based practice' to a member of your staff.

AC 1.2 Critically review approaches to outcome-based practice

Key term

A critical review provides a summary of a book or text and evaluates it. In undertaking a review you need to read the text in depth and also look at other texts that are related to the same subject. You are then able to make a more reasoned judgement.

Several approaches to outcome-based practice have been identified. These include the following:

- **Results-based accountability** is also known as outcomes-based accountability. It uses data-driven decision making processes to help problem solving and is a way of thinking and acting that improves the lives of the community. It has been developed to improve the performance of an organisation's services.
- **Outcomes management** is the means to help patients and providers make care-related choices based on knowledge of the effects of these choices may have on the patient's life.
- **Outcomes into practice** focuses on the outcomes people value.
- **Logic model** is a logical framework and theory of change used by funders, managers and evaluators of programmes to evaluate effectiveness.

Whichever model is used, the basic premise is that outcome-based practice is a new way of working which replaces the needs-led approach that tended to focus on the immediate situation and support requirements that would be provided by the care professional.

A different approach

The idea of 'outcomes' in care was seen focused on achievement and was seen as a more meaningful way to assist with care.

In using this approach, the care worker takes on the role of assisting the client to identify immediate, medium-term and long-term goals. Rather than leading the client's care, the health professional:

'steers, guides, (and) pronounces the identification of "needs" and the proposed "intervention" towards practice driven by the service user, who is encouraged and facilitated to identify their "outcomes", a set of immediate, medium- and long-term goals that they wish to achieve. The focus on outcomes overcomes many of the deficiencies of the "needs" model described above.'

Qureshi *et al.* (2000), quoted in Barnes and Mercer (2004)

Care work becomes target driven and specific, with a goal in mind and it is the service user in this type of care who sets review dates and monitors their achievement, thus moving away from the care professionals' 'assessment of the service user's needs'.

The client then remains in complete control of the entire process, from the identification of outcomes, to their achievement and evaluation of the success or failure of the venture. In this type of approach, the role of the care professional is to assist the service user in the achievement of their outcomes only.

While this approach would seem to provide the ultimate in person-centred care, it is not without its critics and a critical evaluation of the approach by Qureshi *et al.* in 2000 for York University highlighted some of the issues with it.

Care professionals seemed to struggle with the concept of outcomes as they lacked understanding of what the outcomes' focus actually was.

A further area of concern was with the notion of 'expert power'. Putting the service user at the centre of the assessment process, identifying their own aims and objectives in negotiation with care professionals meant that the professional felt their role had been reduced to one of facilitator as the control and responsibility for the achievement sat very much with the service user. For some professionals this did not sit well with the belief that as experts, they should have a bigger part in the decision-making process.

This somewhat radical approach to care meant that professionals needed to change their perceptions

In practice

1.2 Approaches

Consider the needs-led and the outcome-based approach to care and provide an in depth evaluation of the two approaches. Show examples of how you have used the latter approach in your own care. In a critical review, you should summarise the pros and cons of each approach and determine how they differ.

of care and embrace a newer way of working. The move to using the term 'outcome' rather than 'need' was one which helped to change perceptions, although the research showed this was not easy.

The role of the care professional

Further issues with this type of approach seemed to stem from the care professional's need to reach a service solution instead of listening to the client's desired outcomes. This was reported as a need to take responsibility on the part of the professional and was also linked to pressure of work. A number of professional practice issues have been noted in the research and the challenge of introducing an outcomes approach has been raised. These were:

- the tendency of the care professionals to fall back into a provider service mode instead of thinking and acting creatively with service users
- the inability of care staff to grasp the outcomes concept.

Interestingly, the research showed that service users valued the outcomes approach and 'appear comfortable with setting goals and working towards them'.

AC 1.3 Analyse the effect of legislation and policy on outcome-based practice

The Department of Health published its 'Transparency in outcomes: a framework for quality in adult social care' paper in The 2012/13 Adult Social Care Outcomes Framework in 2012. The document describes a set of outcome measures, which demonstrates the achievements of adult social care both nationally and locally, and

further developed moves to a more outcome-based system of practice.

Historically, the NHS and Community Care Act 1990 (Section 47(1)) required local authorities to carry out assessments of need for community care services with individuals who appeared to need them and developed the use of a 'needs-led approach'. This legislation with respect to outcome-based practice is part of the personalisation agenda so favoured by health professionals and government over the last 40 years or so.

In the 1980s and 1990s, there was a move towards a more individualistic, consumer-led approach to social care and away from the 'dependency culture.'

Other changes have included:

- The Social Security Act of 1986 replaced Supplementary Benefit with Income Support.
- The Disabled Persons Act (1986) brought about assessment of needs for disabled persons and the Independent Living Fund (ILF), which aimed to increase choice and control in order to promote independent living, was brought in in 1988 and removed in 2015.
- The 1988 Griffiths Report advised the use of a variety of providers to prevent a 'monopoly' on the provision of care and support and the concept of the 'mixed economy of care' was introduced.
- The 'Caring for people' White Paper (1989) paved the way for community care and care management in social work.
- In the late 1990s, direct payments were introduced as a result of the Community Care and Direct Payments Act 1996.
- In 2003 'individual budgets' were introduced and brought about a new model of social care provision.
- The 'Valuing People' White Paper (2001) (Figure 8.1) made direct payments available to more people with a learning disability and it is in this paper that we first officially came across the term 'person-centred planning'. In 2009, this paper was redrafted and the 'Valuing People Now: A Three Year Strategy for People with Learning Disabilities, Making It Happen for Everyone' was released updating the personalisation and budget plans.

- *Improving the Life Chances of Disabled People* (2005) meant the introduction of individual budgets to improve choice and control over the mix of care and support.
- *Independence, Wellbeing and Choice* (2005) obligated social care services to help people to maintain their independence by 'giving them greater choice and control over the way their needs are met'.
- *Our Health, Our Care, Our Say: A new direction for community service* (2006) introduced the concept of personalised care.
- *Putting People First: A shared vision and commitment to transformation of adult social care* was a commitment to enable people to manage and control their own support through individual/personal budgets.
- *Care, Support, Independence: Shaping the future of care together* (2009) provided a consultation on how personalised social care and support could be delivered and funded.
- The introduction of the personal health budget to allow people to have more choice, flexibility and control over the health services and care they receive was introduced as a result of the White Paper *Personal Health Budgets: First steps* (2009).
- The White Paper *A Vision for Adult Social Care: Capable communities and active citizens* (2010) set out the plans for a new direction for adult social care, putting personalised services and outcomes centre stage.

The Care Act 2014

The Care Act 2014 brings the personalisation agenda right up to date and although there is still some discussion about needs-led care, it requires local authorities to:

'consider the person's own strengths and capabilities, and what support might be available from their wider support network or within the community to help in considering what else alongside the provision of care and support might assist the person in meeting the outcomes they want to achieve.'

The Care Act 2014

Additionally, it introduced the idea of a 'strengths-based approach' in which an individual's strengths – personal, community and social networks – are

Reflect on it

1.3 Legislation and your practice

Write a reflective account that shows how your own practice, with respect to outcome-based practice, has been affected by legislation.

Research it

1.3 Government documents

Research some of the government documents discussed and explain how they have affected outcome-based practice in your setting.

maximised to 'enable them to achieve their desired outcomes, thereby meeting their needs and improving or maintaining their wellbeing' (SCIE – see http://www.scie.org.uk/care-act-2014/assessment-and-eligibility/process-map/).

AC 1.4 Explain how outcome-based practice can result in positive changes in individuals' lives

Outcome-based care puts the person firmly at the centre of the care service and delivers meaningful individual outcomes. This has created a results-based accountability culture, which relies on data-driven decision-making processes to help to improve the lives of citizens and the community as a whole. Being accountable in this way means evidence is provided for the outcomes achieved for service users and in this way services can be judged as to whether service users are better off as a result of the services input.

The key benefits of such care are:

- Services users can choose care preferred and needed to improve their quality of life.
- They can have more flexibility in choice and any changes to need can be responded to more quickly.
- Care workers can work closely with service users to enable them to become more independent.
- It strengthens partnership working.

- Evaluating the effectiveness of services is easier where outcome measures are set out.

In practice

1.3, 1.4 Legislation, outcome-based practice and positive changes

How have changes in legislation and policy improved outcome-based practice? Prepare an account showing an example from your setting.

What are the positive changes that can come about with outcome-based practice that are not apparent in a service-led approach? Compare the two approaches.

LO2 Be able to lead practice that promotes social, emotional, cultural, spiritual and intellectual well-being

AC 2.1 Explain the psychological basis for well-being

A subjective view of psychological well-being would be to say that we are happy or satisfied with our lives. But this is fraught with difficulty since what makes you happy is unlikely to be the same for service users or other care workers. So although our emotions and how we feel are a part of psychological well-being, it is not enough. In order to feel really good and to have fulfilling lives, we need to experience purpose and meaning, in addition to positive emotions. Psychologist Carol Ryff has developed a clear model of psychological well-being that breaks it down into six key parts:

1 Self-acceptance.
2 Positive relations with others.
3 Autonomy.
4 Environmental mastery.
5 Purpose in life.
6 Personal growth.

These are explained in detail in ACs 2.2 and 2.3.

Source: From Ryff's 1989 Psychological Well-being Inventory

If we are to lead practice that promotes social, emotional, cultural, spiritual and intellectual well-being, we need to be aware of the factors that can contribute to this.

Psychological well-being is about enabling service users to experience a well-rounded and balanced life and the emotions that go with this.

The Care Act 2014 definition of well-being

The DOH (2014) Care and Support Statutory Guidance; Issued under the Care Act 2014 defines well-being as a broad concept, relating to the following areas:

- personal dignity (including treatment with respect)
- physical and mental health and emotional well-being, protection from abuse and neglect
- control by the individual over day-to-day life (including care and support)
- participation in work, education, training or recreation
- social and economic well-being, which refers to being actively engaged with life and with other people and having a positive standard of living based primarily on financial security
- domestic, family and personal issues
- suitability of living accommodation
- the individual's contribution to society.

Ensuring well-being of service users

Ensuring the 'well-being' of our clients and even our staff requires us as managers to determine how we might measure the state of well-being. When things are not going well and our joy with life and general sense of calm is lacking, we start to experience stress, worry and anxiety. Our psychological well-being becomes compromised and this will inevitably lead to our quality of life being reduced. For the people in our care, this can lead to depression and its subsequent effects on physical well-being and health.

Maslow in his hierarchy of needs outlined the things that contribute to a person's well-being – see Figure 8.1.

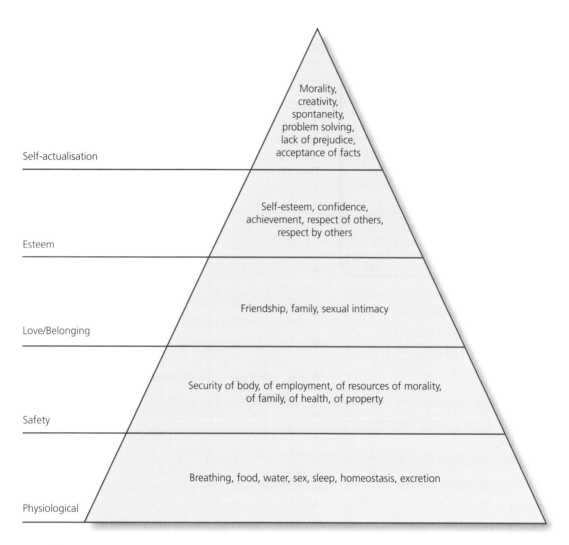

Figure 8.1 Maslow's hierarchy of needs

In practice

2.1 Psychological basis for well-being

Explain the psychological basis for well-being.

The concept of holistic health and well-being incorporates several different facets, including:

- physical
- intellectual/mental
- emotional
- social
- spiritual
- sexual.

Source: Ewles and Simnett, 1999

You will also need to consider cultural aspects.

Briefly define each of the terms and say how you promote psychological well-being in your clients.

AC 2.2, 2.3 Promote a culture among the workforce of considering all aspects of individuals' well-being in day-to-day practice and review the extent to which systems and processes promote individual well-being

Key term

Culture is the behaviour, values, thoughts and norms of an organisation – the unspoken rules. In a health and social care setting, this refers to the staff's beliefs about care and how these might affect the way in which they work.

In order to promote psychological well-being, let's take as our starting point Ryff's 1989 Psychological Well-being Inventory. In engendering a culture that promotes well-being in our day-to-day practice, as managers we need to ensure we have an awareness of the aspects of well-being and what it is service users may need.

By valuing the concept of positive well-being for service users as a manager, you can ensure that staff are reminded about the need for positive outcomes for people in their care. Training and ongoing staff development during supervision can also ensure that staff fully appreciate the need to constantly raise their awareness about how well-being for service users can be improved.

There are certain factors you should consider to promote a culture of well-being in day-to-day practice:

Self-acceptance

The way we view our lives and ourselves is a major source of well-being. Self-acceptance is about coming to terms with what we can't change or control. If we are satisfied with who we are, and can live with our experiences without bitterness or regret, we can find contentment with our current situation.

Positive relations with others

Loving relationships and friendships in which care and trust are apparent are so important to all of us and yet there may be a tendency to forget this in the workplace. Just as we value closeness and support of others, so too will our service users, but this can be neglected when we merely attend to physical needs. The need to be able to connect with others and have the opportunity to make friendships is just as important in long-term care for service users (who may not see family or friends daily) as it is to us who can return home to our families every night.

Autonomy

Being free to make choices and our own decisions is a liberating feeling. Being in control of our destiny is what autonomy refers to. When a person goes into a care home or is ill for a long period of time, often choice is removed from them and well-meaning care workers may think this is the right thing to do. As unique people with our own identity, values and goals in life, we need to be able to maintain the ability to think and act for ourselves and as care workers we must empower our clients to do the same.

Mastery

Autonomy is about making decisions for ourselves and keeping control of our lives. Being masters of our own environment and adapting to and modifying our situations in order to progress and achieve what we need is a vital part of this concept. In long-term care this may seem to be difficult to achieve, but as care professionals it is imperative to keep the lines of communication open and to access the service user's desires as to how they wish to live and what they need to do to control their circumstances as much as possible. This in turn will give them confidence and belief in our abilities, which brings with it a sense of pride and success.

Purpose in life

Can you imagine a life without a purpose? Some service users may feel that once they are in long-term care or have a disability that prevents them from living the way they used to, life is not worth living. They need to be empowered to feel that there is something to strive for, even in changed circumstances. By enabling the client to continue to use their strengths and talents, to develop relationships and to pursue their goals, they can find real purpose in living.

Personal growth

We never stop learning so long as we are willing to be open to new experiences and seek out our potential. Service users may be elderly or in long-term care, yet we as care professionals need to encourage them to continue to be curious about aspects of life and to seek out opportunities to grow as a person.

The whole concept of well-being is about being comfortable in our lives where everything has come together. But the question is, how can you enable the people you care for to feel this way?

Systems and processes

The systems and processes, such as training for staff, supervision and evaluating care, you have in place for managing care may seem to be counter-productive to promoting the things we have just discussed. How, for example, are you able to allow service users to have mastery over their own environment when that environment is one in which a number of constraints operate with respect to the way it is managed and the procedures it operates? Or how much autonomy can a person have if they live in a care home?

Overcoming constraints

We recognise there are constraints to enabling clients to live full and purposeful lives when it comes to service delivery, and of course some things may be difficult to achieve. But a positive outcome for an individual is possible only if they are fully involved in deciding what that positive outcome will be. In planning our service users' care, we need to have systems in place which allow the client to be at the centre of that care and be an equal partner in the decisions made.

In the last activity you may have referred to the following sorts of things:

- Systems which do something more for the client than simply allowing them to have choice are those in which the person is valued, has dignity and is treated as the unique person they truly are.

In practice

2.2, 2.3 Well-being

In your own care setting, how do you promote a culture among the workforce which shows consideration of all aspects of individuals' well-being? Write a case study which shows the systems and processes in place that promote individual well-being.

Reflect on it

2.2, 2.3 How systems and processes promote well-being

Reflect on the culture of well-being in your organisation. Say how the systems and processes promote individual well-being and provide evidence of this.

- Respect for the person is shown when care staff take the time to really get to know the person and take into account all their cultural and religious choices, and values and preferences.
- There should be equality in a relationship and support for the client to live the life they want in the circumstances they find themselves in. It's about them, not us!

LO3 Be able to lead practice that promotes individuals' health

AC 3.1 Demonstrate the effective use of resources to promote good health and healthy choices in all aspects of the provision

'Improving England's Mental Health: The First 100 Days' was published in 2015 and sets out a number of practical actions the government will take to ensure mental and physical health are valued equally.

Budgets and funding

With poor mental health costing £105 billion annually in England, and businesses losing £26 billion due to mental ill health issues every year, the report highlighted the need to ensure that resources by means of increased funding were made available.

Research has shown poor mental health as a contributor to wider health inequalities being associated with increased health-risk behaviours and increased morbidity and mortality from physical ill health. Promoting good mental health, therefore, has significant potential benefits – not only the improvement to health outcomes and life expectancy, but also improving educational and economic outcomes.

Research it

3.1 Mental Health: The First 100 Days

Take a look at the following link to see the document: http://nhsconfed.org/resources/2015/05/the-first-100-days-and-beyond

Look at the five priority areas for action and say how you might use these in your setting.

Your staff

The biggest resource at your disposal are your staff and by ensuring they are well equipped in terms of the training they require to promote good health and healthy choices for service users, you will be able to lead a practice that promotes health.

Care work requires research in terms of well-trained staff and budget being used appropriately. In planning, care staff must be aware that the promotion of good health and giving service users information to help them to make healthier lifestyle choices is as important as managing long term chronic conditions

AC 3.2 Use appropriate methods to meet the health needs of individuals

Services for our clients are provided by a range of professionals and in a variety of ways. In planning care for positive outcomes, the care worker needs to work with the client to ensure that the best services are offered to meet the needs of the client. Care planning is about what the client needs and wants, not about what the care worker can arrange for them. Sometimes this may lead to conflict. For example, we, as care professionals, recognise that obesity can cause health issues and we may believe that it is in the service user's best interests to change their diet.

However, the choice remains with them and we can only investigate services that may be of use to them; we are not at liberty to insist they use them.

Some of the things you may be asked to help with are outlined below:

- **agreed therapeutic/development activities** as requested by the services user.
  The service user may require help with the **assistive technology** for example in order to improve their communication and we may need to source help for them in this area of our work.
- **regular health checks** required by medical staff. Service users who are unable to visit the GP or other health professional may require assistance to set up an appointment for health checks, for example, or may just require help to get to an appointment.
- **administering prescribed medication/treatment** Any medication prescribed for the service user will need to be administered at the correct time but occasionally it may be in a form that is difficult for the service to take so we can help by accessing easier ways in which medication might be administered.
- **promoting/supporting healthy lifestyle choices** Service users may need additional help to undertake changes to their lifestyle and as health care workers we should be able to give information as to how change may be effected. such as providing information about diet, smoking and exercise.

Standard Two of the National Framework for Elderly People outlines person-centred care and gives us guidance as to how we should go about meeting the health needs of the elderly.

The essential factors in any care planning and provision is to adopt a holistic approach, recognising that all service users – young, older or those with disabilities (either physically or with a learning disability) – are individuals with needs which impact upon their lives. It is important to give individuals choice and doing so requires you to have information about services which are available. **Assistive technology** (AT) is improving all the time and we need to be up to date with what is available for our service users. For example for older people, simply introducing amplification devices may make communication with everybody more effective. Those individuals with mobility issues may benefit from having a scooter so they can travel over distances. AT is anything that helps an individual to actively undertake daily activities on their own allowing them to live more independently.

Your staff must be aware of all the options available and need to be able to give out that information in an unbiased way. You may be asked, 'What would you do or what would you choose?' In most cases the answer has to be, 'I am not you and it is for you to decide.'

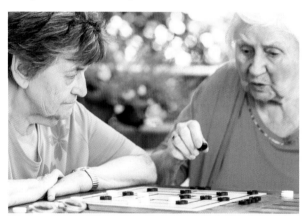

Figure 8.3 Care workers should use appropriate ways to meet the care needs of individuals

In practice

3.2 Appropriate methods

Supervise a member of staff carrying out a care assessment and evaluate the extent to which the member of staff used appropriate methods to meet the health needs of individuals.

How might they improve on the assessment and how can you ensure as a manager that all staff are fully aware of what is required of them with respect to the essential standards for your own setting?

AC 3.3 Implement practice and protocols for involving appropriate professional health care expertise for individuals

The manager's role is to ensure that guidelines for practice are available for staff which highlight the care for service users to ensure that seamless care is provided. Decisions about the care to be given are made during the assessment process with the service user and are then translated into treatment plans, procedures, medical notes and care plans. Care plans are provided to ensure that care given is standardised to reduce the risk of variation throughout the day. For example, a staff member on a night shift who may not have been involved in the initial assessment needs to be aware of how a service user is cared for during the day and how they wish to be treated so that the same care can be continued. Practice protocols are there for guidance and as a manager you are responsible for ensuring they are upheld and also implemented. Sometimes it may be necessary to involve other members of the wider disciplinary team to provide a different area of expertise so staff need to know how the referral to other professionals can be made.

AC 3.4 Develop a plan to ensure the workforce has the necessary training to recognise individual health care needs

Managers are responsible for planning for the future and this will require you to estimate what you will require in terms of staffing, and training for example, so that the service is ready for any changes on the horizon. Your plan will be invaluable for this purpose since it will identify how the service intends to meet the needs of the health provision for its service user and how it will develop the service provision for the future.

Your planning for the future needs to ensure that the staff are fully aware of how training will impact upon the care they give to service users. We occasionally lose sight of the value of updating our knowledge and may neglect to attend training because we are too busy. Staff must be aware that the organisation values training which upskills their staff and enables them to recognise individual health care needs.

AC 4.4 Develop a plan to ensure the workforce has the necessary training to support individuals to achieve outcomes

Service users must be able to make their own decisions with respect to the care they need and want so the staff should be prepared to ensure they are able to do this. It will require the staff to understand and fully adopt the use of an outcome-based approach. Occasionally they may find it difficult to step back from simply giving care where they, the staff, deem it necessary, disempowering the service user in the process. As a manager you will need to support your staff in this. You may need to develop a plan of action to ensure that staff are able to access training to ensure they fully appreciate all the issues surrounding outcome-based care.

See the 'Legislation' and 'Useful resources' sections at the end of the unit, which will be relevant to your understanding of ACs 3.3, 3.4 and 4.4.

In practice

3.3, 3.4, 4.4 Practice, protocols and plans

For your portfolio, list and evaluate the policies and protocols for involving appropriate professional health care expertise for individuals in your work setting.

Develop and implement staff training to ensure the workforce is able to recognise individual health care needs and can support individuals to achieve outcomes.

How will you ensure that your staff have the necessary training to support individuals to achieve outcomes? Show how you intend to develop staff with respect to the personalisation agenda.

LO4 Be able to lead inclusive provision that gives individuals choice and control over the outcomes they want to achieve

AC 4.1 Explain the necessary steps in order for individuals to have choice and control over decisions

In any decision being made, the person who is at the centre of making that decision has to feel they are actively doing so. Too often a client may feel they are merely a passive attendant at a meeting, with little say in what goes on. We take for granted the work we do, with all its related administration, meetings and bureaucracy. For service users, this may seem rather overwhelming and it would take a lot of confidence on their part to question anything you may put forward. The following steps may help:

Step 1

The client needs to be clear about who they want involved in their care and about the choices they have but may rely on you to help them to identify the specialist help. For example, a service user who is being cared for at home by their spouse may not realise that special equipment such as hoists for bathing to help her and her husband cope is available and so they may fail to realise they have a choice.

Step 2

Monitor the process of the care arrangements as you go along and check that the client is clear about what has happened so far. It is important that the communication method is suitable for service users. If, for example, service users have trouble reading small print, you need to ensure that they have access to large-print versions of documents. Service users may also need extra assistance if English is not their first language and interpreters may be required at each meeting.

Step 3

It may be that service users have previous case notes with another agency and in this step, you need to obtain your client's consent to obtain those notes. **Service users need to be informed of all aspects of their care, including the need to contact others for additional information.**

Step 4

Recording the above step is necessary and your client may be asked to sign to confirm that they have agreed for certain information to be released. If at any point your client does not give consent for any action, this must be respected.

Step 5

Obtain feedback. Just as you need to monitor the process throughout, you must also ensure that feedback from the client and family and friends is

In practice

4.1 Choice and control

Show how the assessment in In practice 3.2 enabled the client to exercise choice and control over decisions.

Provide the care plan with annotations to show where each step has been accomplished.

Research it

4.1 Service users in your setting

How inclusive is the provision in your setting?

Undertake a short survey of staff, service users and others such as family members and other professionals to determine their views on how much choice and control over outcomes individuals in your setting have.

forthcoming regularly. Positive feedback will mean that, of course, the process is working well. However, any concerns must always be dealt with in an efficient and non-judgemental way. If the service user wishes to make a complaint, it is up to you to support them in accessing the correct procedures to do so.

AC 4.2, 4.3 Manage resources so that individuals can achieve positive outcomes and monitor and evaluate progress towards the achievement of outcomes

Resources
Funding and services

To ensure that our service users have positive outcomes we need to be clear about the resources at our disposal and how they will be used. Any plan of care produced needs to be resourced in terms of finances, as well as the availability of services, which of course may change over time. This is why there needs to be a continual check on what is happening with the service user's care.

Funding may be reduced or demand for a particular service may increase, thus making it more difficult for your client to access the service. Adjustments to the plan should be made in accordance with how it is progressing.

In practice

4.2, 4.3 Resources and progress

1 Give an example of how you have managed resources so that individuals can achieve positive outcomes in your setting.
2 How does your organisation monitor the resources and evaluate progress towards the achievement of outcomes for your clients? Write a reflective account of the process undertaken and place copies of relevant documentation into your portfolio.

Monitoring and evaluating

When we audit or monitor a provision we make a judgement as to how the resources have been used and whether there has been a positive impact on the service user. For example, we may have decided that by 'inputting' more funding into a community outing (output) services users will experience improved quality of life which will result in a positive 'outcome'. The resources here would be seen to be well used and effective in improving an outcome.

We may also monitor the effects of the way in which the programme of activities we have planned for the service users has improved their well-being. By structuring a simple evaluation questionnaire we can gain feedback as to how the services users enjoyed a session to determine whether we would repeat it.

In answer to the above activity, it is likely that you have in place an evaluation system to enable everyone involved in the care to comment and document how that care is working.

Monitoring and evaluating through feedback

Lay carers, the client themselves and the service care providers all need to provide regular feedback about the circumstances of the care package and any need for adjustment. At the start of the whole care planning process, you will have put into place a means for providing feedback. You will also have identified some key people in the process:

● individual receiving the care
● family and friends involved in the care

- health care professionals
- the service provider.

Individual receiving the care

Being the central figure in the care process, there needs to be a clear process for service users to record how they experience the care receive. This can be achieved by the use of a checklist, perhaps on a weekly or monthly basis, regular contact via email, telephone or meetings with the care manager or the person facilitating the care, and recording the care given on a daily basis on the care plan.

Family and friends involved in the care

Feedback from these individuals is valuable, but form filling can be laborious and time consuming. They may feel overwhelmed with having to provide a regular feedback form, so you need to be able to obtain their views in different ways. Perhaps a weekly phone call may be the solution.

Health care professionals

By agreeing what will trigger contact at the start of the care process with other health care professionals, you can ensure that contact is maintained and care is monitored. For example, you may agree to notify them only if the client's condition changes.

Any problems with taking medication or medication being ineffective may mean you need to contact other health care professionals such as GPs. If mobility problems change or the service user starts to refuse certain aspects of the care, this will also be a sign that the health care professional should contact the care manager. In between regular review meetings, these instances will ensure the seamless delivery of care and that the client is not at risk of inadequate care.

The service provider

As the care manager, you are in the best position to monitor the client's care and to notice any change. You can tell whether a service requires changing or increasing by being in close contact with the client on a daily basis.

AC 4.5, 5.2 Implement systems and processes for recording the identification, progress and achievement of outcomes and implement systems, procedures and practices that engage carers, families and significant others

The whole process of monitoring and evaluating the care package is about recognising and documenting changes to circumstances. You will already have systems in place that record the care to be provided and to evaluate that care. As a service provider, you are also duty bound to regularly ask for feedback from clients and their family about how well you do in the delivery of your service.

Records should monitor the progress of the service user towards their outcome so that all staff are able to observe progress and gain information. In order to record the progress there must be a clear statement of the outcome, a plan of how the outcome will be achieved and regular feedback about progress.

Systems, procedures and practices that engage carers, families and significant others

It is most important that we do not underestimate the input from carers, family and others in the care of an individual. Should a carer become ill themselves making them unable to continue in the caring role for a while then there must be a procedure in place to ensure that care for the service user can be continued in the way it has been planned.

As a manager you need to be able to engage with families to ensure that they feel included in the care planning process and that they have somebody they can access should they ever feel the need to. Families and other carers can sometimes experience great isolation socially so it is useful if there are systems in place that can ensure they are informed of groups and help they can expect when they feel this way.

One system that might be implanted could be for carers to have access to a monthly meeting to discuss the progress of the care being given

In practice

4.5, 5.2 Implementing systems, processes, procedures and practices

Collect together the documentation you use to show how you go about recording progress in care and the achievement of client outcomes.

What systems and practices are in place to address the needs of family and other carers?

to the service user and to suggest and changes should they feel these are needed. There might also be a system in place whereby a carer can telephone a direct number to speak to a staff member who can help them with queries regarding the care.

LO5 Be able to manage effective working partnerships with carers, families and significant others to achieve positive outcomes

AC 5.1 Analyse the importance of effective working relationships with carers, families and significant others for the achievement of positive outcomes

In analysing the importance of effective working relationships, it is necessary to look closely at the way in which we interact with each other and to determine how this might affect positive outcomes.

In the course of our working life, we interact with many people and the quality of these interactions can have a profound effect, not only on our own health and well-being, and our enjoyment of work, but also for those with whom we interact. For our client and their carers, we have a responsibility to ensure that these working relationships promote their best interests and work towards positive outcomes in their care package.

To remind ourselves of the role of the health and social care worker, we turn to Standard One in the Common Induction Standards, which clearly outline the responsibilities and limits of your relationship with an individual in your care.

Citing the General Social Care Council's Code of Conduct, your responsibilities are to:

- protect their rights and promote their interests
- establish and maintain their trust and confidence
- promote their independence and protect them as far as possible from danger or harm
- respect their rights and ensure their behaviour does not harm themselves or other people
- uphold public trust and confidence
- be accountable for the quality of your work and take responsibility for maintaining and improving your knowledge and skill.

While you may feel confident that you do all of the above and maintain good working relationships with all individuals you come into contact with, we need to be mindful of the actual relationship between health care professionals and those requiring care and their carers. For example, look at the language the standards use and note the use of the word 'their'. This seems to imply a passive relationship in which the health professional is 'doing something' to the individual. For us, it conjures up a relationship in which the health professional takes on the responsibility of ensuring that the individual is 'cared for' rather than a major part of their own care.

The difficulty we believe is in the hierarchical nature of the relationship between health professional and the client which, try as we might to diminish, is still prevalent and has the potential to affect the outcome of care. The power the health care professional possesses in terms of knowledge and expertise, the language used in care work, professional autonomy and the environment in which we work will all have an effect on the relationship if not carefully handled. It is the transfer of the power to the client and their carer which is fraught with difficulty and one that needs to be worked on constantly.

Positive benefits come from effective team work and by seeing the client as the central figure in the team working towards their own care package, the relationship forged will be effective. The Health Care Commission in 2006 outlined the characteristics of a good team as having the following in place:

- clear objectives
- close working relationship towards those objectives

- regular meetings to discuss ways of improving and outcomes achieved
- no more than 15 members.

Although these characteristics are more often applied to teams in health care settings, we make no apologies by applying them to the team that makes up the care providers for the client. By adopting this sort of strategy, we can expect the working relationship between all parties to be improved.

AC 5.3 Use appropriate approaches to address conflicts and dilemmas that may arise between individuals, staff and carers, families and significant others

In Unit LM1c we looked at Thompson's (2006) RED approach to managing conflict and we revisit it here.

R – Recognise the conflict; do not sweep it under the carpet.

E – Evaluate the conflict to see how detrimental it would be if it was allowed to develop.

D – Deal with the conflict; keep open communication.

Appropriate ways in which to deal with any barriers and conflicts which arise can be on a one-to-one basis or in group discussion. Providing information to enable service users and the team involved in their care to make informed decisions may also help the process and reduce the conflict. Conflict may sometimes be the result of lack of information, which causes distress and may lead to angry outbursts.

We might also instigate contracts between people to highlight expectations with respect to roles and behaviour. This can then help to resolve potential conflict areas.

Another way in which conflict may be managed is through a mentoring system. By allocating a mentor to each staff member, conflicts can be brought to them for discussion and mediation.

The way in which you deal with and resolve conflict comes from your favoured leadership approach. The skills approach developed by Mumford *et al.* (2000) lists within its five components social judgement skills as one of the competencies required in dealing with conflict. The capacity to understand people and social systems serves to enable leaders to work with others to solve problems and to implement change. Part of this competency is *social performance* and this refers to the skill in persuasion in communicating with others. Any conflict can be resolved if the leader acts as a mediator in the process.

AC 5.4, 5.5 Explain how legislation and regulation influence working relationships with carers, families and significant others and implement safe and confidential recording systems and processes to provide effective information sharing and recording

Legislation and regulation

From April 2015, under the Care Act carers for those with health and social care needs are entitled to an assessment of needs and support will be offered if carers meet the eligibility criteria. These changes improve existing legislation, putting carers on an equal legal footing to those they care for and putting their needs at the centre of the legislation. (See the Care Bill explained: Including a response to consultation and pre-legislative scrutiny go to www.carers.org/sites/default/files/care_act_briefing_june_2014.pdf)

This act puts carers' needs firmly into perspective and highlights their needs as being highly important in the care process.

The Data Protection Act (1998) is also worth revisiting here. The act protects information kept on an individual and also regulates how information must be stored and kept. See Unit SHC 51 for more information.

5.4, 5.5 Legislation and confidential recording systems

1 How do legislation and regulation influence your working relationships with carers, families and significant others?

2 Complete a case study to show how you deal with clients' and carers' confidential information with respect to person-centred care and positive outcomes.

Legislation

See AC 1.3, which provides the legislation in detail. The laws relevant to ACs 3.3, 3.4 and 4.4 are listed here:

- The Care Act 2014
- Carers and Disabled Children's Act (2000) www.opsi.gov.uk
- Disability Discrimination Act (1995) www.opsi.gov.uk
- Human Rights Act (1998) www.opsi.gov.uk
- Mental Health Act (2007) www.dh.gov.uk
- Mental Health (Care and Treatment) (Scotland) Act (2003) www.opsi.gov.uk
- NHS and Community Care Act (1990) www.opsi.gov.uk

Assessment methods

LO	Assessment criteria and accompanying activities	Assessment methods *To evidence these assessment criteria you could:*
LO1	1.1 In practice (p. 160)	Write a short piece to show what you understand by 'outcome based practice' and explain it to a staff.
	1.2 In practice (p. 161)	Compare the needs-led and the outcome-based approach to care. You can include a table to show the similarities, differences, pros and cons. Show examples of how you have used the latter approach in your own care.
	1.3 Reflect on it (p. 162)	You could write a reflective account. Discuss with your assessor how your own practice, with respect to outcome-based practice, has been affected by legislation.

LO	Assessment criteria and accompanying activities	Assessment methods *To evidence these assessment criteria you could:*
	1.3 Research it (p. 162)	Access some of the government documents discussed and explain to your assessor how they have affected outcome-based practice in your setting.
	1.3, 1.4 In practice (p. 163)	Discuss the questions outlined with the team and with team. Following this meeting, prepare a written account addressing the questions
LO2	2.1 In practice (p. 164)	Prepare a hand-out for staff which covers the questions in the activity.
	2.2, 2.3 In practice (p. 166)	Discuss the activity with your assessor. You might also write a case study which shows the systems and processes in place that promote individual well-being. Include the systems and processes in place that promote individual well-being.
	2.2, 2.2 Reflect on it (p. 166)	Write a reflective account and place the evidence in your portfolio.
LO3	3.1 Research it (p. 166)	You might like to take a look at the link in the activity and discuss with your assessor or team the five priority areas for action. Ask staff to identify how you might use these in your setting and reflect on their comments.
	3.1 In practice (p. 167)	Preparing a hand-out or leaflet. Alternatively you could show the accounts to your assessor which demonstrate how you put your resources, both staff and budgets, to effective use with respect to this aspect of well-being.
	3.1 Reflect on it (p. 167)	Write a short reflective account for your portfolio.
LO4	3.2 In practice (p. 168)	You could undertake observation. Or you could speak with a staff member about how they could improve on the assessment, and ask your assessor to witness an interview. Discuss the points in the activity with your assessor .
	3.3, 3.4, 4.4 In practice (p. 169)	Use the suggestions in the activity.
	4.1 In practice (p. 170)	You might prepare a short piece to show how the assessment in In practice 3.2 enabled the client to exercise choice and control over decisions. You could also provide the care plan with annotations to show where each step has been accomplished.
	4.1 Research it (p. 170)	Discuss points in the activity with your team. Undertake a short survey of staff as suggested.
	4.2, 4.3 In practice (p. 170)	Follow the points in the activity.
	4.5, 5.2 In practice (p. 172)	Follow the points in the activity. You could provide demonstrate this to your assessor.
LO5	5.1 In practice (p. 173)	Provide a case study as suggested in the activity.

→

LO	Assessment criteria and accompanying activities	Assessment methods *To evidence these assessment criteria you could:*
	5.3 Reflect on it (p. 173)	Discuss with your assessor, a real example of conflict you had to deal with and say how you managed it.
	5.3 In practice (p. 173)	Write a short account addressing the points in the activity.
	5.3 Research it (p. 173)	Prepare a table which compares the models.
	5.4, 5.5 In practice (p. 174)	Write an essay or complete a case study to address the points in the activity.

References

Barnes, C. and Mercer, G. (eds) (2004) *Disability Policy and Practice: Applying the social model.* Leeds: The Disability Press.

Department of Health (1989) *Caring for People: Community care in the next decade and beyond.* London: HMSO.

Department of Health (2000) *National Service Framework – for Older People.* London: HMSO.

Department of Health (2005) *Independence, Wellbeing and Choice: Our Vision for the future of social care for adults in England.* London: HMSO.

Department of Health (2006) *Our Health, Our Care, Our Say: A new direction for community service.* London: HMSO.

Department of Health (2009) *Personal Health Budgets: First steps.* London: HMSO.

DOH (2012) *Transparency in Outcomes: A framework for quality in adult social care. The 2012/13 Adult Social Care Outcomes Framework.* Crown.

Harris, J., Foster, M., Jackson, K. and Morgan, H. (2005) *Outcomes for Disabled Service Users.* York: Social Policy Research Unit, University of York.

HM Government (1990) *The NHS and Community Care Act 1990.* London: HMSO.

HM Government (2005) *Improving the Life Chances of Disabled People.* A joint report with Department of Work and Pensions, Department of Health, Department for Education and Skills, Office of the Deputy Prime Minister. London: HMSO.

HM Government (2009) *New Horizons: A shared vision for mental health.* London: HMSO.

Kishida, Y., Kitamura, T., Gatayama, R., Matsuoka, T., Miura, S. and Yamabe, K. *Ryff's Psychological Well-Being Inventory: Factorial structure and life history correlates among Japanese university students.* Department of Psychiatry, Kumamoto University School of Medicine, 1-1-1 Honjo, Kumamoto, Kumamoto, 860–8556, Japan. kitamura@kaiju. www.medic.kumamoto-u.ac.jp

Maclean, I., Maclean, S. and Pardy McLaughlin, L. (2002) *A Handbook of Theory for Social Care. Volume Two.* London: City and Guilds.

Mumford, M. D., Zaccharo, S. J., Connolly, M. S. and Marks, M. A. (2000) 'Leadership skill: conclusions and future directions,' *Leadership Quarterly*, 11(1), 155–70.

Qureshi, H., Patmore, C., Nicholas, E. and Bamford, C. (1998) *Overview: Outcomes of social care for older people and carers, Outcomes in Community Care Practice No. 5.* York: Social Policy Research Unit, University of York.

Qureshi, H., Bamford, C., Nicholas, E., Patmore, C. and Harris, J. (2000) *Outcomes in Social Care Practice: Developing an outcome focus in care management and user surveys.* York: Social Policy Research Unit, University of York.

www.carers.org/sites/default/files/care_act_briefing_june_2014.pdf

http://www.scie.org.uk/care-act-2014/assessment-and-eligibility/strengths-based-approach/care-act-video-eligibility-approach.asp

Useful resources and further reading

Department of Health (2010) *New Horizons: Confident communities, brighter futures: a framework for developing wellbeing*. London: HMSO http://webarchive.nationalarchives.gov.uk/+/www.dh.gov.uk/en/Healthcare/Mentalhealth/NewHorizons/index.htm

DOH (2014) *Care and Support Statutory Guidance; Issued under the Care Act 2014*. Crown Publishing.

Ewles, L. and Simnett, I. (1999) *Promoting Health: A practical guide to health education* (4e). Edinburgh: Harcourt.

Northouse, P. (2010) *Leadership Theory and Practice* (5e). Thousand Oaks, CA: Sage.

Tilmouth, T., Davies-Ward, E. and Williams, B. (2011) *Foundation Studies in Health and Social Care*. London: Hodder & Stoughton.

Websites relevant to your understanding of ACs 3.3, 3.4 and 4.4:

National policies on learning disabilities

Equal Lives (Northern Ireland) https://equallives.org.uk/

Fulfilling the Promises (Wales) www.wales.gov.uk

The Same as You (Scotland) www.scotland.gov.uk

Valuing People (England) https://www.gov.uk/government/publications/valuing-people-a-new-strategy-for-learning-disability-for-the-21st-century

Law on consent to treatment

Office of the Public Guardian: Mental Capacity Act (2005) www.publicguardian.gov.uk

Northern Ireland: Guidance on Consent to Treatment (2003) www.dhsspsni.gov.uk

Scottish Executive: Adults with Incapacity Act (2000) www.scotland.gov.uk

Unit P1

Safeguarding and protection of vulnerable adults

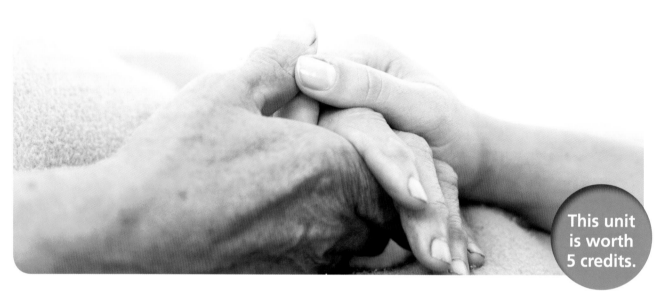

This unit is worth 5 credits.

The purpose of this unit is to enable you to engage with issues related to the protection and safeguarding of vulnerable adults and to manage staff to enable them to have a greater understanding of this area of work. The unit will introduce you to the legal framework and the best practice with respect to handling situations where abuse may be suspected as well as systems and processes that safeguard vulnerable adults. One of the key steps in safeguarding is to work in partnership with other organisations in order to achieve the best possible outcomes and this unit will help you to address this area of your work.

Learning outcomes

By the end of this unit you will:

1 Understand the legislation, regulations and policies that underpin the protection of vulnerable adults.
2 Be able to lead service provision that protects vulnerable adults.
3 Be able to manage inter-agency, joint or integrated working in order to protect vulnerable adults.
4 Be able to monitor and evaluate the systems, processes and practice that safeguard vulnerable adults.

LO1 Understand the legislation, regulations and policies that underpin the protection of vulnerable adults

AC 1.1 Analyse the differences between the concept of safeguarding and the concept of protection in relation to vulnerable adults

Key term

Safeguarding, according to the CQC, means 'protecting people's health, well-being and human rights, and enabling them to live free from harm, abuse and neglect. It is fundamental to high-quality health and social care'.

Safeguarding and protection, while often used synonymously, are different concepts and since the introduction of the personalisation agenda perceptions have changed. The main difference between the two concepts is that protection implies decisions are made by care professionals rather than allowing individuals to safeguard themselves and make choices as to the risks they take. If the service user has the capacity to make decisions about their care, then they should be enabled to safeguard themselves and to make calculated risks if they choose to do so.

A vulnerable adult is defined as an individual aged 18 or over who depends on others for assistance with respect to the performance of basic functions or who has a severe impairment in the ability to communicate and therefore a reduced ability to protect themselves from assault, abuse or neglect. But there is a debate about the differences in definitions which seem to surround this subject.

The Department of Health's definition of vulnerable adults refers to persons who:

'may be in need of community care services by reason of mental or other disability, age or illness; and who is or may be unable to care for him or herself, or unable to protect him or herself against significant harm or exploitation.'

DOH (2000), pp. 8–9

In practice

1.1 Safeguarding, protection and vulnerable adults

Discuss with your staff the concepts of safeguarding, protection and what constitutes a vulnerable adult. What is their understanding about the term?

This definition does seem to identify groups of people such as the elderly as being vulnerable and we may find this unacceptable. It is, after all, the situation in which the person finds themselves that makes them vulnerable, not the actual individual, necessarily. There are many elderly people who would be most upset to be termed vulnerable just by virtue of the fact that they happen to be aged over 65, for instance.

CSCI, in its 2008 document *Raising Voices: Views on safeguarding adults*, further addressed the definition debate, going as far as commenting that such a lack of clarity with respect to the terms used also led to confusion over the roles and responsibilities of care workers responding to concerns (McKibbin et al., 2008).

There does not seem to be a commonly accepted definition for 'safeguarding adults' and as such, your own policies need to clarify the terms for your staff in order to ensure that a shared understanding is at least possible for your workplace.

AC 1.2, 1.3 Evaluate the impact of policy developments on approaches to safeguarding vulnerable adults in own service setting and explain the legislative framework for safeguarding vulnerable adults

Legislative framework
Our work in the care system is governed by the legal system and you will be familiar with the laws under which we work.

The Care Act 2014
With the passing of the Care Act 2014, adult safeguarding became an important part of public services, with the key responsibility put on local authorities in partnership with the police and the NHS.

This was a major move to put adult safeguarding into a legal framework.

Under the Care Act 2014 LAs are responsible for:

- setting up local Safeguarding Adults Boards (SABs), with core membership from the local authority, the police and the NHS Clinical Commissioning Groups and other relevant bodies
- arranging independent advocates to represent and support adults who are the subject of a safeguarding enquiry or Safeguarding Adult Review (SAR)
- following up any concerns about actual or suspected adult abuse.

The key message of the new legislation highlights six principles of safeguarding:

- **Empowerment** – the key here is the emphasis on person-led decisions and informed consent.
- **Prevention** – taking action before harm occurs.
- **Proportionality** – the need to risk assess and apply proportionate and least intrusive responses.
- **Protection** – support and advocacy for those with the greatest needs.
- **Partnerships** – to seek local solutions through services working with their communities.
- **Accountability** – accountability and transparency in delivering safeguarding.

In line with the personalisation agenda this law advocates a person-centred approach and a move away from the process-led care. In addition, there is a recognition of the key role of carers in relation to safeguarding.

The whole concept of partnership working in order to achieve safety for vulnerable adults is very much the highlight of this act recognising that safeguarding people requires joint working with police, NHS and other key organisations as well as awareness of the wider public. The statutory guidance also introduces Designated Adult Safeguarding Managers (DASMs) in organisations concerned with adult safeguarding.

Historically, the laws provided guidance as to the rights and requirements for service provision, but there was limited mention of protection until the Care Standards Act was published in 2000, which led to the development of the National Minimum Standards. This Act set out the Protection of Vulnerable Adults (POVA) scheme, which was then implemented on a phased basis from 26 July 2004.

Other acts you may be aware of and which are relevant to protection and safeguarding include:

- National Assistance Act 1948
- Theft Act 1978
- Mental Health Act 1983
- Mental Health Bill 2004
- Mental Capacity Act 2005 (see unit 10 for more information. Section 44 highlights abuse/ill treatment and neglect)
- Chronically Sick and Disabled Persons Act 1986
- Disability Discrimination Act 1995
- Public Interest Disclosure Act 1998
- NHS Community Care Act 1990
- Criminal Justice Act 2003
- Sexual Offences Act 2003
- Safeguarding Adults 2005 in which the term safeguarding was introduced, allowing individuals to take more control of risks and choices.
- Safeguarding Vulnerable Groups Act 2006
- Fraud Act 2006
- Adult Support and Protection Act (Scotland) 2007
- Deprivation of Liberty Safeguards 2008
- Equality Act 2010
- Law Commission Review of Adult Social Care (2011), which sought to promote the well-being of the individual and focus on their needs rather than those of the local authority or service provider and was accepted in 2012 by government
- Statement of Government Principles on Adult Safeguarding 2011 and the introduction of the six principles of empowerment, protection, prevention, proportionality, partnership and accountability, which are now enshrined in the Care Act 2014.

These laws have developed over a number of years and came about as a response to cases of concern being highlighted in the media.

> **Research it**
>
> **1.3** Legislation
>
> Research the various pieces of legislation. How do they affect your role in your setting?

The Human Rights Act 1998

This aimed to protect adults from abuse and if we have a role in the public sector, we have responsibility to comply with this Act.

Health and Social Care Act 2012

This introduced the role of the Care Quality Commission, set up to ensure the Essential Quality Standards were being implemented and regulated. Safeguarding and protection of individuals are specifically mentioned in these laws to address concerns about abuse.

Policy documents

Our Health, Our Care, Our Say (2006) and Putting People First (2007)

In January 2006 the White Paper 'Our Health, Our Care, Our Say' set a new direction for the whole health and social care system. With a radical move in the way services were delivered, there was a keen effort to ensure that a more personalised service was available, giving people a stronger voice to enable them to become the major drivers of service improvement.

In 2007 this was taken a step further with the Putting People First: A Shared Vision and Commitment to the Transformation of Adult Social Care document. Recognising that the key elements of a reformed adult social care system in the UK had been outlined in several papers since 2000, this paper intended to set out a care system that addressed the demographic changes presented by an ageing population who would depend on long-term care way into the future. In implementing the guidance, targets for 2011 were set for local councils to provide a wide range of personalised services to improve the lives of people who need care and support at all levels. You would be correct in observing that the idea of individualised care is nothing new, but the 'Putting People First' paper represented a shift in culture, responding in a more radical way to the changing demands of an ageing society.

The 'personalisation agenda' outlined in the paper supported this shift by recognising the need to view people as unique individuals rather than group them together and define them as a 'vulnerable client group'. The impact of these policies has therefore been to fully implement the personalisation agenda to ensure that individualised care and choice became a major step to more positive outcomes for service users.

No Secrets and In Safe Hands

No Secrets (2000) was a government publication introduced as a response to the ever increasing media coverage of adult abuse. The guidance ensured that local authorities were responsible for coordinating the development of policy to protect the vulnerable individual through multi-agency working and setting up Safeguarding Adults Boards and Vulnerable Adults Safeguarding policies and procedures, all of which have now been enshrined in the Care Act 2014.

The Welsh assembly also published its guidance, In Safe Hands, Implementing Adult Protection Procedures in Wales (July 2000), as a response to the Welsh White Paper Building for the Future (1999), which identified the protection and promotion of the welfare of vulnerable adults as a priority and reinforcing the Welsh Assembly's respect for human rights and the provisions of the Human Rights Act 1998. The Safeguarding Adults 2005 developed the 'No Secrets' agenda further.

The Care Standards Act of the same year (2000) set out the Protection of Vulnerable Adults (POVA) scheme, which was rolled out on a phased basis and fully implemented by 2004. These policies support wholeheartedly the protection of vulnerable adults and have had an impact on the way abuse is to be dealt with.

Vetting and Barring Scheme/Independent Safeguarding Authority from the Safeguarding Vulnerable Groups Act (2006) and DBS

Changes to the reporting system by way of the Vetting and Barring Scheme ('the Scheme') were introduced following the publication of the Bichard Inquiry (2004), which recommended a new scheme under which everyone working with children or vulnerable adults should be checked and registered. The Bichard Inquiry was commissioned following the well-publicised murders of Holly Wells and Jessica Chapman and revelations that certain checks had been missed.

Criminal Records Bureau and the Vetting and Barring Scheme

It was the POVA scheme set out in the Care Standards Act 2000 and implemented in 2004 that went further to protect those in care from abuse by care providers. Central to the POVA scheme is the POVA list of care workers who have harmed vulnerable adults in their care. In appointing people to care work, it became a legal requirement from July 2004 to undertake checks through the Standard or Enhanced Disclosure application process from the Criminal Records Bureau (CRB).

Recognising the need for a single agency to vet and register individuals who want to work or volunteer with vulnerable people, the Independent Safeguarding Authority (ISA) was set up and the CRB was made responsible for managing the system and processing the applications for ISA registration. The inquiry led to the Safeguarding Vulnerable Groups Act 2006 ('the Act') and the Safeguarding Vulnerable Groups Order (Northern Ireland) 2007 ('the Order'), which set up the scheme.

Whilst these policies have been instrumental in ensuring that all people working with children and vulnerable adults undergo strict checks if they are to work with these groups it has been criticised for being expensive to undertake and time consuming leading to adverse impact on the voluntary sector. It has led in some cases to potential staff in these sectors deciding not to volunteer as the checks required are too onerous and costly to undertake.

The Disclosure and Barring Service replaced the Criminal Records Bureau (CRB) and Independent Safeguarding Authority (ISA). The DBS helps employers make safer decisions regarding recruitment and prevent unsuitable people from working with vulnerable groups, including children. It acts as a central access point for criminal records checks for all those applying to work with children and young people.

Local Safeguarding Adults Boards

Local Safeguarding Adults Boards are in place to safeguard adults with care and support needs by ensuring that local safeguarding arrangements are in place and that the safeguarding practice offered is person-centred and outcome-focused. They are a collaborative group comprised of various agencies led by social services.

Other useful policy documents
Modernising Social Services

The government's White Paper *Modernising Social Services*, published at the end of 1998, sought to provide better protection for individuals needing care and support, but it was with the express intention of addressing the need for greater protection for victims and witnesses of abuse that the government actively implemented the measures proposed in *Speaking Up for Justice*, a report on the treatment of vulnerable or intimidated witnesses in the criminal justice system.

Valuing People: A new strategy for learning disability in the 21st century

This was published in 2001 and was a landmark White Paper for people with learning disabilities. It set out ways in which services would be improved, highlighting four main principles: civil rights, independence, choice and inclusion.

Quality of care for vulnerable adults was set to improve in a marked way because of these new initiatives, not least because of the changes to staff training, quality controls and the response by professional bodies to address codes of practice to bring them into line with National Minimum Standards.

> **Key term**
>
> **White Paper** is a government report which highlights information or proposals on an issue and then asks for comment.

> **In practice**
>
> **1.2, 1.3 Impact of policy documents and legislation**
>
> All of the above legislation and guidelines changed the way in which care was being delivered, recognising the real threat of abuse and its impact.
>
> Evaluate the impact of the legislation and policies on your work in the care setting and how it affects the standards by which you work.

AC 1.4 Evaluate how serious case reviews or inquiries have influenced quality assurance, regulation and inspection relating to the safeguarding of vulnerable adults

In May 2011 the BBC *Panorama* programme aired a documentary showing shocking undercover footage of abuse and humiliation carried out by a team of carers at the Winterbourne View Hospital. As a result of this programme, a serious case review was undertaken, leading to 11 employees being charged and the closure of Winterbourne View, as well as criticism of the CQC for its failure to act when complaints had been made. Lessons learned from this serious breach of human rights led to a review of management structures by the providers of the care at Winterbourne as well as the launch of a new strategy for quality.

Orchid View was a nursing home registered as a care home with nursing for up to 87 people in the categories of old age and dementia. Opened in November 2009, it closed in October 2011 following revelations of a number of safeguarding alerts and investigations and possible criminal offences. In October 2013 an inquest found that five people had 'died from natural causes attributed to neglect' and that several other people 'died as a result of natural causes' with 'insufficient evidence before me to show that this suboptimal care was directly causative' of their deaths. ... This suboptimal care caused distress, poor care and discomfort to residents and the families of people who were not the subject of the Inquest' (Orchid View Serious Case Review, June 2014).

These two cases highlight the need for quality assurance, regulation and inspection procedures

to be in place and monitored to ensure that safeguarding is foremost in our care giving.

Efforts to address such abuse has been ongoing for a number of years. The House of Commons Report of 2003–2004 on elder abuse highlighted the plight of the elderly and other vulnerable groups with respect to addressing issues of abuse. Abuse occurring in institutional settings and in the home by care staff, relatives and friends, (in the form of sexual and financial abuse, abuse of medication to control and sedate, physical abuse, neglect and behaviour designed to degrade and humiliate), was fast becoming known through media coverage and reporting as a result of the changes brought about by the No Secrets document.

The Francis Report (2010) also highlighted the experiences of the patients at the Mid Staffordshire NHS Trust and recommendations for change were made.

These reviews highlight shortcomings in the management in the setting and also the training of staff. As a manager you may find that you are expected to run a service with smaller budgets and perhaps fewer staff and this is where there is potential for good practice to suffer. Your role, then, is to be vigilant and to challenge poor practice before it results in abuse or neglect.

Key term

Serious case review takes place after a person is seriously injured or dies, particularly if abuse or neglect is thought to have been a causative factor. It looks at what we might learn from the occurrence in order to help prevent similar incidents from happening in the future.

In practice

1.4 Influence of serious case reviews or inquiries

Without doubt the serious cases reported in various research have moved government and health care organisations to address the issues relating to the vulnerable person in care.

You can read the Francis Report 2010 at http://webarchive.nationalarchives. gov.uk/20150407084003/http://www. midstaffspublicinquiry.com/report.

Write 500 words for your portfolio on how this report has influenced quality assurance, regulation and inspection relating to the safeguarding of vulnerable adults and how you have addressed these aspects in your care setting.

AC 1.5 Explain the protocols and referral procedures when harm or abuse is alleged or suspected

Abuse may consist of a single or repeated act and may be physical, verbal, sexual, psychological, or an act of neglect or an omission to act. If a vulnerable person is persuaded to enter into a financial or sexual transaction to which he or she has not consented, or cannot consent, this is also abuse.

The *Action on Elder Abuse* (2006) document defines abuse as:

> *'a single or repeated act or lack of appropriate action, occurring within any relationship where there is an expectation of trust, which causes distress and harm to an older person.'*

Protocols and referral procedures

The protocols and procedures for reporting abuse will already be part of your role and will be set out in policy and for which you will already have undergone training.

Table 9.1 has been compiled from Standards 6, 7, 8 and 9 of the Safeguarding Adults (2005) document.

> **Key term**
>
> **Abuse** is defined in *No Secrets* as 'a violation of an individual's human or civil rights by any other person or persons'.

Table 9.1 Guidelines from the Safeguarding Adults document

Action	Time frame
Alert Report concerns of abuse or neglect which are received or noticed within a partner organisation. Any immediate protection needs should be addressed. Ensure the individual is safe. Seek medical attention if needed.	**Alert** Immediate action to safeguard anyone at immediate risk.
Referral Ensure other agencies are given information and made aware of the concern.	**Referral** Within the same working day.
Decision Deciding whether the 'Safeguarding Adults' procedures are appropriate to address the concern.	**Decision** By the end of the working day following the one on which the safeguarding referral was made.
Safeguarding assessment strategy Formulate a multi-agency plan for assessing the risk and address any immediate protection needs.	**Safeguarding assessment strategy** Within five working days.
Safeguarding assessment Coordinate the collection of the information about abuse or neglect that has occurred or might occur. This may include an investigation, e.g. a criminal or disciplinary investigation.	**Safeguarding assessment** Within four weeks of the safeguarding referral.
Safeguarding plan Coordinate a multi-agency response to the risk of abuse that has been identified.	**Safeguarding plan** Within four weeks of the safeguarding assessment being completed.
Review Review the plan.	**Review** Within six months for first review and thereafter yearly.

Reflect on it

1.5 Protocols and referral procedures

Think about the protocols and referral procedures when harm or abuse is alleged or suspected in your own work setting and write an account of how you would deal with a suspected case.

In practice

1.5 Protocols and referral procedures

In your own setting, what are the protocols and referral procedures you follow when harm or abuse is alleged or suspected?

In answering the above, you may have highlighted the safeguarding policy you have in place, together with the complaints procedure. In both cases these protocols need to be accessible and publicised to enable individuals ease of use. If anyone, care worker or client, suspects abuse, they should be encouraged to use the protocols.

The standard in the *Safeguarding Adults* document also recommends:

- the appointment of safeguarding managers who receive specific training and support for the role
- that the worker who first becomes aware of concerns of abuse or neglect needs to ensure that emergency assistance, where required, is summoned immediately
- that if there is evidence of criminal activity, the police are contacted
- any information given directly by the adult concerned is listened to and recorded carefully, but the person is not questioned at this stage. Such questioning may create unnecessary stress and can also risk the contamination of evidence.

A referral to the multi-agency 'safeguarding adults' process should be made, along with a record of the abuse, with the person making the report stating their name clearly, and signing and dating it. Local authorities should be informed of any decisions made. You should also ensure that the person who is suspected of causing the abuse is kept away from the individual who has been harmed or allegedly harmed.

It is your responsibility to ensure that your staff are clear about how the reporting of such instances is to be undertaken and who needs to be informed in such cases. A clear line of responsibility and procedures should be in place and staff need to be trained in these protocols.

Confidentiality and consent

Confidentiality needs to be assured for all parties involved, and all complaints need to be taken seriously. The following checklist will be of help:

- Is everybody in your organisation aware of the existence of the policy?
- Is it located in an easily accessible place?
- Is it clearly written and available in other languages or other formats if necessary?
- Does it describe what will happen and the responses the person may expect?

If the adult who is experienceing the abuse is deemed mentally capable, they are asked to give consent to being referred to other agencies and a clear and concise report is compiled before any further action is taken.

LO2 Be able to lead service provision that protects vulnerable adults

AC 2.1 Promote service provision that supports vulnerable adults to assess risks and make informed choices

Underpinning all service provision should be the recognition of human rights as laid out in the Human Rights Act, particularly in relation to Article 2, 'the Right to Life', Article 3, 'Freedom from Torture' (including humiliating and degrading treatment), and Article 8, 'Right to Family Life'. These rights mean that a person is afforded the opportunity to make choices according to their needs.

The personalisation agenda has brought into sharp focus risk management and this has an impact on your care provision. Your workplace should have in place a comprehensive risk assessment strategy which identifies risks relating to the workings of the organisation, how it provides its services, together with its delivery of

2.1 Supporting vulnerable adults to assess risk

Obtain and read a copy of your organisation's risk assessment and safeguarding procedure.

How do you ensure you promote a service that supports vulnerable adults to assess risk and make informed choices?

individual activities and any strategy associated with its guardianship responsibility. See unit M1 for more information on risk.

Together with the policies on risk management on-going discussions and assessment of the service users in your care will inform you as to how they like to be supported in their decisions and how they can make informed decisions where they are fully aware of the consequences.

AC 2.2 Provide information to others on: indicators of abuse, measures that can be taken to avoid abuse taking place, steps that need to be taken in the case of suspected or alleged abuse

Indicators of abuse

Abuse is about the misuse of power and control that one person has over another which results in harm to be caused, together with the impact of the harm (or risk of harm) on the individual.

According to the SCIE, Adult Safeguarding Resource, abuse can be:

- physical
- emotional
- sexual
- neglect and acts of omission
- financial

Key term

Indicator is anything that might lead us to suspect that something may be wrong with a person. Signs and symptoms (which may vary) may be the obvious indicators, although they may not always mean abuse has occurred.

- discriminatory
- institutional.

Source: www.scie.org.uk/publications/elearning/adultsafeguarding/resource/2_study_area_3_4.html

Additionally we might include such things as domestic abuse, enforced marriage and prostitution as forms of abuse.

The NHS 'Choices: Your health, Your Choices' website clearly details indicators of abuse in vulnerable adults while recognising that it is not always easy to spot the symptoms. Reporting abuse is no easy thing to do and due to embarrassment or fear, a vulnerable person may not wish to speak out. They may make excuses for why they have bruises or why they are always short of money. As the NHS website shows, waiting for the person to share their concerns with you may only delay matters and allow the abuse to continue.

There are, of course, behavioural signs to consider and these include:

- becoming quiet and withdrawn
- being aggressive or angry for no obvious reason
- looking unkempt, dirty or thinner than usual
- sudden changes in their normal character, such as appearing helpless, depressed or tearful
- physical signs of abuse, such as bruises, wounds, fractures and other untreated injuries
- the same injuries happening more than once
- not wanting to be left on their own or alone with particular people
- being unusually light-hearted and insisting there's nothing wrong.

Source: www.nhs.uk/CarersDirect/guide/vulnerable-people/Pages/vulnerable-adults.aspx

Also, changes in the individual's financial circumstances which result in debts arising or financial documents going missing should alert the care worker to something being amiss. We need to ensure that information about how to recognise signs of abuse is made available to staff, carers and family.

Measures that can be taken to avoid abuse taking place

It is a difficult task to take care of a vulnerable adult where there is a variety of needs and this increases the risk of abuse, both intended and unintended. By being aware of the situation and the needs of the vulnerable adult, the care professional can be forewarned as to the risk factors.

The responsibilities and demands of care giving can be extremely stressful, leading to mental and physical health problems in the person undertaking the care role. Among carers, significant risk factors for abuse of vulnerable adults to occur might include the carer displaying the following:

- inability to cope with the stress of the situation
- depression
- lack of support from others within the family or in a care organisation
- substance abuse.

Family and carers who can feel isolated in looking after vulnerable adults may be offered support in the form of financial help and physical help from professional carers coming into the home and these can be measures that can be put into place to prevent the potential for abuse.

For staff in care settings, inadequate resources or lack of other staff for support and heavy workloads are indicators that also need to be addressed to prevent abuse. Staff should be able to voice their concerns to management about the need for additional help without fear of repercussions and steps should be taken to address these issues.

The Care Quality Commission (2007) identifies factors that can help to prevent abuse from happening:

- Operating a culture of openness and dignity. This enables the families and clients in care homes to raise any concerns they have about their care.
- Visible and clear complaints procedures. Clients must be able to understand that they

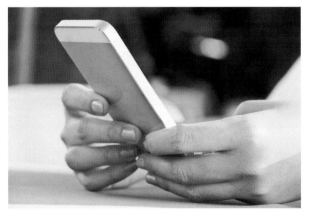

Figure 9.1 Carers may need support to cope with difficult situations

have a right to complain and that they will not be coerced or intimidated in any way.

- Roles and responsibilities of staff and managers are clear with respect to handling complaints.
- Training for all staff in adult protection and providing information about this.

Steps that need to be taken in the case of suspected or alleged abuse

Any suspicion of abuse or discovery of abuse happening must be dealt with immediately. It may also transpire that an individual approaches you or a member of your staff and tells you/them that they are being abused. Your complaints procedure may be a way in which abuse is reported and should therefore be taken seriously.

This is called 'disclosure' and you are duty-bound to believe what you are being told and act on it. If the person wants to tell you in confidence, you need to inform them that if they are at risk of harm, then you have a duty to put a stop to it and will need to inform others in order to help them. You cannot keep abuse a 'secret'. In addition, reviewing care plans and assessments may highlight issues with respect to care and may raise questions as to potential neglect and abuse.

If you are put in such a position, you will need to ensure that you:

- reassure the person
- do not take a detailed report just yet but listen and avoid questioning
- report the disclosure immediately to a senior person
- access the procedures in your workplace for dealing with suspected abuse
- write down when the report was made to you, date, who was involved, names of witnesses, what happened and the facts of the conversation
- do not discuss the incident further
- keep the report safe until it can be investigated further
- keep the individual who reported the abuse safe.

This is also covered in Unit M1.

Staff, family and others must be informed about the steps that need to be taken if abuse is suspected.

The flow chart shown in Figure 9.2 highlights the stages involved in responding to concerns about abuse.

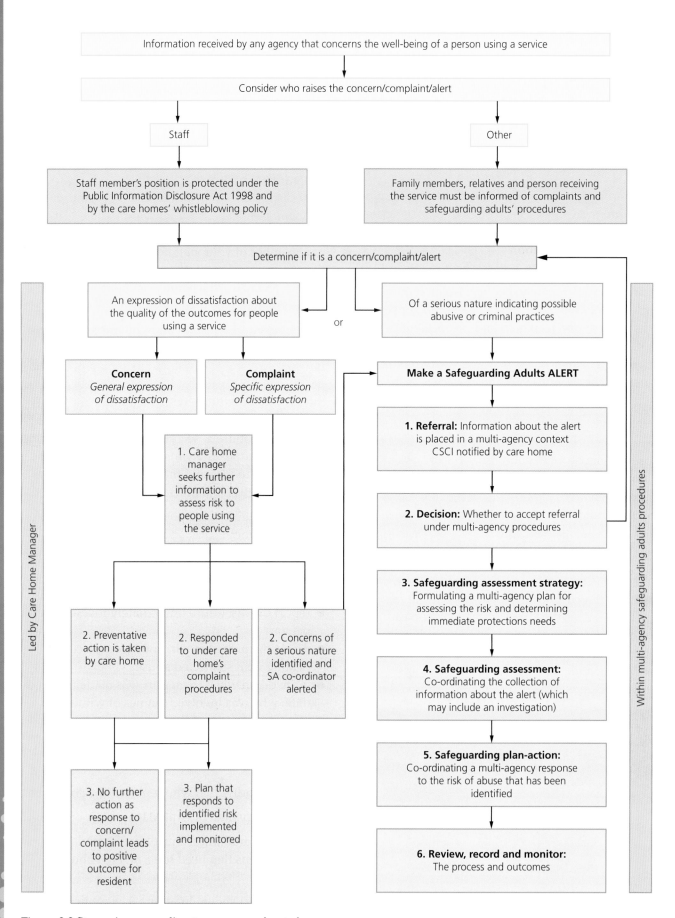

Information received by any agency that concerns the well-being of a person using a service

Consider who raises the concern/complaint/alert

Staff

Other

Staff member's position is protected under the Public Information Disclosure Act 1998 and by the care homes' whistleblowing policy

Family members, relatives and person receiving the service must be informed of complaints and safeguarding adults' procedures

Determine if it is a concern/complaint/alert

An expression of dissatisfaction about the quality of the outcomes for people using a service

or

Of a serious nature indicating possible abusive or criminal practices

Concern
General expression of dissatisfaction

Complaint
Specific expression of dissatisfaction

Make a Safeguarding Adults ALERT

1. Care home manager seeks further information to assess risk to people using the service

1. Referral: Information about the alert is placed in a multi-agency context CSCI notified by care home

2. Decision: Whether to accept referral under multi-agency procedures

2. Preventative action is taken by care home

2. Responded to under care home's complaint procedures

2. Concerns of a serious nature identified and SA co-ordinator alerted

3. Safeguarding assessment strategy: Formulating a multi-agency plan for assessing the risk and determining immediate protections needs

4. Safeguarding assessment: Co-ordinating the collection of information about the alert (which may include an investigation)

3. No further action as response to concern/complaint leads to positive outcome for resident

3. Plan that responds to identified risk implemented and monitored

5. Safeguarding plan-action: Co-ordinating a multi-agency response to the risk of abuse that has been identified

6. Review, record and monitor: The process and outcomes

Led by Care Home Manager

Within multi-agency safeguarding adults procedures

Figure 9.2 Stages in responding to concerns about abuse
(Flow chart developed by CSCI)

In practice

2.2 Providing information to others

Using your own workplace and if possible a case study, highlight how you as a manager address the cases of suspected abuse. Be sure to detail the measures that you take with your staff to avoid abuse taking place as well as the steps taken in the case of suspected or alleged abuse. How do you make sure that you provide information on all of these areas to individuals, staff and families?

Write a short piece to show your understanding about this crucial area of work.

Reflect on it

2.3 Policies in your setting

Review the policies now and reflect on how you might need to change them in light of legislation such as the Care Act 2014 or the Equality Act 2010.

AC 2.3 Identify the policies and procedures in own work setting that contribute towards safeguarding and the prevention of abuse

One of the policies your workplace will have is a risk assessment specifically for examining potential cases of abuse and a safeguarding policy. (There will also be policies for induction, training and CPD and an equal opportunities policy to ensure recruitment procedures are adhered to, for example.)

A risk assessment of this type will examine the potential causes of harm to vulnerable adults, staff, volunteers or others in your organisation with respect to the activities and services provided, as well as the interactions with and between vulnerable adults and the wider community.

In your organisation's risk assessment there should be details of the risk of harm that might be posed in different situations such as:

- threatening behaviours or intimidation
- behaviours which might result in injury, neglect or exploitation by self or others
- the use and misuse of medication
- the misuse of drugs or alcohol
- aggression and violence
- suicide or self-harm
- the type of impairment or disability of individual in your setting
- the potential for accidents, for example while out in the community or participating in a social event or activity.

Each local authority has established a multi-agency partnership to lead 'safeguarding adults' work and the set of standards outlines the multi-agency framework within which planning, implementation and monitoring of 'safeguarding adults' work should take place, including a list of suggested partner agencies. Your organisation will have a copy of that policy and as a manager you need to be aware of its contents.

AC 2.4 Monitor the implementation of policies and procedures that aim to safeguard vulnerable adults and prevent abuse from occurring

As a manager you will need to ensure that checks to monitor safeguarding are undertaken regularly to ensure best practice is being implemented. Staff must be under no illusion as to their role in completing paperwork and records correctly and any issues of concern must be reported to you as the manager.

AC 2.5 Provide feedback to others on practice that supports the protection of vulnerable adults

Feedback may be gained through a variety of means. This may include:

- staff meetings
- appraisals
- supervision.

These are also useful ways in which to share updated information and to monitor the implementation of policies and procedures. Safeguarding could be scheduled for discussion at each team meeting.

The following activity will provide you with the evidence you need for these outcomes.

2.3, 2.4, 2.5 Policies, procedures and practice

1 What policies are in place in your setting to ensure safeguarding procedures and prevention of abuse are addressed?

2 Undertake a small-scale study to audit and evaluate how these policies are being implemented and write a report to show how your own area is responding to the protection of vulnerable adults. Ensure the report is published to all staff and any recommendations being made are acted upon.

Research it

2.4 Protecting vulnerable adults

Serious case reviews show the results of abuse and neglect in substandard care provision. Carry out secondary research on protecting vulnerable adults and ensure you have a clear understanding of the terms and your role in how to lead a service devoted to this.

LO3 Be able to manage inter-agency, joint or integrated working in order to protect vulnerable adults

AC 3.1 Follow agreed protocols for working in partnership with other organisations

Multi-agency working was summarised in the *No Secrets* (2000) and also the *Safeguarding Adults* (2005) documents and resulted in local authority planning and the development of Safeguarding Adults Boards and safeguarding procedures. The statement of government policy on Safeguarding 2011 further built on these documents and highlighted principles for care.

Local Safeguarding Adults Boards are made up of the local social services authority, the police, the NHS and all groups involved in protecting at-risk adults. In order to ensure that the public are able to have a say in decision making, the boards also include members of the local community.

The Standards outlined in the Safeguarding Adults national framework specifically detail how the

partnerships should work and be set up. The onus is on the local authority to establish a multi-agency partnership to lead 'safeguarding adults' work and to include representation from all the appropriate statutory agencies such as adult social services, housing, welfare rights/benefits, education services, legal services, primary care trusts, other NHS care trusts, the Commission for Social Care Inspection, the Health Care Commission, the Strategic Health Authority and the Department for Work and Pensions.

Boundaries are in place in care work to ensure there is clarity about what your role and responsibilities are. With clear boundaries all members of staff in the partnership will be clear about where their roles begin and end.

- **Information sharing and recording information**- In partnership, there must be a safe way of sharing information and confidentiality must not be breached. Systems need to be in place to ensure that all partners are aware of how they may accomplish this. Record keeping should also be standardised where possible across the partnership so that records are consistent

- **Limits of authority**- As with boundaries, all partners must know where their authority ends and is taken up by another service.

- **Decision making** - Clarity with respect to who makes final decisions in certain areas of the service should be drawn up at the outset of the partnership.

- **Areas of responsibility** - Like boundaries each partnership member needs to be clear about what they are responsible for with respect to the care the service user requires. You will need to have an understanding of all of these.

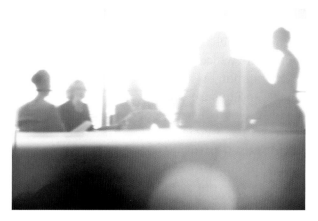

Figure 9.3 You will need to agree ways of working when working in partnership

190

Research it

3.1 Agreed protocols

Research the agreed protocols for working in your partnerships.

The established partnership then brings together an executive management team to oversee strategic development of the work in the form of a strategic/forward plan. The strategic plan includes:

- safeguarding adults policy – development and review
- safeguarding adults procedures for reporting and responding to concerns of abuse or neglect – monitoring, development and review
- equal access strategy
- information-sharing agreement – development and review
- training strategy for all staff and volunteers
- training strategy for service users and carers
- strategy to disseminate information about adult abuse and 'safeguarding adults' work to staff, volunteers, service users, carers and members of the public
- a commissioning strategy for services for people who are at risk of or have experienced abuse or neglect
- a commissioning strategy for responses to and services for perpetrators of abuse/neglect
- strategies for reducing risk of abuse and neglect across a range of settings, including care settings and the community
- review of the strategic plan and publication of an annual report.

Source: From Safeguarding Adults – A National Framework, October 2005

AC 3.2 Review the effectiveness of systems and procedures for working in partnership with other organisations

Partnerships require working with a varied number of people from different types of sectors. For example, you may find yourself working with people from the police service or housing section of the council as well as other health care professionals. The effectiveness of the work you do with these partners depends upon having shared aims and objectives and goals with all parties working together to achieve the same ends.

Reflect on it

3.2 Systems and procedures

Reflect on one aspect of the systems and procedures used within your partnership and comment upon the effectiveness of them. What have you learned about how partnerships work as a result of this?

In practice

3.1, 3.2 Working with other organisations

Obtain a copy of the protocols for working in partnership with the organisations you deal with and write a short review of how effective the systems and procedures are. You need to evaluate the performance of your own organisation and that of your partners and make an assessment of how you might improve the service for your clients.

See Unit M2c on working in partnership for more information.

Without this, breakdown in communication is likely to occur so there needs to be shared policies, procedures and, in some cases, resources that are implemented and used effectively.

LO4 Be able to monitor and evaluate the systems, processes and practice that safeguard vulnerable adults

AC 4.1 Support the participation of vulnerable adults in a review of systems and procedures

Good practice and personalisation demand that the service user is the 'central' part in the process of care and is part of the decision-making process. A review of the No Secrets document in the SCIE 'Report 47: User involvement in adult safeguarding' (2011) made a firm recommendation for the involvement of service users in strategic planning. They highlighted the notion that service users and their representatives should be seen as key partners in safeguarding and strategic planning with all views being taken into account. The review further recommended the involvement of service users in training staff and in making staff appointments. In 2001/2, the Department of Health reviewed social work education, consulting people who used such services. This review found that service users were able to state what they wanted from social workers, emphasising qualities such as empathy, respect and non-judgemental attitudes as being important. As a result, the DOH brought in a new requirement for social workers to be educated to degree level and for user and carer involvement to be integrated into the design and delivery of the degree programme (SCIE, 2011).

The Care Act of 2014 takes the process further:

'It signals a major change in practice – a move away from the process-led, tick-box culture to a **person-centered** *social work approach which achieves the outcomes that people want. Practitioners must take a flexible approach and work with the adult all the way through the enquiry and beyond where necessary.'*

Source: Page 2 Briefing: Care Act implications for safeguarding adults, SfC

One Stop contact point

An adult protection helpline has been set up, which members of the public can ring to express a concern or simply to obtain advice or information with regards to adult abuse. The helpline has a direct link to the Adult Protection Unit and is advertised in local magazines and through distribution of contact cards and leaflets.

Source: From Safeguarding Adults – A National Framework of Standards (2005)

In practice

4.1 Participation of vulnerable adults

How might you involve service users in your own setting?

Undertake the support of vulnerable adults in your care and describe the process. How could you have improved the process?

An example of good practice has been supplied in the Safeguarding Adults document (see below). Perhaps your own area has a similar example.

AC 4.2 Evaluate the effectiveness of systems and procedures to protect vulnerable adults in own service setting

We talked earlier about how the complaints process in your setting is one way of monitoring systems and you need to ensure that you are aware of others. For example, involving service users in reviewing processes can help to highlight areas of concern.

In evaluating how effective systems and procedures are you need to be collating evidence from such things as satisfaction surveys and also be able to show evidence of how you actually deal with any complaints received. At all stages of care there will be a trail of evidence which shows how effective the protection of your vulnerable service users is.

In practice

4.1, 4.2 Effectiveness of systems and procedures

How effective are the systems and procedures in your setting? Audit the complaints procedure and the staff in your area to determine whether changes need to be made.

AC 4.3 Challenge ineffective practice in the promotion of the safeguarding of vulnerable adults

Unfortunately, as managers you may come across practice that is not only ineffective but also unsafe and you will be expected to challenge this. Reporting any concerns about practice is known as 'whistle-blowing' and all staff are protected by means of the Public Interest Disclosure Act of 1998, which clearly encourages people to report poor practice without fear of reprisals should they do so.

Procedures and systems to address

When unsafe practice is uncovered you need to resort to the system you have in place to address it and you must be familiar with your organisation's safeguarding policy. It would be useful also to refer to the CSCI flow chart shown on page 188 to determine whether to deal with the issue as a:

- complaint
- concern
- alert.

A complaint or a concern, according to CSCI, is a 'general expression of dissatisfaction' and may serve as an alert to an issue of a serious nature which might indicate potential abuse.

Record accurately

Any information you have been given must be carefully recorded, using the words and phrases of the person who is disclosing the information, and recording facts only and not your opinions.

You also need to record the event as soon as possible and sign, date and give timings of what has happened.

Actions to be taken

If the situation means an allegation is made against a member of staff, then your action must be swift and you need to determine whether or not the police need to be involved and the member of staff suspended from duty. In doing so, it needs to be clear to the staff member and those who work with them that this is termed a 'neutral activity' and in no way implies guilt of any kind. It is only following an inquiry that action against staff may need to be taken using the disciplinary framework or capability procedures.

Case study

4.3 What is poor practice?

But what actually constitutes poor practice? Look at the following scenarios and then say which you think are unsafe in terms of safeguarding vulnerable adults.

1 Joan refuses to take her medication and staff have decided to mix it in with her food.
2 A member of staff has recently become an agent for a cosmetics company. She brings in the catalogue for the elderly clients and often takes orders from them.
3 The staff are very busy and often leave some of the more ill service users until the last minute. This occasionally results in having less time to complete the dressings effectively. Occasionally a wet bed is also the result of having to wait for the care staff.
4 A non-English-speaking service user is accompanied to outpatients for her regular diabetic check-ups and staff communicate through her husband. They notice bruising on her arm and comment on it, only to be told she is clumsy due to her condition.
5 Jim wants to watch the football on TV but there is a planned trip to the local shopping centre. He does not wish to go and has always said he dislikes shopping, but the staff encourage him to do so since he would not be able to stay behind.

How would you challenge the staff in each of these cases?

Although some of the above situations may seem particularly unsafe or potentially abusive, namely 3 and 4, all of the others would also require challenging. In situation 1, the hiding of medication in food is a breach of rights, and refusal to take the medication must be discussed with the client and their family to try to deal with the problem in another way.

Situation 2 puts the clients in a difficult situation and they may feel obliged to buy from the member of staff. They may believe that not doing so may jeopardise their care in some way. The last situation is a case of staff meeting their own needs and not Jim's. It will be difficult if Jim is the only person who does not wish to go shopping, but they need to respect his views and by persuading him otherwise, this is not happening.

In *all* of the situations the staff are not providing good care and should be challenged. To do this you need to make sure that you are in possession of the facts about the incident and that you can show the member of staff policy or procedure which they may be in breach of. Could it be that they are experiencing some personal issues which may be impacting upon their judgement and decision making?

Whatever it is, you can be clear about the way forward to help the situation.

In practice

4.3 Challenging ineffective practice

How would you go about challenging ineffective practice? Give an example.

AC 4.4 Recommend proposals for improvements in systems and procedures in own service setting

In recommending proposals for improvements to systems and procedures, you may for example start by taking a look at how you process complaints, what happens with the incident and accident reports and how care plans are used. You need to first of all ensure they are up to date and are useful for determining how well your safeguarding procedures are working.

In all the aforementioned activities you will have accessed the policies and procedures you use in your organisation and may have identified areas that require improvement. Complete the following activity and then say how you would address any of the issues your research has raised with respect to safeguarding vulnerable adults.

In practice

4.4 Recommending proposals for improvement

The following website has an excellent set of training film clips which might be used for staff training: www.nmc-uk.org/Nurses-and-midwives/safeguarding-film-one-an-introduction/.

Review these now and determine where you might use them to help staff to understand more fully safeguarding issues for vulnerable adults.

Report on how you might improve the safeguarding process within your own organisation and ensure these recommendations are made known to staff and management.

Research it

4.4 Systems, processes and practice

Research another setting's systems, processes and practice that safeguard vulnerable adults and compare their work to your own setting.

Reflect on it

LO3, 4.4 Joint working and recommending proposals

Reflect on the issues that have arisen with managing inter-agency, joint or integrated working in order to protect vulnerable adults.

Reflect on the issues that have arisen as a result of the above recommended proposals for improvement in systems and procedures in your own setting. (4.4)

Legislation

In this unit we have highlighted a number of laws and guidance papers with respect to safeguarding:

- National Assistance Act 1948
- Mental Health Act 1983
- Mental Health Bill 2004
- Mental Capacity Act 2005
- Chronically Sick and Disabled Persons Act 1986
- Disability Discrimination Act 1995
- NHS Community Care Act 1990
- Safeguarding Vulnerable Groups Act 2006
- Adult Support and Protection Act (Scotland) 2007
- Public Interest Disclosure Act 1998
- The Care Act 2014

Assessment Methods

LO	Assessment criteria and accompanying activities	Assessment methods *To evidence coverage of the ACs, you could:*
LO1	1.1 In practice (p. 179)	Ask your assessor to witness a discussion with your staff about the points in the activity. Or at a team meeting ask staff about their understanding of the term.
	1.3 Research it (p. 180)	Prepare a hand-out which details the various pieces of legislation and show how they affect your role in the setting.
	1.2, 1.3 In practice (p. 182)	Discuss the points in the activity with your assessor. Write a short piece which evaluates the impact of the legislation and policies as suggested in the activity.
	1.4 In practice (p. 183)	For this AC you need to understand how serious cases reported in various research have moved government and health care organisations to address the issues relating to the vulnerable person in care. You will find it useful to read the link in the activity. Write 500 words for your portfolio as suggested in the activity.
	1.5 Reflect on it (p. 185)	Discuss with the team the points in the activity. Provide a written account.
	1.5 In practice (p. 185)	Provide a written account addressing the points in the activity.
LO2	2.1 In practice (p. 186)	Complete the activity and discuss with your assessor. Provide a written account.
	2.2 In practice (p. 189)	Produce a case study or write a short piece showing how you as a manager address the cases of suspected abuse. Be sure to detail the measures that you take with your staff to avoid abuse taking place as well as the steps taken in the case of suspected or alleged abuse. You could also discuss this with your assessor.
	2.3 Reflect on it (p. 189)	Complete the activity. Provide copies of the policies for your portfolio.
	2.3, 2.4, 2.5 In practice (p. 190)	Explain to a member of your staff the points in question 1. Undertake a small-scale study and address the points in question 2.
	2.4 Research it (p. 190)	You could carry out secondary research on protecting vulnerable adults as instructed in the activity. Test your understanding of this by discussing this with staff at a team meeting. Explain to them your role in how to lead a service devoted to this. Write a report to show how your own area is responding to the protection of vulnerable adults. Ensure the report is published to all staff and any recommendations being made are acted upon.
LO3	3.1 Research it (p. 191)	Explain to your assessor the agreed protocols for working in your partnerships.
	3.2 Reflect on it (p. 191)	Write a short reflective account.
	3.1, 3.2 In practice (p. 191)	Complete the activity. You could discuss this with your assessor.

➔

LO	Assessment criteria and accompanying activities	Assessment methods *To evidence coverage of the ACs, you could:*
LO3/LO4	4.1 In practice (p. 192)	Interview a client from your setting and ask them to comment upon how they feel they could be more involved in the setting? Ask them what support vulnerable adults in your care require and describe the process How could you have improved the process?
	4.1, 4.2 In practice (p. 192)	Undertake a short survey of staff and clients to ascertain how effective the systems and procedures in your setting are. Audit the complaints procedure and the staff in your area to determine whether changes need to be made.
	4.3 Case study (p. 193)	Study the scenarios and then say which you think are unsafe in terms of safeguarding vulnerable adults. Alternatively get the staff involved and use these as a staff training exercise.
	4.3 In practice (p. 194)	Discuss with your assessor the way in which you go about challenging ineffective practice? Give an example. Produce a written account of how you would you challenge ineffective practice according to your organisation's safeguarding of vulnerable adults policy.
	4.4 In practice (p. 194)	Review the website in the activity. Write a short piece addressing the points in the activity.
	4.4 Research it (p. 194)	Undertake an observation within another setting or interview a member of staff from another setting and look at their systems, processes and practice that safeguard vulnerable adults. Draw up a table which compares their work to your own setting.
	LO3, 4.4 In practice (p. 194)	Using any documents available in your setting comment upon issues that have arisen with managing interagency, joint or integrated working in order protect vulnerable adults. Provide a reflective account.

References

Action on Elder Abuse (2006) www.elderabuse.org.uk/

ADSS (2005) *Safeguarding Adults: A National Framework of Standards for good practice and outcomes in adult protection work*. London: ADSS.

www.adass.org.uk/images/stories/Publications/Guidance/safeguarding.pdf

CSCI (2005) *Safeguarding Children: The second joint Chief Inspectors' Report on arrangements to safeguard children. A summary*. London: CSCI.

CSCI (2008) *Raising Voices: Views on safeguarding adults*. London: CSCI.

DOH (1999) *Building for the Future: A White Paper for Wales*. London: HMSO.

DOH (2001) *Valuing People: A new strategy for learning disability in the 21st century*. London: HMSO.

DOH (2006) *The White Paper Our Health, Our Care, Our Say: A new direction for community services: A brief guide*. London: HMSO.

DOH (2007) *Putting People First: A shared vision and commitment to the transformation of adult social care*. London: HMSO.

DOH (2011) *Statement of Government Principles on Adult Safeguarding*. London: HMSO.

Home Office (1989 and 2004) The Children Act 1989. London: HMSO.

Home Office (1999) Action for justice (implementing the Speaking up for justice report on vulnerable or intimidated witnesses in the criminal justice system in England and Wales). London: HO Communication Directorate.

DOH and the Home Office (2000) *No Secrets: Guidance on developing and implementing multi-agency policies and procedures to protect vulnerable adults from abuse*. London: DOH and the Home Office www.dh.gov.uk/en/Publicationsandstatistics/ Publications/PublicationsPolicyAndGuidance/ DH_4008486

House of Commons (2005) Elder Abuse – Second Report of Session 2003–04. www.publications. parliament.uk/pa/cm200304/cmselect/ cmhealth/111/111.pdf.

Lee-Treweek, G. (2008) 'Bedroom Abuse: The Hidden Work in a Nursing Home' in Johnson, J. and De Souza (eds) *Understanding Health and Social Care: A Reader*. London: Sage Publications, in association with the Open University.

SCIE (2011) Report 47: User involvement in adult safeguarding. London.

Souza, C. (eds) *Understanding Health and Social Care: An introductory reader* (2e). London: Sage.

The West Sussex Adult Safeguarding Board (WSASB) (2014) Orchid View Serious Case Review.

Law Commission (2011) Adult Social Care. London: HMSO, www.lawcom.gov.uk/reforming-the-law-for-adult-social-care/.

Legislation. Gov.Uk (2006) Safeguarding Vulnerable Adults Act www.legislation.gov.uk/ ukpga/2006/47/notes/division/2.

http://www.nhs.uk/Conditions/social-care-and-support-guide/Pages/vulnerable-people-abuse-safeguarding.aspx

Useful resources and further reading

McKibbin, J., Walton, A. and Mason, L. (2008) *Leadership and Management in Health and Social Care for NVQ/SVQ Level 4*. London: Heinemann.

Unit P3

Lead and manage group living for adults

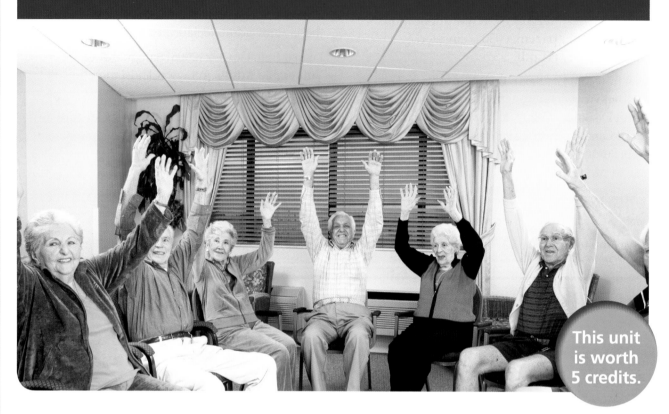

This unit is worth 5 credits.

In this unit we look at the skills and knowledge required for managing group living. Group living refers to the facilities and services provided for individuals with particular needs such as those found in residential and care homes, sheltered accommodation, rehabilitation services as well as shared community services for those with mental health and special learning needs. By undertaking the activities, you will build upon your knowledge base to enable you to lead group living environments that provide individuals with the opportunities to achieve positive outcomes.

Learning outcomes

By the end of this unit you will:

1 Be able to develop the physical group living environment to promote positive outcomes for individuals.
2 Be able to lead the planning, implementation and review of daily living activities.
3 Be able to promote positive outcomes in a group living environment.
4 Be able to manage a positive group living environment.

LO1 Be able to develop the physical group living environment to promote positive outcomes for individuals

AC 1.1 Review current theoretical approaches to group living provision for adults

The emphasis on person-centred care has seen a rise in a number of initiatives to enable people to live as independently as possible. There are, however, some groups of people who may require support of a more substantial nature and who therefore need to move into residential accommodation and group-living arrangements.

Housing and group-living provision

Today there are various options for care, not only for elderly adults but also for children and young people. From small residential homes for the elderly or young people with learning disabilities to sheltered accommodation or extra care housing, there are numerous options available now for group living. As an alternative to residential accommodation, extra care housing is becoming increasingly popular. Individuals can buy or rent accommodation which is self-contained but has the option of communal living arrangements where shared restaurant facilities offer the chance for the community to meet. There are also care facilities on hand to ensure that residents have extra help should they require it. You may be familiar with other terms used to describe the various types of housing with care for the older adult and these include 'very sheltered housing', 'enhanced sheltered housing', 'supported housing', 'integrated care', 'extra care' 'and 'assisted living'.

Theoretical approaches

A literature review by Croucher *et al.* (2006) entitled *Housing with Care for Later Life* suggests that the numerous definitions we see today reflect the way in which housing with care has developed in the UK within the past 20 years. It shows the response by housing providers to the changing needs of the tenants in their sheltered housing schemes.

Key terms

Residential accommodation is usually a care home providing housing for a group of individuals who may require care on a daily basis.

Extra care housing is a type of supported housing for older people to enable them to live independently for as long as possible with access to services that are responsive to their particular needs.

Nursing home is similar to residential care but with additional medical facilities on site.

Shared community is living in a shared house and sharing facilities but with one's own private room. Some support from care workers may be available.

More recently, health and social care professionals have become more interested in housing with care models, in order to reduce the need for residential care and to facilitate the maintenance of independence, highlighting the differences in the schemes with regard to the types of needs being met and the services that residents can access and the levels of dependency that can be accommodated (see, for example, Greenwood and Smith, 1999).

A committee chaired by Paul Burstow for Demos (2014), 'A vision for care fit for the twenty-first century' Commission on Residential Care at www.demos.co.uk, undertook a year-long investigation into the future of the housing with care sector, gathering evidence which demonstrated what good housing with care can achieve but also recognising challenges the sector faces and the need for all parties involved in social care to help overcome them.

'Assisted living', 'housing with care' and 'very sheltered housing' are all terms that have been used to describe 'extra care housing'. A paper published in 2015, 'Cost Model: Extra Care Housing' supports this view and further points out the features of this type of living as being 'self-contained homes to enable self-care and independent living' but with the addition of 'extra care'.

Hughes (2015) a contributor to the paper, pointed out that 'the key factor that differentiates extra care from sheltered housing or retirement housing is the 24-hour presence of care staff on site. Care is not brought in on a visiting basis' (www. housinglin.org.uk/_library/Resources/Housing/ Support_materials/Reports/CostModel_ECH_ April15.pdf).

Promoting independence

The primary function of any housing scheme or group living for adults is the promotion of independence, but the major difference to that of the residential care home is that residents are tenants or owners, with their own front door, living in barrier-free environments with use of assistive technologies should they require them. These are clearly meant to be an alternative to residential or institutional models of care, with the emphasis on housing rather than the care.

They do, however, share certain common features with residential care settings in that there is the provision of a meal, together with communal facilities or shared spaces, all residents are from one age group, and there is 24-hour staffing.

Your role as a manager requires you to be up to date about latest discussions surrounding group living, so knowledge of the theoretical models will improve best practice in your area.

Reflect on it

1.1 Group living provision in your setting

Reflect on the group living provision for your clients. How does it compare to what you have learned so far?

In practice

1.1 Current theoretical approaches

Compare your own setting with a sheltered housing or extra care facility setting and write a short piece showing the differences.

How does your setting differ from the one you have looked at? What are the benefits and drawbacks of both settings?

AC 1.2 Evaluate the impact of legal and regulatory requirements on the physical group living environment

Historical background

Historically, the delivery of health care in this country has had an uncomfortable journey through the years, from the terribly dehumanising regime and the institutionalisation of people who were disabled or who had mental health problems or learning disabilities, to the civil rights movement of the 1960s and 1970s when the closure of psychiatric institutions and former asylums (see Figure 10.1) became a major government issue, particularly when there were media reports of inhumane treatment in such places.

The move towards a more individualistic, consumer-led approach to social care in the 1980s and 1990s saw the Conservative government suggesting that a 'dependency culture' was in evidence.

The Disabled Persons Act (1986) brought about the movement of people out of long-term institutions, together with provision of an Independent Living Fund (ILF). In the late 1980s the concept of the 'mixed economy of care' was introduced and the 1988 Griffiths Report on Community Care advised that social services should use a variety of providers to prevent a 'monopoly' on the provision of care and support.

The 1989 *Caring for People* White Paper paved the way for community care and care management

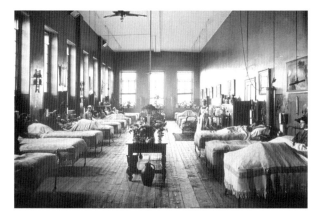

Figure 10.1 Asylums and Nightingale-style wards

in social work and this gathered momentum with the NHS and Community Care Act (1990). The emphasis was to be on providing flexible care in people's own homes so that they might live 'as normal a life as possible'.

More recently

In 2000 the Care Standards Act 2000 (CSA) was published, identifying minimum standards for care. The DOH (2010) Paper *Healthy Lives, Healthy People: Our strategy for public health in England* made recommendations about 'designing communities for active ageing and sustainability'. In this paper there is a commitment to:

> *'make active ageing the norm rather than the exception, for example, by building more Lifetime Homes, protecting green spaces and launching physical activity initiatives.'*

Recently the Care Act 2014 extended the personalisation agenda and increased the focus on well-being. The intention is to enable local authorities and partners to have a wider focus on the whole population in need of care. For people who need care and support, and their carers, there will be:

- access to information, advice, preventative services and assessment of need
- an entitlement to care and support
- a new fee model of paying for care, with a cap on the care costs for which an individual is liable
- a common system across the country (national eligibility threshold) – see 'Fact sheet: Overview of the Care Act' at https://www.gov.uk/government/publications/care-act-2014-part-1-factsheets/care-act-factsheets

This act now repeals a number of previous acts:

- National Assistance Act 1948
- Chronically Sick and Disabled Persons Act 1970
- NHS and Community Care Act 1990
- Choice of Accommodation Directions 1992
- Delayed Discharges Regulations 2003
- NHS Continuing Healthcare (Responsibilities) Directions 2009
- Charging for Residential Accommodation Guidance (CRAG) 2014
- Transforming Adult Social Care (LAC(2009)1)

In practice

1.2 Impact of legal and regulatory requirements

Show how your care setting has responded to the changes in law in the development of a person-centred group living environment by evaluating the impact of legal and regulatory requirements.

In evaluating the impact of this, you might assess the positive and negative changes that have come about as a result of the new laws and regulations.

- Fair Access to Care Services (FACS) guidance on eligibility criteria 19 Guide to the Care Act 2014 and the implications for providers
- No Secrets: Guidance to protect vulnerable adults from abuse
- DOH 2000.

The impact of the legislation and the guidance provided has been to ensure care has developed into a more humane and personalised provision.

AC 1.3 Review the balance between maintaining an environment that is safe and secure and promoting freedom and choice

Both **risk assessment** and **risk management** are an essential part of adult social care and reassure us that we are acting in the best interests of the service user. Often, though, it is difficult to balance empowerment with the duty of care we owe our clients. If individuals are to be enabled to lead independent lives, they need to be able to take the risks they choose, but this constantly needs to be weighed against the likelihood of significant harm arising from that choice.

Key terms

Well-being is a subjective state of being content and healthy.

Risk assessment is the way in which we evaluate the potential risks in an activity.

Risk management is the evaluation of risk together with the procedure to minimise or avoid the impact of that risk.

You are also bound by law as stated in Section 3(1) of the Health and Safety at Work etc. Act 1974, which clearly states:

'It shall be the duty of every employer to conduct his undertaking in such a way as to ensure, so far as is reasonably practicable, that persons not in his employment who may be affected thereby are not thereby exposed to risks to their health or safety.'

Unfortunately, this can make us risk averse and will undoubtedly lead to a lack of choice for the clients, together with a loss of control and independent living, leading to an adverse effect on care.

Care settings and housing vary in type and the risks associated with them will differ. The rights of individuals in our care can occasionally be in conflict with health and safety issues and we need to be prepared to address such occasions. While the client is clearly not imprisoned in the home, occasionally we may have concerns as to the client's safety when they are not in our care. The CSCI document *Rights, Risks and Restraints: An exploration into the use of restraint in the care of older people* (2007), although concerned mainly with how some older people have been restrained in some care settings, makes some useful points and may be worth referring to.

Balancing maintaining a safe environment with providing choice and independence

Respecting people's basic human rights to dignity, freedom and respect underpin good quality social care. People may need support in managing their care and making decisions but they have the right, whether in their own home or in a care home, to make choices about their lives and to take risks.

Our attitudes to risk are likely to be different when it comes to risking our personal safety, but as care professionals we have a duty of care to our clients and this is likely to change our attitude to risk management. We may be more careful when dealing with clients and take the view that as 'vulnerable adults' they need to be protected in some way. We may occasionally take a 'safety first approach' and focus upon what the client cannot do.

This type of approach focuses on the person's physical problems and disability and tends to ignore other needs. Treatment of this kind may lead to loss of self-esteem and denies the right to choice and an increase in independence. In this way, there is a danger that the care worker becomes more controlling of the client and person-centred approaches become less of a reality.

Risk in this instance is thought of in terms of danger, loss, threat, damage or injury and the positive benefits of risk taking are lost. A more balanced approach therefore needs to be adopted.

The Department of Health agrees with this. In its paper of 2007, Independence, Choice and Risk: A Guide to Best Practice in Supported Decision making, it makes the point that a 'safety first approach' may 'not be necessarily the best option for the person and may be detrimental to quality of life and a risk to maintaining independence'.

In Titterton's '**Positive Risk** Approach', risk is seen as positive and enhancing, and recognises the needs of individuals. It demonstrates that choice and autonomy are important and promotes the rights of vulnerable people.

Risk management is covered in Unit M1 (Chapter 4).

Key term

Positive risk taking refers to looking at the potential benefits and harm of carrying out one choice of action over another and developing a plan that reflects the positives and stated priorities of the service user. It demands a well-thought-out plan for a specific course of action.

In practice

1.3 Safety, security and freedom of choice

Undertake a review of your risk policy and write a short piece outlining how you maintain an environment that is safe and secure but still manage to promote freedom and choice.

What are your views on positive risk taking and keeping service users safe but happy with their choices?

AC 1.4, 1.5 Explain how the physical environment can promote well-being and justify proposals for providing and maintaining high quality decorations and furnishings for group living

The environment and well-being

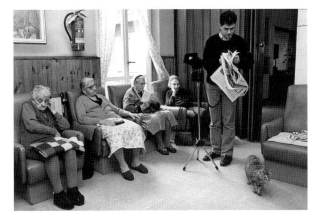

Figure 10.2 Old school: the traditional style care home set-up

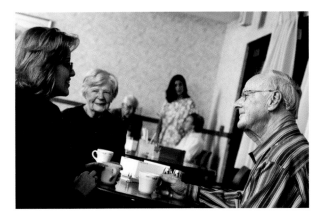

Figure 10.3 New school: a more modern approach to life in a care home

Look at Figures 10.1 and 10.2. Which setting do you prefer? There can be little doubt that the picture showing a more vibrant and modern set-up is going to enhance the quality of life of those who live there. The somewhat sterile picture of previous types of care settings we would hope is very much a place of the past. The Mind website offers the following insight:

'Good quality, affordable, safe housing is essential to our well-being. Poor housing or homelessness can contribute to mental ill health or can make an episode of mental distress more difficult to manage.

This may also be compounded by the fact that poor housing and homelessness are often linked to other forms of social exclusion, such as poverty.'

Source: www.mind.org.uk/help/social_factors/housing_and_mental_health

Although this particular quote mentions homelessness and housing, it can be applied to the care setting. A poor setting with respect to the accommodation in a care home may lead to mental distress and does little to promote independence and high self-esteem.

Design, decorations and furnishings

Judd *et al.* (1997) in their work *Design for Dementia* point out two main principles for designing care homes which can be applied to all settings, not just those dealing with dementia.

1 The design should encourage independence, confidence and raise self-esteem. It should welcome relatives and reinforce personal identity.
2 Key design features should include familiar, domestic, homely styles, with single rooms enabling the individual to bring personal belongings to their living space. Furniture and fittings should be age-appropriate and encourage residents to take part in various activities in different spaces.

With respect to the internal state of decoration and furnishings, the National Minimum Standards 19–26 are specific in their guidance (DOH, 2001). In the preamble to this set of standards, they write:

'The links between the style of home, its philosophy of care and its size, design and layout are interwoven. A home which sets out to offer family-like care is unlikely to be successful if it operates in a large building with high numbers of resident places. It would need special design features – being divided into smaller units, each with its own communal focus, for example, to measure up to its claim to offer a domestic, family-scale environment. On the other hand, someone looking for a "hotel"-style home may prefer a large home with more individual facilities than could be offered by the small family-style home.'

The text goes on to describe various differences and changes that would need to be made to the accommodation to enhance the living space for individuals with special needs.

It firmly places the onus on the home owners and proprietors to make clear which clientele their homes are aimed at and to make sure the physical environment matches their requirements. The philosophy of care is therefore an important consideration in determining how you might go about designing and decorating the home.

AC 1.6 Develop an inclusive approach to decision making about the physical environment

Decision making about the day-to-day running of the home and the general state of repair and decorations should not only be the decision of the staff but should include the residents in discussion as well. Most care establishments now run a weekly or monthly service user meeting in which such things can be discussed.

LO2 Be able to lead the planning, implementation and review of daily living activities

AC 2.1 Evaluate the impact of legislation and regulation on daily living activities

In health care we use the term 'daily living activities' to refer to daily self-care activities such as:

- personal hygiene
- dressing and undressing
- self-feeding
- mobility and transfers (getting from bed to wheelchair, or the ability to get on or off toilet, etc.)
- bowel and bladder management.

As professionals, we must assess our clients to determine their ability or inability to perform these daily living activities. By measuring in this way, we gain knowledge of the client's functional status and can determine how independent a client is. This has been impacted by law, which requires us to practise in safe and humane ways.

Legislation and regulation

Government policy and law have identified the need to assess individuals as to the care

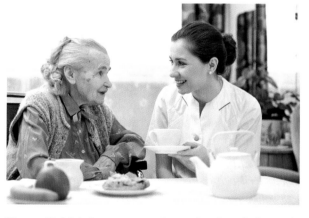

Figure 10.4 It is important to determine how independent a client is

2.1 Legislation, regulation and daily living activities

Show how legislation and regulation on daily living activities has changed your practice in the care setting over the last five years or so. How have you developed the assessment process to take into account any changes in the law?

they require. From as far back as the National Assistance Act in 1948, local authorities were required to promote the welfare of individuals with sensory, physical or mental difficulties by making an accurate assessment of their needs. This practice was further implemented in the 1986 Disabled Persons Act, the NHS and Community Care Act (1990) and the Care Standards Act (2000).

The Care Act 2014 has brought all this together and addresses local authorities' duties in relation to assessing people's needs and their eligibility for funded care and support. It also requires authorities to offer carers increased support in their roles. As a result, we are now duty and legally bound to ensure that the needs of services users and their carers are treated with the utmost importance.

AC 2.2 Support others to plan and implement daily living activities that meet individual needs and preferences

Your management role with respect to supporting others to plan and implement daily living activities requires you to ensure that you and the staff are clear about what the service user needs from you and that they are provided with well-trained staff to meet these needs. Staff may require additional training or mentoring to undertake this.

AC 2.3 Develop systems to ensure individuals are central to decisions about their daily living activities

The systems you have in place to ensure that the personalisation agenda is met in your setting need to show regard for the service users' views and their needs. Your systems must hold the service

user at the centre of the decision making if this is to work. Care planning is a good example of a system we have in place to ensure that care is individualised. The development of these puts the service users at the centre of the process.

AC 2.4 Oversee the review of daily living activities

One of your main responsibilities as a manager is to ensure that best practice for care is the main goal in your own setting and you can only know that you and your staff are achieving this if you audit the systems in place and monitor the service. This requires regular feedback from all who use or work in the service, as well as families, and other care professionals who are part of the multidisciplinary team. By eliciting their feedback about the performance of the service with respect to daily living activities and acting upon the information received, you will be able to ensure that your overseeing of the daily living activities will highlight areas for improvement to ensure the care standards remain high.

Reflect on it

2.4 Oversee review of daily activities

Write a reflective piece to show the effect of the systems you have in place and comment on the strengths and weaknesses of the whole process.

2.2, 2.3, 2.4 Daily living activities

Using a case study approach and working with a staff member, undertake the assessment of daily living activities for one client and evaluate the approach.

1 How will you support a member of staff in planning and implementing daily living activities to meet an individual's needs and preferences?
2 Show how the systems you have in place for ensuring that the client remains the central figure in the assessment process.
3 After one week, return to the client and review the process. Prepare an evaluative account of the whole process.

LO3 Be able to promote positive outcomes in a group living environment

AC 3.1, 3.2 Evaluate how group living can promote positive outcomes for individuals and review the ways in which group activities may be used to promote the achievement of individual positive outcomes

The effects of living alone

Service users that we may be caring for may be elderly. The ageing process brings with it challenges with respect to every aspect of our lives. Elderly people may find that they are unable to move as freely as they once did, or they may develop a disability which brings with it restrictions of varying types. Younger adults with a learning disability may find they require a lot more help if they are to continue to live as independently as they can. It may be that the daily living activities become increasingly stressful or difficult to undertake alone. Such difficulties bring with them the possibility of isolation. If the person is unable to move freely, they may opt to stay at home, becoming more socially isolated. The resulting loneliness can then lead to depression and helplessness. In addition, the worry about safety and being alone at home is a problem for some individuals. With limited mobility, the potential to fall is very real to some people and this can cause stress and anxiety.

There is some support from research to suggest that living alone is linked with the experience of different emotions, including anger, loneliness and depression. Russell (2011) in Distress in Context Ph.D. thesis suggested that people living alone expressed more loneliness, particularly when they suffered physical limitations making it difficult to leave the house to meet others. Spending a great deal of time alone also means social support is lost and this can lead to depression. For those who have been recently widowed and live alone for the first time in years, depression becomes a very real threat. A study by Bright *et al.* (1999) found that mutual support groups were generally just as effective as trained therapists in alleviating moderate levels of depression. Roberts *et al.* (1999) also found that individuals with serious mental health problems taking part in mutual support groups showed improved psychosocial adjustment over the course of the study.

How group living and activities can promote positive outcomes

There is little doubt that support groups for various conditions have positive outcomes for those in attendance, not only in the advice or support received but also because they can give support to others in the same position.

Group living for such individuals will thus pay dividends with respect to their health and happiness. Having an active social life and being able to take part in in-house and external activities is vital to well-being, whereas being alone for much of the time can be a recipe for depression. By enabling our service users to develop friendships and perhaps even to take part in certain duties we are engaging them in activities that develop skills that are vital for raising self-esteem and promoting well-being. This may be what brings clients to the care setting – the opportunity to make friends and the offer of facilities with a range of social and recreational activities.

We can also turn to research within the educational field to show how group activity can promote the achievement of personal outcomes. Cooperative learning theory posits the view that people working together to achieve shared goals are more successful in attaining outcomes than those who strived independently to complete the same goals. If this is indeed the case, then group activities in which there is a cooperative environment will motivate the individual within the group to succeed. Working together as a group engenders a feeling of belonging and is also a huge motivator.

Research it

3.1, 3.2 Group living and positive outcomes

Undertake a small piece of research within the care setting to determine how group living has promoted positive outcomes for your clients. Develop a questionnaire or interview the clients to evaluate how you have measured the outcomes for the client. In addition, show how group activities have been used to promote the achievement of individual positive outcomes.

In practice

3.3 Supporting individuals with relationships

What policies and procedures are in place in your care setting that show that the organisation ensures individuals are supported to maintain and develop relationships?

Write a short account of how you have helped somebody to develop good relationships within the home.

In practice

3.1, 3.2 Group living, activities and positive outcomes

1 How do you promote positive outcomes for your service users? How can group living promote positive outcomes?
2 What group activities do you encourage in your setting to promote the achievement of individual positive outcomes?

Reflect on it

3.3 Supporting individuals

Think about what support an elderly person in a group living environment might need and reflect on how your own positive outcomes could be promoted.

AC 3.3 Ensure that individuals are supported to maintain and develop relationships

Relationships are an integral part of our lives and create an interdependent state of dependence between two or more people. This sort of dependence therefore impacts on individuals and can lead to conflict if the relationship should falter at any time. From early childhood we are subject to interactions with various people and groups, and these interactions may be of an intimate nature or friendly or part of family life. We learn how to relate in different ways in relationships and also identify those with whom we do not get on and those sorts of people we like.

In your work setting, the people you care for will be interacting with staff and other clients, family, friends and visitors and will be forming attractions and likes and dislikes. As we grow older, friendship networks decrease, so encouraging the development of relationships with others will help to reduce potential feelings of isolation.

As a professional care worker, though, you need to ensure that all relationships between staff and clients within the care setting have integrity and are based on the values and attitudes that underpin best practice. By asking about the client's family or making reference to certain events and their plans for the future, you deepen the relationship; such interest shown in the client can also make you seem more human.

A research study by Hubbard *et al.* (2003) entitled 'Meaningful social interactions between older people in institutional care settings' showed the important influence of social relationships in older age on the health dimensions of the quality of life, including life satisfaction and emotional, subjective and psychological well-being.

In the literature review, the study also revealed reports that institutional care settings occasionally lack high levels of social interaction and social activity and cited the work of Bowie and Mountain (1993), Godlove *et al.* (1982); and Mattiasson and Andersson (1997). Even in care, the individual may feel isolated. Other literature showed caring relationships between residents, in addition to conflict. Reference is made to the lack of understanding about sexuality and intimate relationships in care settings (Berger, 2000), the predominate view being that:

'older people in institutional care settings are without sexual interests, identities, needs or capabilities, and that expressions of sexuality among residents ought to be repressed.'

Source: Brown (1989); Glass *et al.* (1986)

AC 3.4 Demonstrate effective approaches to resolving any conflicts and tensions in group living

Occasionally conflict may arise in a group setting. Hubbard *et al.* (2003) found that within care settings there was open hostility among residents, leading to angry exchanges and conflict. The research highlighted some of the following disagreements among service users:

- Some residents disliked one another and informed each other of this.
- The behaviour of some residents aroused anger.
- Some made threats due to annoyance of requests for toileting help.
- Some were annoyed at the sound of others' voices.
- Some showed deep hostility to the behaviour of others and subsequently labelled them as 'idiots', 'stupid', 'clowns', 'funny types', 'mental' and 'confused'.
- Some isolated themselves to reduce interaction with residents with whom they did not want to socialise.
- Other residents placed gates on their doors to prevent others from entering.

We cannot hope to get on with everybody we come into contact with and it is the same for service users. There are, however, certainly ways in which such conflict can be dealt with and we can salvage any relationships which may be under threat. Conflicts in the setting may highlight shortcomings in our policy, so we may need to look at these again. With respect to handling conflict, we have covered this in units SHC 51, M2c, LM1c, LM2c, M3 and P3 but to recap, here are the principles for dealing with conflict:

- Maintain a mutual respect.
- Keep the lines of communication open.
- Aim to gain the viewpoint of all parties involved.
- Keep an open mind.
- Be willing to compromise and negotiate.

In practice

3.4 Approaches to resolving conflicts

Prepare a flow chart to show how you would deal with resolving conflicts and tensions in group living.

LO4 Be able to manage a positive group living environment

AC 4.1 Evaluate the effects of the working schedules and patterns on a group living environment

As the manager of a care service you are responsible for ensuring that the service user receives the best possible experience in that setting and that means ensuring that the team delivering the care are well qualified and have the resources to carry out their role. The work schedule of the team is also an important aspect of this part of your role and you need to be aware of the needs of the service users at any given time in order to schedule staff with the correct experience and skills to work the shift. For example, a change in the condition of a service user may require you to assign a more experienced member of staff to their care and this may have an impact on the rest of the team work.

Working schedules such as the off-duty rota are bound to have an effect on the relationships between carer and client and the continuity of care within the environment. Carers are not at work for 24 hours a day and unless there has been careful planning with respect to care, clients may be left in a difficult position.

For continuity to exist, care must be experienced as connected and coherent. For clients and their families, the experience of continuity of care demonstrates that the care provider knows about the client's care and is familiar with everything about them, and this leads to confidence in the care others will be supplying when the key worker is off duty.

AC 4.2 Recommend changes to working schedules and patterns as a result of evaluation

Occassionally you may need to make changes to the way the team is working in order to improve the effectiveness of the service. For example, you may need to check in with staff during supervision sessions about their workloads and how they are performing. Also feedback from staff and others in the setting may reveal that

In practice

4.1, 4.2 Effects of working schedules and recommending changes

Analyse the rota system in place in your care setting and evaluate the effect this has on the continuity of care in the environment.

Collect evidence from clients and staff as to how they view the system and how it impacts on the care given and the relationships within the group living environment.

Make recommendations as to changes you wish to make, then implement those changes.

levels of staff needed on shift are insufficient to meet current service needs and require change. Evaluating what is happening at the ground level can reveal how effective the work schedules are.

AC 4.3 Develop a workforce development plan for the group living environment

The Social Care Institute for Excellence (SCIE) tells us that workforce planning is about addressing two basic premises in terms of the workforce: how many and what sort of staff. As manager you will be well aware of the need to determine what skills each staff member has and to ensure that during a span of duty you have the right people in place for the care that needs to be given.

In developing your **workforce development plan**, you will need to:

● analyse your current workforce and identify the skills mix required in your setting to deliver the sort of service you provide
● ensure staff receive any training that is required to meet service user needs.

It is not only about your current provision, though. You need to be aware that changes in the future to

Key term

Workforce planning is the process whereby the staff with the necessary skills are allocated to the task when they are needed in order to deliver organisational objectives.

the type of service user or the number of service users coming to your setting will need to be considered so that your plan can highlight gaps to be filled.

When the Care Standards Act 2000 came into force, a lot of care homes failed to plan for the training of staff and this resulted in a number of homes being closed due to the lack of qualified staff as set out by the Act. As an employer of staff, you are bound by the National Minimum Standards for Care Homes to show that you make appropriate plans for your workforce.

In developing your plan, it is useful to consider the stages outlined by SCIE.

Audit of current provision

You need to have up-to-date records of all staff working in your setting, with details such as working hours, training undertaken, retirement ages and turnover. You would also do well to look at the diversity of your staff to see whether the workforce matches that of the clientele you have. If not, you may wish to plan for future campaigns to bring in more diverse staff.

The context of your service

In this section of the plan you make reference to the trends in the business: whether it is expanding or otherwise; the changing needs of service users; new regulations or legal initiatives that may change the service delivery.

Forecasting

This refers to the identification of gaps in the service that you have identified from stages one and two. You may have realised that with the growth of the elderly population in your area, not only will more staff be needed but there may be a need to recruit qualified nurses if these clients come with chronic conditions requiring nursing care.

Planning

Three areas are necessary in this part of your plan:

● recruitment and succession planning (i.e. replacing staff who leave or retire)
● career development plans for staff and retention plans
● changes to remuneration packages or benefits to staff.

In practice

4.3 Workforce development plan

Develop a workforce development plan for your setting. Start by detailing the following:

- Forecast of what is needed in the next year in terms of staff and their development.
- A clear plan of upcoming staff changes (e.g. are any staff nearing retirement or seeking promotion?).
- Budgetary forecasts.
- Number of staff and the skills and training they have.
- A copy of the strategic plan.

Implementation

In this stage, the plan needs to be integrated into the strategic plan of the organisation and should then be reviewed in line with it (adapted from SCIE).

Workforce development helps to identify current trends and forecast future workforce structures to meet service delivery requirements. The health care system is concerned with productivity and outcomes, and with changing structures in health and social care, workforce development planning is critical to maintaining a good service and achieving positive outcomes for people.

AC 4.4 Support staff to recognise professional boundaries whilst developing and maintaining positive relationships with individuals

Boundaries are the framework within which the care worker and the client relationship occurs and they ensure that the carer and the client remain in a safe situation underpinned by the law within the codes of conduct and professional frameworks in which we work. These are then translated into policy and procedure.

Staff may be unaware of the sorts of boundaries under which professional carers operate and it

Key term

Professional boundary describes the appropriate interaction between professionals and the public they serve and the policies that are in place to protect both parties.

Reflect on it

4.4 Professional boundaries

What systems do you have in place to support your staff in recognising professional boundaries?

should be part of their induction and training to ensure these boundaries are clear. Issues such as personal disclosure, the use of touch and the limits to that, and the general tone the professional relationship may take should be clear to all workers. Uppermost in our minds should always be that any relationship has to be with the best interests of the client in mind.

In order to protect the carer–client relationship, the following checklist may be useful:

- As a care professional you are obliged to maintain healthy professional boundaries and not to cross the social barrier. The professional role is one that ensures professional caring and social relationships are not confused.
- Crossing a boundary constitutes a risk to a service user and could result in abuse. We could ask ourselves: could my conduct in this instance be construed as anything less than professional?
- Romantic or sexual relationships are not allowed during the course of a professional relationship.
- In dealing with vulnerable people in care, any discomfort expressed about a relationship with a carer must be taken seriously and investigated.
- If a boundary has been crossed, then staff need to be aware that this will constitute professional misconduct and that it must be reported to protect client care.
- A professional carer must be made aware that they are not to receive personal gain of any kind at the client's expense, even if the client has expressed that they wish this to be so. They need to seek advice from you, the manager, if this happens.

AC 4.5 Use appropriate methods to raise staff awareness of the group dynamics in a group living environment

We all exhibit certain characteristics in our interactions and, in a group setting, our behaviour can help or hinder the way in which the group works. Anyone who is working in a setting where there are groups will benefit from looking at the ways in which groups operate.

A group consists of two or more people interacting in such a way that each individual influences and is influenced by another. You can see how this might affect the way in which the care setting operates. In the health and social care setting, group dynamics might be quite diverse and include relationships between individuals, relationships between members of staff, and relationships between staff and individuals as well as with those outside of the setting.

One of your aims in a group living setting is to make everyone feel comfortable and happy. It is crucial that all in the setting are involved in the activity and general day-to-day running of the environment. The levels of involvement will vary, of course, with some clients being more active and willing to participate in all activity offered, while others may be more withdrawn and reluctant to do so. There are factors that will affect participation:

● The **physical** environment – is it a comfortable physical or social space?
● The **psychological** atmosphere – is it non-threatening, i.e. are staff and other group members friendly and approachable?
● The client's **personal thoughts and preoccupations** – is there anything worrying the client and therefore preventing them from taking a more active part in group living?
● The **level of interaction** – is information provided which everyone understands?
● **Familiarity** – do clients know each other sufficiently well to feel safe and valued in the environment?

Group dynamics

The theory of group dynamics came about as a result of the work of Lewin (1951) in his research field theory and refers to the collective interactions that take place within a group. Lewin's work concerned the types of leadership he observed and the effects of 'democratic, autocratic and *laissez-faire*' methods/styles of leadership on group structure and the behaviour of group members.

The results were interesting since they expressed how groups work under such leadership.

For example, the democratic leader gained superior group results from the team as change was more easily accepted. The encouragement within this leadership style to allow all individuals to participate and therefore become an identifiable part of the group was seen to be part of that success. The more authoritarian group structures, and the rigidity of the approach, led to dysfunctional decision making, which seemed to reduce creativity. Inefficiency was noticed with the groups that had *laissez-faire* styles of leadership.

This is interesting as it appears that the type of leader we may be will undoubtedly affect the ways in which the groups we lead and manage will function. Of the three leadership styles, it is the democratic leaders who can expect a more friendly setting in which groups can function. Autocratic and *laissez-faire* leadership-style groups seem to engender feelings of discontent, hostility, scapegoating and aggression (Daniels, 2003).

We would hope in our care setting to encourage friendships to develop among the clients and for everyone to get along well, but friendships might actually affect the rest of the group. On the positive side, strong friendships mean that there is communication going on, but on the other hand, friendships may exclude others, with the development of so-called cliques and subgroups damaging the group's cohesion.

Raising staff awareness of group dynamics

In raising awareness about group dynamics, staff need to be familiar with the way in which groups are formed and how they function. One of the main areas in which groups may not get along – and this can apply to teams of professionals and your clients – is poor communication. Communication within a group deals with verbal and non-verbal communication and your staff should be aware of the explicit and the implied messages that can be seen if they pay attention to the person.

Groups are formed for various reasons. For your clients, the group they have been assigned to is not necessarily their own choice and so they will need to have some help to establish good relationships for a harmonious living environment. Being able to share experiences and gain some support and reassurance from others is a good starting point and group discussion can help this along.

When people move into the care setting, they bring much of their own experience with them and this can have a major effect on group dynamics. For example, clients bring their past experiences, with their own perceptions, attitudes and values, which can sometimes cause contention. They may also come with a particular set of expectations about the setting and how they will be living and these expectations can influence the manner in which the group develops over a period of time.

As a manager, you need to ensure staff are aware of the way in which they can help the group to work in harmony, and that they need to make a conscious effort to not only understand what is happening within the group but also be aware of how their personality may affect the status quo. For example, you may have noticed that there are some issues with the group in the setting and that not everyone wants to participate in some of the pre-arranged activities and that some show little interest. A potential cause might be that some of the clients are being intimidated by others and feel insecure simply because of stronger members in the group.

You might also notice that some of the clients are consistently ignored when they voice their opinions or try to join in activities and this may be due to others being nervous of their contribution. Perhaps their educational background is different and others feel threatened.

Staff need to be aware of the personalities of everyone in the setting in order to be able to promote a harmonious and welcoming atmosphere for all. There will be dominant personalities – those with ideas and those who take on the role of the joker or the clown, for example. You will also have people who always take the alternative view and constantly act as devil's advocate, never agreeing with the group. All these are roles that people play in groups and care professionals need to be able to handle these types of clients in a meaningful and sympathetic manner.

Appropriate methods

Through staff meetings and in individual supervision and appraisals we can raise staff awareness with respect to these things.

In practice

4.4, 4.5 Professional boundaries and group dynamics

Prepare a staff training session on group dynamics to raise their awareness of the group dynamic in your group living setting. Evaluate the preservation and check that learning has occurred.

What are the professional boundaries that exist for staff in this setting with respect to relationships with service users and group living? Prepare a staff training session on group dynamics to raise their awareness of the group dynamics in your group living setting.

Evaluate the presentation and check learning has occurred.

AC 4.6 Review the effectiveness of approaches to resource management in maintaining a positive group living environment

Budgets and financial resources

Effective businesses need business plans and as a manager you will have been asked to prepare such a document. The Department of Health requires all care establishments to have business and financial plans in place for external inspection.

You may have been asked to present financial accounts to the Care Standards Commission to demonstrate that clients' fees are being used in an effective way towards their care and that you are providing the best value in your service delivery. In order to do this, you need to be aware of how to set budgets and also monitor the expenditure of your own department. This expenditure is likely to be in relation to supplies, staffing, equipment and overhead expenses.

A budget refers to the allocation of finances for specific purposes and will form a part of your action plan for the future. If you are part of a large organisation, you will be allocated a small part of the overall financial income and will be expected to audit the expenditure you undertake and to keep within the limits of your budget for a specific length of time, usually known as the financial year. If, however, you work within a small care home and are in total control of the whole income and outgoings, then you need to ensure that the budget is carefully allocated to various areas and to avoid overspending.

Budgeting is a continuous process and to manage the process effectively requires the ability to see beyond the barriers of the yearly divisions and to project future trends with respect to the business. In preparing a budget, the expected income for the year needs to be predicted, along with the predicted expenditure for the year.

Whichever way you choose to set your budget, variations may occur – the cost of services may be far more expensive than it was last year, for instance – and you need to be aware of the potential to overspend. Accuracy is the key to managing the finances effectively.

You may also need to undertake a cost–benefit analysis, which is weighing the effectiveness of the resources and services you wish to purchase against alternatives. For example, you may have decided that the setting needs to be updated and decorated and new furniture purchased. However, if the washing machine breaks down and a new one is needed, you might have to change the plans or at least re-assess the needs with respect to the decorative update. Planning therefore needs to be on both a long-term and a short-term basis.

The flow chart in Figure 10.5 may be helpful in the planning process.

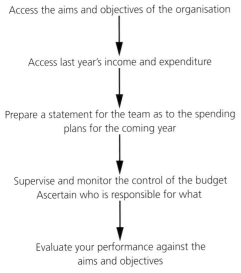

Figure 10.5 The planning process

Regular review and monitoring of the budget is essential as the amount you spend throughout the year is likely to vary. In the winter time, the expense of heating and lighting is likely to be

much more than during the summer months, so seasonal fluctuations need to be taken into account, for example. Such planning for this is called budgetary profiling and if you do not take this into account, you are likely to introduce cash flow problems, which can be most stressful. Your staff may not understand how the budget is set and why sometimes they are unable to purchase certain items or undertake activities with clients. It is important therefore to ensure that the team is aware of how the budget functions. You will need to discuss changes with your team and clarify the costs of any changes. For example, some staff may not understand why they are now being asked to finance their own university courses when in the past these costs have been met by the organisation. Clear discussions in an open and transparent manner can help to clarify this for them.

Maintaining a positive group living environment requires shrewd budgetary and resource planning. How effective it has been will depend on whether it has a positive impact upon the service users and the setting.

Legislation

The Care Act 2014 is the most up-to-date law that requires review here.

Assessment methods

LO	Assessment criteria and accompanying activities	Assessment methods *To evidence coverage of the assessment criteria, you could:*
LO1	1.1 Reflect on it (p. 200)	Write a short reflective piece addressing the points in the activity.
	1.1 In practice (p. 200)	Write a short piece showing the differences of your own setting with a sheltered housing or extra care facility setting and what the benefits and drawbacks of both settings are. Undertake an observation in a sheltered housing setting and compare it to your own. Reflect on how the group living provision for your clients differ. Alternatively interview a member of staff who has knowledge of such a setting and ask them to detail the differences.
	1.2 In practice (p. 201)	Write a short piece to Show how your own care setting has responded to the changes in law in the development of a person-centred group living environment. Or you could discuss with your assessor the differences and the changes you have made as a result of changes in law.
	1.3 In practice (p. 202)	Undertake a review of your risk policy and write a short piece addressing the points in the activity. At a team meeting ask staff what their views on positive risk taking are and how they keep service users safe but happy with their choices?
	1.4, 1.5 Research it (p. 204)	Access the link in the activity. Complete the task, and explain it to you assessor. You could give photographic evidence of the actual living arrangement in your setting to make your point.
	1.4, 1.5 In practice (p. 204)	Complete the activity. Again photographs could be used here
	1.6 In practice (p. 204)	Have a professional discussion with your assessor and manager about the points in the activity. Complete the activity. You could provide a written account, for example.
LO2	2.1 In practice (p. 205)	Prepare a staff training session, and provide a written account to document the activity.
	2.4 Reflect on it (p. 205)	Write a reflective piece.
	2.2, 2.3, 2.4 In practice (p. 205)	Complete the activity. You could discuss this with your assessor.
	3.1, 3.2 Research it (p. 207)	Undertake a small piece of research within the care setting to determine how group living has promoted positive outcomes for your clients by interviewing service users. Or you could develop a questionnaire for the clients to evaluate how you have measured the outcomes for the client. In addition, show how group activities have been used to promote the achievement of individual positive outcomes.
LO3	3.1, 3.2 In practice (p. 207)	Complete the activity. Discuss with your team. Write a report on the discussion.
	3.3 In practice (p. 207)	Complete the activity. Collect together policies and procedures. Highlight the policies and discuss with your assessor. Provide a short written account as instructed.

LO	Assessment criteria and accompanying activities	Assessment methods *To evidence coverage of the assessment criteria, you could:*
	3.3 Reflect on it (p. 207)	Prepare a checklist or a short reflective account.
	3.4 In practice (p. 208)	Prepare a flow chart as instructed.
LO4	4.1, 4.2 In practice (p. 209)	Complete the activity, provide a written account and place the documents in your portfolio.
	4.3 In practice (p. 210)	Develop a workforce development plan for your own setting.
	4.4 Reflect on it (p. 210)	Discuss this with your assessor or provide a written account.
	4.4, 4.5 In practice (p. 212)	Prepare a staff training session on group dynamics as instructed. Or you might prefer to write an essay which demonstrates your understanding of group dynamics.
	4.6 In practice (p. 213)	Complete the activity. If you are able to, obtain a copy of last year's financial activity from your manager (ensuring that this does not breach or disclose any confidential information). You could complete a case study to review the effectiveness of your approach to resource management. You could discuss this with your assessor.
	LO4 Research it (p. 213)	Complete the activity. Present a report to your manager.

References

Baker, T. (2002) *An Evaluation of an Extracare Scheme – Runnymede Court*. Estover, Plymouth: Hanover Housing Association.

Berger, J. (2000) 'Sexuality and intimacy in the nursing home: a romantic couple of mixed cognitive capacities,' *Journal of Clinical Ethics*, 11(4), 309–13.

Bowie, P. and Mountain, G. (1993) 'Using direct observation to record the behaviour of long-stay patients with dementia,' *International Journal of Geriatric Psychiatry*, 8, 857–64.

Bright, J. I., Baker, K. D. and Neimeyer, R. A. (1999) 'Professional and paraprofessional group treatments for depression: a comparison of cognitive-behavioural and mutual support interventions,' *Journal of Consulting and Clinical Psychology*, 67(4), 491–501.

Brown, L. (1989) 'Is there sexual freedom for our aging population in long-term care institutions?' *Journal of Gerontological Social Work*, 13(3/4), 75–93.

Croucher, K., Hicks, L. and Jackson, K. (2006) *Housing with Care for Later Life*. University of York: Joseph Rowntree Foundation.

Daniels, V. (2003) *Kurt Lewin Notes*. Sonoma State University.

DOH (2000) *No Secrets: Guidance on protecting vulnerable adults in care*. London: HMSO.

DOH (2001) *Care Homes for Older People. National Minimum Standards; Care Homes Regulations*. London: TSO (The Stationery Office).

DOH (2010) *Healthy Lives, Healthy People: Our strategy for public health in England*. London: HMSO.

Glass, J., Mustian, R. and Carter, L. (1986) 'Knowledge and attitudes of health-care providers toward sexuality in the institutionalized elderly,' *Educational Gerontology*, 12, 465–75.

Greenwood, C. and Smith, J. (1999) *Sharing in ExtraCare*. Staines: Hanover.

Hubbard, G., Tester, S. and Downs, M. G. (2003) 'Meaningful social interactions between older people in institutional care settings,' *Ageing*

& Society, 23, 99–114. Cambridge: Cambridge University Press.

Judd, S. Marshall, M. and Phippen, P. (1997) *Design for Dementia*. London: Hawker Publications.

Lewin, K. (1951) *Field Theory in Social Science: Selected theoretical papers*, Cartwright, D. (ed.). New York: Harper & Row.

Mattiasson, A. and Andersson, L. (1997) 'Quality of nursing home care assessed by competent nursing home patients,' *Journal of Advanced Nursing*, 26, 1117–24.

Oldman, C. (2000) *Blurring the Boundaries: A fresh look at housing and care provision for older people*. Brighton: Pavilion Publishing in association with JRF.

Roberts, L. J., Salem, D., Rappaport, J., Toro, P. A., Luke, D. A. and Seidman, E. (1999) 'Giving and receiving help: interpersonal transactions in mutual-help meetings and psychosocial adjustment of members,' *American Journal of Community Psychology*, 27(6), 841–68.

Russell, D. (2011) 'Distress in context,' Ph.D. thesis, www.psychologytoday.com/experts/david-russell-phd.

Smith, K., Hughes, D. and Porteus, J. (2015) 'AECOM. Cost Model: Extra Care Housing', www.housinglin.org.uk/_library/Resources/Housing/Support_materials/Reports/CostModel_ECH_April15.pdf.

www.mind.org.uk/help/social_factors/housing_and_mental_health.

www.scie.org.uk/workforce/Peoplemanagement/leadership/workforcedev/index.asp.

https://www.gov.uk/publications/care-act-2014-part-1-factsheets/care-act-factsheets

www.sonoma.edu/users/d/daniels/lewinnotes.html.

Useful resources and further reading

Haggerty, J. L., Reid, R. J., Freeman, G. K., Starfield, B. H., Adair, C. E. and McKendry, R. (2003) 'Continuity of care: a multi-disciplinary review,' *BMJ*, 327, 1219–21.

Unit P5

Understand safeguarding of children and young people (for those working in the adult sector)

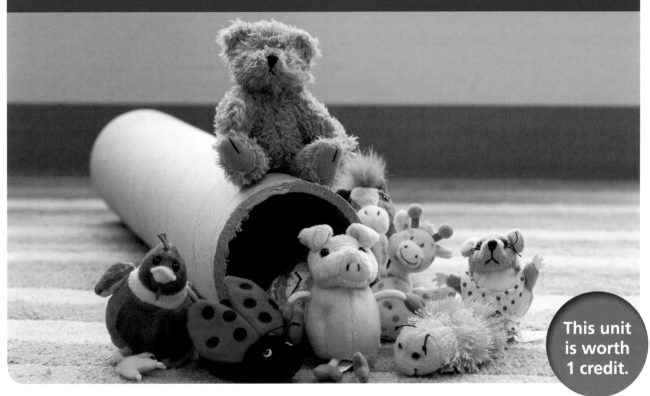

This unit is worth 1 credit.

As a health and social care professional you may not work directly with children but you will come across children, families and carers in your work and as such, you are required to have some understanding of the safeguarding protocols and procedures when working with children. In this unit you will be introduced to the policies and procedures for safe working with children and the ways in which to respond to evidence of abuse and harm in children.

Learning outcomes

By the end of this unit you will:

1 Understand the policies, procedures and practices for safe working with children and young people.
2 Understand how to respond to evidence or concerns that a child or young person has been abused or harmed.

LO1 Understand the policies, procedures and practices for safe working with children and young people

AC 1.1 Explain the policies, procedures and practices for safe working with children and young people

Legislation and policies underpinning procedures and practice

It was following the horrific murders of Jessica Chapman and Holly Wells by a school caretaker in 2002 that the issue of safeguarding children came under the spotlight once again. Prior to this event, the Children Act of 1989 and subsequently 2004 highlighted the obligations of professionals working with children to report suspected abuse. However, following some serious incidents, most notably the death of Victoria Climbié in 2000, a public inquiry was set up to address the failure of the law to uphold the protection of vulnerable children. As a result of the inquiry carried out by Lord Laming into Victoria's death, major changes in child protection policies came about.

The following legislation has changed the safeguarding agenda for children:

- The Children Act 1989 and 2004 introduced the principle of 'Paramountcy' meaning that the welfare and safety of the child must be paramount or a priority when making decisions and working with children and families. It also brought about new parental responsibilities revising physical punishment. The importance of partnership working in safeguarding children was also highlighted. The 2004 Act introduced the 'Every Child Matters' agenda and Local Safeguarding Children's Boards.

- The Every Child Matters (ECM) initiative was launched by the government in 2003 and has become one of the most far-reaching policy initiatives to be released in recent years. Covering children and young adults up to the age of 19, or 24 for those with disabilities, it led to changes in the Children Act as shown in the 2004 version and provided a detailed framework for working with children within multi-agency partnerships.

Since 2010, there has been a move away from the terminology of 'Every Child Matters'.

- The Children's Plan of 2007 set out five principles to improve the care of children in this country to provide more support for parents and families and to ensure that all children were able to succeed. Additionally, services were to be improved to be more responsive to children and not simply designed around professional boundaries. The main drive was to see that children and young people enjoyed their childhood growing up prepared for adult life (DfCSF, 2007).

- In 2009 the Department for Children, Schools and Families (DfCSF) published practice guidance on safeguarding children with. The guidance recognised that children with disabilities have additional needs but also the same human rights as non-disabled children. It called for health and education practitioners to act upon the issues that influence the safety of disabled children, especially regarding placement on child protection registers and protection plans. (https://www.gov.uk/government/publications/safeguarding-children-and-young-people-from-sexual-exploitation-supplementaryguidance)

- 'Working Together to Safeguard Children: A Guide to Inter-agency Working to Safeguard and Promote the Welfare of Children' was first published in 2010 and was revised in 2015. It details the overarching responsibility local authorities have for safeguarding and promoting the welfare of all children and young people in their area and highlights a number of statutory functions and specific duties in relation to children in need and children suffering, or likely to suffer, significant harm, regardless of where they are found. Although local authorities play a lead role, safeguarding children and protecting them from harm is everyone's responsibility. It also provides a summary of the nature and impact of child abuse and neglect, and how to operate best practice in child protection procedures. It gives details of the role of LSCBs, and the process to be followed when there are concerns about a child together with the roles and responsibilities of different agencies and practitioners.

- The Special Educational Needs and Disability Act 2001 (SENDA) established legal rights for disabled students in pre- and post-16 education, ensuring that disabled students were not discriminated against in education, training and any services provided wholly or mainly for students.

- The Children and Families Act 2014 seeks to ensure that all children and young people can succeed, no matter what their background. The law gives greater protection to vulnerable children and enables children to have better support when parents are separating. Adoption is also included, with reforms to the speed with which a child can be placed. For children in care the law gives them the choice to stay with their foster families until their 21st birthday.

- SEND Code of Practice 2014: Part 3 of The Children and Families Act includes a new Special Educational Needs and Disabilities (SEND) Code of Practice. This supercedes the Code of Practice from 2001 (but it does not replace the Special Educational Needs and Disability Act 2001). Under this code of practice, local authorities will draw up education health and care (EHC) plans for children identified as SEND. They are also required to publish a 'local offer' of services and offer a personal budget to meet the EHC plan. 0-25 year olds with SEN and SEND will have a plan covering things like education, health and social care. Two years olds who received disability living allowance will receives free early education

- The Counter Terrorism and Security Act 2015 places a duty on all schools and children's homes to prevent people being drawn into terrorism. Statutory guidance has been published stating that school leaders (including governors) must have robust safeguarding policies that identify children and young people at risk, intervening where appropriate, and a need to provide staff with training so they understand the 'Prevent Duty'. This duty places a requirement on specified authorities to 'have due regard to the need to prevent people from being drawn into terrorism.' You can find more information at http://www.legislation. gov.uk/ukdsi/2015/9780111133309/pdfs/ ukdsiod_9780111133309_en.pdf.

One of the main criticisms of the services for children in the past had been the failure of professionals to understand each other's roles or to work together in a multi-disciplinary manner. This was highlighted by the Laming Inquiry and

Key terms

The Paramountcy Principle underpins all new legislation with respect to the child. Any decision made on behalf of a child must reflect that the child's welfare is of 'paramount' concern or consideration (Children Act 2004).

Safeguarding includes well-being and encourages a preventative approach to meet the needs of children before problems occur.

Child protection forms a small part of safeguarding.

the ECM initiative sought to change this. Despite huge changes being made to the way in which professionals were to work with children and to safeguard them, the murders of Jessica Chapman and Holly Wells prompted a further inquiry. The Bichard Inquiry recommended a new scheme under which everyone working with children or vulnerable adults should be checked and registered.

Checks and vetting

The Vetting and Barring Scheme (the Scheme) focused public attention on the way that people who work with children are screened as to their suitability and led to the Safeguarding Vulnerable Groups Act 2006 and the Safeguarding Vulnerable Groups Order (Northern Ireland) 2007.

The Disclosure and Barring Service (DBS) helps employers make safer recruitment decisions and prevent unsuitable people from working with vulnerable groups, including children. It replaces List 99, the Criminal Records Bureau (CRB) and Independent Safeguarding Authority (ISA). The DBS acts as a central access point for criminal records checks for all those applying to work with children and young people. See unit P1 ACs 1.2 and 1.3 for more information on ISA, CRB and DBS. It needs to be stressed that although these systems have improved the safeguarding of children, the need for employers to have robust recruitment procedures remains paramount.

The 'Munro Review of Child Protection: Final Report; A child-centred system 2011' provided guidance to move to a child protection system that keeps a 'focus on children'. Munro called for a 'move from compliance to a learning culture' to give 'more scope to exercise professional judgment in deciding how best to help children and their families' (DfE, 2011, The Munro Review).

The statutory guidance *Working Together to Safeguard Children* (2015) replaced the former role of Local Authority Designated Officer (LADO) with the Designated Officer which is a local authority role responsible for managing and overseeing concerns relating to staff and volunteers in childcare cases. This officer is responsible for managing allegations of abuse against adults who work with children (teachers, social workers, church leaders, youth workers, etc.).

Local Safeguarding Children Boards (LSCBs) have been set up to ensure that agencies and professionals in their area promote the welfare of children. In the event of the death or serious injury of a child, a Serious Case Review is initiated to identify failings and improve future practice.

There have been cases of abuse which may have been prevented or stopped had health and social professionals and the public worked together in a more coherent way. The importance of partnership working in protecting and safeguarding children therefore cannot be over-emphasised.

Research it

1.1 Legislation and policy documents

Further policy documents you need to be aware of are *Working Together to Safeguard Children 2006* (updated in 2010) and *The Protection of Children in England: A progress report* (Laming, 2009), which continue to promote the sharing of data between those working with vulnerable children.

You will also need to have an understanding of other legislation relevant to safeguarding children. See the legislation section on page 225.

See Unit M1 on health and safety, which will also be useful in the reading of this unit.

Reflect on it

1.1 Differences between safeguarding children and adults, and mental capacity

Think about the various policies in place for children and reflect upon the similarities with safeguarding adults. How does the issue of mental capacity affect the service offered?

In practice

1.1 Policies, procedures and practice

Write short notes on the policies shown in this section to demonstrate your understanding of safe working with children and young people.

LO2 Understand how to respond to evidence or concerns that a child or young person has been abused or harmed

AC 2.1 Describe the possible signs, symptoms, indicators and behaviours that may cause concern in the context of safeguarding

Your local safeguarding board will have guidance in place which details the sorts of signs and symptoms of abuse that you need to be aware of. Another useful organisation to which you can turn for information is the NSPCC and we encourage you to look at this website now: www.nspcc.org.uk/inform. The fact sheet compiled by NSPCC Consultancy Services offers guidance for individuals who work in voluntary, community and commercial organisations and provides information on how they can recognise the signs of child abuse, so that they can alert the appropriate authorities.

Any maltreatment of a child, whether it is direct or indirect, constitutes abuse and must be remedied. Children are vulnerable to abuse from adults and other children and we should be aware of this.

Working Together to Safeguard Children (2015) is a revised version of the previous guidance from 2010 and 2013. It incorporates recent legislation or statutory guidance. It provides a definition of serious harm for the purposes of serious case reviews (see Unit P1, page 183 for definition). This includes cases where the child has sustained, as a result of abuse or neglect, a potentially life-threatening injury, a serious and/or likely long-term impairment of physical or mental health, or physical, intellectual, emotional, social or behavioural development.

Source: www.gov.uk/government/uploads/system/uploads/attachment_data/file/419595/Working_Together_to_Safeguard_Children.pdf

We can identify abuse as being:

1 Physical abuse
2 Emotional abuse
3 Sexual abuse
4 Neglect.

Signs of abuse

Physical abuse

This is any action that results in a child being hurt in a physical manner, such as hitting, shaking, burning, drowning or suffocating, and resulting in harm. The physical signs of abuse may include:

● unexplained bruising or injuries on any part of the body
● multiple bruises – on the upper arm or on the outside of the thigh
● human bite marks
● fractures
● scalds
● multiple burns with a clearly demarcated edge such as those made by cigarettes (cigarette burns).

This may include abuse by parents who fabricate a child's illness, also known as Munchhausen's Syndrome by Proxy.

Changes in behaviour that might indicate physical abuse include the following:

● fear of parents being approached
● cautious or wary of adults
● unable to play
● aggressive behaviour or temper outbursts
● flinching when approached or touched
● reluctance to get changed, for example in hot weather
● depression
● unable to concentrate
● underachieving
● withdrawn behaviour.

Emotional harm

Any action that leaves a child feeling worthless, unloved or inadequate constitutes emotional abuse. This can include not giving the child opportunities to express their views, deliberately silencing them, or 'making fun' of what they say or how they communicate. It is interesting to note what the NSPCC guidelines say about this type of abuse:

'It may feature age or developmentally inappropriate expectations being imposed on children. These may include interactions that are beyond the child's developmental capability, as well as overprotection and limitation of exploration and learning, or preventing the child participating in normal social interaction. It may involve seeing or hearing the ill-treatment of another. It may involve serious bullying (including cyber-bullying), causing children frequently to feel frightened or in danger, or the exploitation or corruption of children. Some level of emotional abuse is involved in all types of maltreatment of a child, though it may occur alone.'

Unfortunately, it is difficult to measure or recognise emotional abuse, but indications such as failure to thrive and grow or developmental issues may indicate problems. It is also the case that children who are well cared for physically may be being emotionally abused by being put down or belittled by parents or other siblings and when it affects development it is abuse. Receiving little attention or love and affection from parents or carers should also alert the care worker to abuse.

Changes in behaviour that might indicate emotional abuse include the following:

● sulking, hair twisting, rocking or behaviour which is neurotic in nature
● being unable to play or unable to relate to others of their own age
● low self-esteem and under-achievement at school
● fear of making mistakes
● speech disorders which develop suddenly
● self-harm such as cutting
● fear of parent being approached or involved in discussion
● developmental delay in terms of emotional progress
● difficulty in forming relationships.

Sexual abuse

This abuse can include forcing a child to take part in sexual activity and may also include non-contact activities, such as involving children in looking at sexual images or encouraging children to behave in sexually inappropriate ways. The child may be unaware of what is happening to them and may therefore be seeming to comply.

Female genital mutilation (FGM), although arguably a cultural practice, is still abusive in nature and would require sensitive handling. Cultural reasons cannot be used as an excuse and any concerns must be addressed, with steps taken to protect a vulnerable child.

Changes in a child's behaviour may cause you to become concerned and physical signs can also be present. Children may tell you about sexual abuse and they do this because they want it to stop. It is important that you listen to them and take them seriously.

The physical signs of sexual abuse may include:

- pain or itching in the genital region
- bruising or bleeding near the genital region
- sexually transmitted disease
- vaginal discharge or infection
- stomach pains
- discomfort when walking or sitting down
- pregnancy.

Changes in behaviour that can indicate sexual abuse include the following:

- becoming aggressive or withdrawn
- fear of being left with a specific person or group of people
- having nightmares
- trying to run away from home
- sexual knowledge which is beyond their age, or sexual drawings or use of sexual language
- bedwetting
- eating problems such as overeating or anorexia
- self-harm or mutilation, or suicide attempts
- saying they have secrets they cannot reveal
- substance or drug abuse
- suddenly having unexplained sources of money or consumer items
- not allowed to have friends (particularly in adolescence)
- acting in a sexually explicit way towards adults or other children.

Neglect

Any failure to meet a child's basic physical and/or psychological/emotional needs is termed neglect and is likely to result in the child's health or development becoming impaired. A pregnant woman who continues to abuse substances during her pregnancy may also be guilty of neglect. Leaving a child in the care of an unsuitable or inadequate carer may constitute neglect.

The physical signs of neglect may include:

- the child being constantly hungry, sometimes resorting to stealing food from other children
- constantly dirty or 'smelly'
- loss of weight, or being constantly underweight
- inappropriate clothing for the conditions, e.g. lack of coat or jumper in winter, etc.

Changes in behaviour that can indicate neglect may include:

- complaining of tiredness all the time and/or looking withdrawn and depressed
- not attending to medical needs and/or failing to attend appointments
- having few friends, being a 'loner'
- mentioning being left alone or unsupervised.

Bullying

For children, bullying can also be a problem and although we may see it as part of physical or emotional abuse, it is not included in many texts as a specific type of abuse.

Under the Children Act (2004), a bullying incident should be addressed as a child protection issue, particularly when there is 'reasonable cause to suspect that a child is suffering, or is likely to suffer, significant harm'. Bullying is deliberately hurtful behaviour and usually takes place over a prolonged period of time. The forms it takes can vary from physical (e.g. fighting, hitting, theft of money or other items), verbal (e.g. racist or homophobic remarks, name calling, threatening behaviour) and emotional (e.g. excluding an individual from the activities and social acceptance of their peer group).

Schools are now required to comply with the new Equality Duty, which was introduced as a result of the Equality Act 2010, which replaced previous anti-discrimination laws. See Unit SHC53 on equality, diversity and inclusion for more information on the Equality Act 2010, discrimination, harassment and equality of opportunity.

Although bullying is not always easy to recognise, a child who exhibits signs of depression, low self-esteem, shyness, poor academic achievement or is constantly on their own and threatens or attempts suicide should alert staff to potential harm. For parents or residential care workers dealing with children, the following may also need to be addressed:

- coming home with cuts and bruises
- torn clothes
- asking for possessions to be replaced because they have 'lost' them
- losing dinner money or reporting not having had any dinner
- falling out with previously good friends
- changes in mood and becoming bad tempered
- wanting to avoid leaving their home and being ill and not wanting to attend school
- aggression with younger brothers and sisters
- doing less well at school or failing
- sleep problems

In practice

2.1 Signs, symptoms, indicators and behaviours

Prepare a staff training session using the above information and give a PowerPoint presentation showing your understanding of the signs, symptoms, indicators and behaviours that may cause concern in the context of safeguarding of children.

Research it

2.1 Signs of abuse

Go to http://nspcc.org.uk/preventing-abuse/signs-symptoms-effects/ for more information on what constitutes abuse.

- anxiety
- becoming quiet and withdrawn.

Source: Adapted from *Working Together to Safeguard Children* (2006)

Children who are in families where domestic abuse occurs are also vulnerable.

Issues such as forced marriage and radicalisation could also fall under the banner of bullying and although it would require a sensitive approach, concerns must be addressed and investigated. Again, cultural reasons cannot be used as an excuse not to explore concerns. This was also highlighted in the Laming Report on the death of Victoria Climbié, which stated that 'there can be no excuse or justification for failing to take adequate steps to protect a vulnerable child, simply because that child's cultural background would make the necessary action somehow inappropriate'.

AC 2.2 Describe the actions to take if a child or young person alleges harm or abuse in line with policies and procedures of own setting

As we have noted in AC 2.1, recognising child abuse is not easy and it is not your responsibility to decide whether or not abuse has taken place or if a child is at significant risk of harm from someone.

But you do have a responsibility and duty of care to act in order that the appropriate agencies can investigate and take any necessary action to protect a child and this will be set out in your organisation's child protection or safeguarding procedures.

When a child makes an allegation, you need to listen to them and ensure they feel that their allegations are taken seriously, they feel reassured and that you believe what they are saying. Following the information you have been given, you will need to decide what to do next (in consultation with other professionals) and whether further investigation is needed.

The DFES guidance entitled *What To Do If You're Worried a Child is being Abused – Summary* supplies useful information on how to deal with such a situation. It highlights the following points that everyone working with children and families should familiarise themselves with:

- Follow your organisation's procedures and protocols for promoting and safeguarding the welfare of children.
- Know who to contact in your organisation to express concerns about a child's welfare.
- Remember that an allegation of child abuse or neglect may lead to a criminal investigation, so do not do anything that may jeopardise a police investigation.
- Do not ask a child leading questions or attempt to investigate the allegations of abuse.
- Ensure that you are aware of who is responsible for making referrals.
- If you are the person who makes the referral, make sure you know who to contact in the police, health, education, school and children's social care.
- Record full information about the child at first point of contact, including name(s), address(es), gender, date of birth, name(s) of person(s) with parental responsibility (for consent purposes) and primary carer(s), if different.
- Keep this information up to date.
- Record in writing all concerns, discussions about the child, the decisions that were made and the reasons for those decisions.

If you are concerned in any way that a child is in danger then you may want to take advice from the NSPCC for example. Whilst we do have concerns about protecting data and maintaining confidentiality you need to ensure that you protect the child in much the same way as you might a vulnerable adult which may mean you have to share information with others. Ensure that you follow your policy about alerting children's services.

Research it

2.2 NSPCC

Access the NSPCC website and familiarise yourself with the guidance it gives on how to deal with abuse. How would you respond to evidence or concerns that a child or young person has been abused or harmed in the light of this new learning?

You could also go to www.nice.org.uk/guidance/cg89/evidence/full-guideline-243694621 and read the NICE guidelines on what to do if you suspect maltreatment.

In practice

2.2 Actions to take

Describe the actions you would take if a child or young person alleged harm or abuse in line with the policies and procedures of your setting. Keep your notes in your portfolio.

AC 2.3 Explain the rights that children, young people and their families have in situations where harm or abuse is suspected or alleged

As we have seen from the preceding text, child abuse is a social problem and as such children need to be protected. Every child has a right to live free of physical and emotional harm, neglect and bullying.

In 1991 the United Nations Convention on the Rights of the Child 1989 was ratified in the UK and included the following rights for children:

- the right to protection from abuse
- the right to express their views
- the right to be listened to
- the right to care and services for disabled children or children living away from home
- the right to protection from any form of discrimination

- the right to receive and share information as long as that information is not damaging to others
- the right to freedom of religion, although they should also be free to examine beliefs
- the right to education.

In June 2010, the Welsh Assembly laid down the Proposed Rights of Children and Young Persons (Wales) Measure. Children are also covered by the Human Rights Act 1998, which incorporates the European Convention on Human Rights. Although children are not specifically mentioned in this Act, it is unlawful for public authorities to act in a manner that is incompatible with the rights and freedoms contained in the Act and these rights include the right to respect for private and family life. Note that there may be changes to the Human Rights Act and it will be important to keep up-to-date with the changes.

The first Children's Commissioner post was created in 2001 as a result of the Children's Commissioner for Wales Act 2001. The aim of this post is to safeguard and promote the rights and welfare of children. Other parts of the UK soon followed with the creation of further commissioners for Northern Ireland (Commissioner for Children and Young People (NI) Order 2003), Scotland (Commissioner for Children and Young People (Scotland) Act 2003) and England (sections 1–9 of the Children Act 2004).

Further rights for children are evidenced in the Education Act 2002, which includes a provision in Section 175 that requires school governing bodies, LEAs and further education institutions to make arrangements to safeguard and promote the welfare of children. In addition, the Adoption and Children Act 2002, which amended the Children Act 1989, included witnessing domestic violence as a further definition of 'harm'.

What the law has done is to give children a voice and this is made clear in the Children Act of 2004, which states that the interests of children and young people are 'paramount' in all considerations of welfare and safeguarding and that safeguarding children is everyone's responsibility. By providing legislation to improve children's lives, there is now a more integrated service delivery to ensure that children are given the services they require for health, education and safety.

Anyone who works with children and young people must recognise that the needs and rights of the child are the main focus and, as the law says, 'paramount', irrespective of what their parents think.

This can cause tension, however, and there is also a need recognise and acknowledge the needs of parents and their right to parent their child.

Where appropriate, the care worker should enable the child to exercise their rights and help them to take decisions. When working with children, you have a duty to safeguard and protect them from harm and occasionally this can mean breaking confidences by sharing information.

Reflect on it

2.3 Your policy

Check your policy on safeguarding and, if your organisation has any connection with children in care, ensure that the policy has a section detailing how you would safeguard children and young people.

In practice

2.3 Children's rights

What rights do children have where harm or abuse is suspected or alleged? Answer with reference to legislation and guidelines.

Research it

2.3 The Children Act 2004

Look at the Children Act 2004 and the guidelines for safeguarding children? How effective have we as a society been in managing to keep children safe? Use some of the serious case reviews you are aware of to inform your answer.

Case study

2.2 Actions to take

You are aware that your work placement student Meena has become withdrawn recently and quite secretive about missing a couple of shifts. This once bright girl has been losing weight and looks constantly troubled. When you sit down for a chat with her one break time she reveals that she is concerned about her mother who is constantly abusing alcohol at home and has lost her job as a result of this. As a single parent this has meant the loss of income and Meena reveals that she and her two brothers are now struggling at home and bills are piling up. She also reveals that food is scarce and that she has been taking food home to help out, for which she is sorry. She has also resorted to shop lifting.

As a manager what actions will you need to take to safeguard Meena and her two brothers?

Legislation

Numerous laws and guidance for the protection and safeguarding of children has been highlighted in this unit. These are listed below:

- United Nations Convention on the Rights of the Child 1989 (see AC 2.3 for more information)
- Health and Safety at Work Act 1974
- Fire Precautions (Workplace) Regulations 1997 (amended 1999), Regulatory Reform (Fire Safety) Order 2005
- Control of Substances Hazardous to Health Regulations (COSHH) 2002, amended 2004
- Care Standards Act 2000
- Manual Handling Operations Regulations 1992
- Reporting of Injuries, Diseases and Dangerous Occurrences Regulations (RIDDOR) 2013
- Health and Safety (First Aid) Regulations 1981
- Food Hygiene Regulations 2006
- Food Information Regulations (FIR) 2014
- Personal Protective Equipment at Work Regulations 1992
- Data Protection Act 1998
- Childcare Act 2004
- Protection of Children Act 1999
- Equality Act 2010
- Race Relations (Amendment) Act 2000
- Safeguarding Children Across Services 2012
- Education Act 2002
- Human Rights Act 1998
- Every Child Matters 2003
- The Children's Plan 2007
- Working Together to Safeguard Children: A Guide to Inter-agency Working to Safeguard and Promote the Welfare of Children 2015
- Working Together to Safeguard Children: A Guide to Inter-agency Working to Safeguard and Promote the Welfare of Children 2010

- Safeguarding Vulnerable Groups Act 2006 and the Safeguarding Vulnerable Groups Order (Northern Ireland) 2007
- Working Together to Safeguard Children 2006 (updated in 2010)
- The Protection of Children in England: A progress report (Laming, 2009)
- The Munro Review of Child Protection: Final Report; A child-centred system (2011)
- Protecting Children – A shared responsibility (Scottish Executive, 1998)
- Co-operating to Safeguard Children (NI, 2002).

Assessment Methods

LO	Assessment criteria and accompanying activities	Assessment methods *To evidence coverage of the assessment criteria you could:*
LO1	1.1 Research it (p. 220)	For this AC, you should be aware of the documents mentioned in the activity. Read these documents and then compile a handout to show your understanding of other legislation relevant to safeguarding children.
	1.1 Reflect on it (p. 220)	Discuss with your assessor the various policies in place for children and reflect upon the similarities with safeguarding adults. Show that you understand how the issue of mental capacity affect the service offered?
	1.1 In practice (p. 220)	Write short notes on the policies shown in the section to demonstrate your understanding of safe working with children and young people. Or prepare a hand-out for staff to enable them to gain a better understanding.
LO2	2.1 In practice (p. 223)	Prepare a staff training session using the above information and give a PowerPoint presentation showing your understanding of the signs, symptoms, indicators and behaviours that may cause concern in the context of safeguarding of children.
	2.1 Research it (p. 223)	Go to the website in the activity for more information on what constitutes abuse and discuss the findings with staff. Alternatively download the signs and symptoms and ensure all staff are aware of these by compiling a hand-out.
	2.2 Research it (p. 224)	Complete the activity and then document or discuss it with your assessor.
	2.2 In practice (p. 224)	Describe to your assessor the actions you would take if a child or young person alleged harm or abuse in line with the policies and procedures of your setting. Keep your notes in your portfolio.
	2.3 Reflect on it (p. 225)	Check your policy on safeguarding and, if your organisation has any connection with children in care, ensure that the policy has a section detailing how you would safeguard children and young people. Place a copy of the policy into your portfolio.
	2.3 In practice (p. 225)	Discuss in a staff training session, the rights children have when harm or abuse is suspected or alleged? Answer with reference to legislation and guidelines. You could also provide a written account.
	2.3 Research it (p. 225)	Complete the activity, you could provide a written account. Use some of the serious case reviews you are aware of to inform your answer.
	2.2 Case study (p. 225)	Use the following case study to show how you as a manager need to respond and what actions will you need to take to safeguard Meena and her two brothers. Alternatively you might use a real life incident.

References

DfCSF (2007) *The Children's Plan – Building Brighter Futures.* London: TSO.

DfE (2011) *The Munro Review of Child Protection: Final Report; A child-centred system.* London: TSO.

DfE (updated in 2010) *Working Together to Safeguard Children: A guide to inter-agency working to safeguard and promote the welfare of children.* London: HMSO.

DfE (2011) *Preventing and Tackling Bullying. Advice for Head Teachers, Staff and Governing Bodies.* London: HMSO.

DfES (2003) *Every Child Matters: Summary.* London: HMSO.

DfES (2006) *What to Do if You're Worried a Child is being Abused: Summary.* London: HMSO.

Home Office (2004) *The Bichard Inquiry. Report HC653.* London: The Stationery Office.

HM Government (2015) *Working Together to Safeguard Children: A guide to inter-agency working to safeguard and promote the welfare of children.* London: Crown. Also available at www.gov.uk/government/uploads/system/uploads/attachment_data/file/419595/Working_Together_to_Safeguard_Children.pdf.

Laming, W. H. (2009) *The Protection of Children in England: A progress report.* London: House of Commons.

NSPCC (2010) *Child Protection Fact Sheet. The definitions and signs of child abuse.* www.nspcc.org.uk.

https://www.nspcc.org.uk/preventing-abuse/child-abuse-and-neglect/?source=ppc-brand&utm_source=bing&utm_medium=cpc&utm_campaign=BND_-_Website_-_[Broad]&utm_term=sitelink_Child_Abuse_and_Neglect&gclid=CJnb54qx28sCFdUZGQodTG4JmQ&gclsrc=ds (Some text in AC 2.1 is adapted from here).

http://www.legislation.gov.uk/ukdsi/2015/9780111133309/pdfs/ukdsiod_9780111133309_en.pdf

Useful resources and further reading

https://www.gov.uk/report-child-abuse

https://www.nspcc.org.uk/preventing-abuse/child-abuse-and-neglect/child-sexual-abuse/research-resources/

http://www.parentsprotect.co.uk/resources.htm

https://www.victimsupport.org.uk/

https://admin.victimsupport.org.uk/help-and-support/young-victims-crime/teachers-and-professionals/useful-resources

Unit HSCM1

Lead person-centred practice

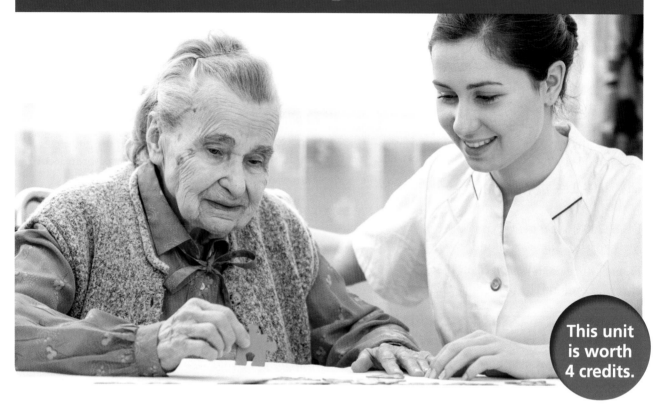

This unit is worth 4 credits.

The purpose of this unit is to enhance the manager's knowledge of the theory and principles, understanding and skills required to promote and implement person-centred practice and to lead the implementation of active participation of individuals.

The Department of Health subscribes fully to the social model of disability and in this unit we will address the changing perceptions about how health and social care must be delivered to improve the quality of life of vulnerable people. From a service-led provision, we look at how the development of the personalisation agenda has changed the face of care in the UK.

We also deal with consent and what this means for clients and address the issues of active participation as a way of working that recognises an individual's right to participate in the activities and relationships of everyday life as independently as possible. The individual as an active partner in their own care or support is given a voice in today's health service and is no longer regarded as a passive recipient and you will be introduced to various models of person-centred practice to enable you to lead and encourage the active participation of your service users.

Key term

Person-centred practice is a process of life planning for individuals based around principles which respect their individuality, rights, choice, privacy, independence and dignity.

Learning outcomes

By the end of this unit you will:

1 Understand the theory and principles that underpin person-centred practice.
2 Be able to lead a person-centred practice.
3 Be able to lead the implementation of active participation of individuals.

LO1 Understand the theory and principles that underpin person-centred practice

AC 1.1 Explain person-centred practice

The Health Foundation (2014) explained person-centred care as:

- giving people dignity, compassion and respect
- offering coordinated and personalised care, support or treatment.
- supporting people to recognise and develop their own strengths and abilities to live independent and fulfilling lives.

It is therefore about making the individual requiring the care the central figure in the process. The government publication *Putting People First: A Shared Vision and Commitment to the Transformation of Adult Social Care* was published in 2007 and outlined its personalisation agenda – the government's vision of enabling individuals to live independently with complete choice and control over their lives.

Personalisation is about allowing individuals to build a system of care and support tailored to meet their individual needs and designed with their full involvement. It is about ensuring that the individual has their choices taken into account and their culture and ethnicity respected, with care given tailored to these factors. Historically, a 'one size fits all' approach to care was in practice and this meant the individual having to fit into and access already existing care services, whether they were appropriate or not.

The term 'person-centred care' is now used to describe care which is user focused, promoting independence and autonomy. Collaborative and partnership approaches to care often use the term 'person-centred' to describe their ethos (Innes, 2006).

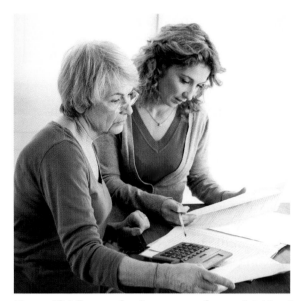

Figure 12.1 A care plan is now user-focused, taking into account individual needs and wishes

AC 1.2 Critically review approaches to person-centred practice

A number of approaches to person-centred care have been identified:

- **Pyschosocial interventions** draw techniques from cognitive behavioural therapies (CBT) and educational theories and can be used for a variety of groups. However, there may be difficulty using these techniques with people who are intellectually impaired.

- The **personalisation agenda**, where everybody receiving support, however it is provided, would have choice and control over that support. Although largely positive, it can lead to conflict amongst staff who may question the way in which care is given and this has the potential to fracture relationships between the staff/carer and the individual. A further issue is that the personalisation agenda may be difficult to meet if budget cuts mean limited choices for service users.

Research it

1.2 Approaches to person-centred practice

Research the reablement approach and biographical or life-story work. Critically review these approaches. What are the advantages and disadvantages of these?

In practice

1.1 Person-centred practice

Explain person-centred practice and describe its benefits.

Historical approaches to care work

We can clearly see the benefits of the philosophy behind person-centred care, but despite extensive support by government, policy makers, practitioners, and clients and their families, there remain difficulties with implementation.

Person-centred practice has resulted from 30 years of investigation into the development of quality care, the origins of which can be traced to changes that took place in the early 1970s as part of a move to 'normalisation' (when long-stay institutions for disabled people began to close down). Normalisation is about 'normalising' the environment, and not the individual, and aims to enable individuals to lead 'normal patterns' of life, rather than forcing them to conform to societal norms.

Unfortunately, the planned changes with respect to moving service users to community care did not have the desired effects. They were expected to fit into the available care services for all and very little personalisation of care was evident at this point in time. In addition to the discrimination and the stigma attached to being a physically or learning disabled person or mentally ill person in the community, the health care system systematically failed these individuals and this led to further criticism of the social care agenda. Research into the problems being encountered at the time revealed major change was needed to the way in which care was being delivered. One critical

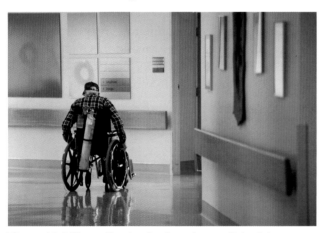

Figure 12.2 Normalisation is about 'normalising' the environment, and not the individual

debate was about two models of care, the Medical Model and the Social Model.

Medical Model vs Social Model

The Medical Model of care described the disabling condition and focused on the impairment the individual suffers and how that impairment reduces the individual's quality of life, causing disadvantage. In this model, the emphasis then was on identifying the disability, understanding it and learning to treat and change its course if possible, or preventing further deterioration.

The Social Model of care took the opposite view and looked at the environment and its disabling impact on individuals. The Social Model supported the notion that society creates disability and that barriers and prejudice, together with the subsequent exclusion by society, are the defining factors for who is disabled and who is not in a particular society. The lack of resources, facilities or the environment which restricted mobility meant that individuals with disabilities were unable to participate in work or education.

This model reflected the view that while physical or mental impairment poses problems, these do not necessarily have to lead to disability unless society fails to accommodate these differences.

This led to a change in the way in which disability was viewed and politicians were forced to address the issues. It was clear that in order to improve care, changes to the way in which it was being delivered would need to be high on the agenda.

Over time, there was marked improvement in how society accepted people with disabilities, those with learning disabilities, as well as people with mental health problems and older people as equal members of the community. The Social Model of care forced the view that society was in fact the problem for such groups because it failed to provide adequate services to meet their needs. The model was hailed as a more person-centred approach to care than the Medical Model.

As we have seen above, the approach to person-centred care has involved a shift in the way in which care is delivered and rather than a 'one size fits all' design, services were designed to fit around the needs of individuals.

The changes haves not only put the person at the centre of the care process but also shifted power towards them, enabling them to have more freedom of choice.

The principles guiding this agenda centre on the notion of equality, choice, independence and inclusion. In order to meet these needs, the services we supply in health care must challenge the unequal power structures that have been evident between service providers and service users. Sanderson (2003, p. 20) talks about this change as being the need to operate from a position where service providers have 'power with' service users rather than 'power over' them.

In trying to implement person-centred care, managers need to be clear about how the support to clients will be delivered; it is not merely a case of including clients and families and asking them what they think or what they want. There are processes to guide practice and six approaches are mentioned below:

1 **The McGill Action Planning System (MAPS)** is a planning process for children with disabilities to enable their integration into the school community. The team in this process includes the child, family members, friends, and regular and special education personnel.

2 **ELP, or Essential Lifestyle Planning**, is detailed plans used to get to know what is important to someone. When using these types of plans the assumptions behind them are that:
   ● the individual will have a lifestyle that works for them
   ● our quality of life depends on how well or badly we achieve that lifestyle.

As care workers we should help people to live their chosen lifestyle – not try to change the person to fit in with our view of life.

3 **Personal Futures Planning** involves getting to know the person to determine what their life is like now and developing ideas about what they would like to do in the future. Action is then taken to help them to implement this, and to explore possibilities within the community to see what needs to change within services (Mount and O'Brien, 1992).

4 **The PATHS (Planning Alternative Tomorrows and Hope)** system was developed by Jack Pearpoint, Marsha Forest and John O'Brien and features a person's dreams for the future (termed 'their north star') and puts it into action, reviewing the plan 1–2 years later.

5 In the **collaborative care and support planning** model, what matters to the person is explored along with the best treatment, care and support. Additionally, the service user is encouraged to set goals and think about actions they can take to reach them.

The charity National Voices has identified four stages of the approach:

● preparing for a discussion
● having the discussion (with the care and support worker)
● writing down the main points from the discussion
● review.

See www.nationalvoices.org.uk/what-care-and-support-planning for more information.

6 In the **person- and family-centred care approach** the focus is on the way in which the care is organised and the way staff interact with patients and their families.

This approach incorporates 'shadowing' patients, in order to develop a knowledge of their perspective and to gain a shared vision for the ideal patient experience, and working through individual improvements.

Go to www.kingsfund.org.uk/projects/PFCC and www.health.org.uk/areas-of-work/programmes/family-patient-centred-care for more information.

We may see the positives in care being given using these approaches. The person is at the centre of decision making and their choice and wishes are paramount. However, negative factors include time to undertake the approach and funding, which may be a scarce resource. Also staff may require additional training to initiate these models.

Health and social care has come a considerable distance in terms of person-centred care. Traditional views of clients as passive recipients of care are now challenged and the way in which the 'needs of the disabled' were determined, without reference to the individual, have largely disappeared. Today, person-centred planning has

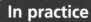
taken centre stage in services, although it has not been fully adopted or implemented across social care provision and there needs to be more work carried out to ensure that it is.

AC 1.3 Analyse the effect of legislation and policy on person-centred practice

Table 12.1 outlines the legislation that affects person-centred care.

Table 12.1 Legislation affecting person-centred care

Date	Act/ Guidance	Purpose and effect
2000	The NHS Plan	Highlighted the need for personalisation and coordination of services, the effect of which was to streamline and improve services and waiting times.
2001	The Valuing People White Paper	Made direct payments available to more people with a learning disability and launched the term 'person-centred planning'. The effect has been movement on the personalisation agenda.
2002 (updated 2008)	The Wanless Report: Securing Good Health for the Whole Population.	Focused on enablement and empowerment, with patients being partners in care.
2005	The Mental Capacity Act	Highlights the patient's right to make choices and have their preferences respected, even if others (advocates) make decisions on their behalf, which has had an effect on enabling people with mental health problems to have greater control.
	SCIE and the Department of Health, Independence, well-being and choice: Our Vision for the Future of Social Care for Adults in England	Report stated that a Social Model approach to care which 'supports people to be independent by ensuring they have the support to live as they wish' was favoured, affecting the way in which care is delivered.
	Improving the Life Chances of Disabled People	Individual budgets to improve choice and control over the mix of care and support.
	Independence, Well-being and Choice	Social care services help people to maintain their independence by 'giving them greater choice and control over the way their needs are met'.
2006	Our Health, Our Care, Our Say: A new direction for community service.	Developed the concept of personalised care.

➜

Date	Act/ Guidance	Purpose and effect
2007	Putting People First: A shared vision and commitment to transformation of adult social care	This was a commitment to enable people to manage and control their own support through individual/personal budgets.
2008	Lord Darzi's report, High Quality Care for All	Highlighted the need to change public expectations of services; included the importance of people being involved in decisions about their care.
2009	The first NHS Constitution in England	Described what people could expect from the NHS and brought policy statements of intent to form a rights framework which reflects the needs and preferences of patients, their families and their carers. Also patients, families and carers would be involved in and consulted on all decisions about their care and treatment.
	Care Support Independence: Shaping the future of care together	This was a consultation on how personalised social care and support can be delivered and funded.
	Personal Health Budgets: 'First steps'	This introduced the personal health budget to allow people to have more choice, flexibility and control over the health services and care they receive.
2010	The Francis Report	The failings in care at Mid Staffordshire NHS Foundation Trust between 2005 and 2009 forced the person-centred care agenda back into the public awareness. It focused sharply on dignity, compassion and respect.
	A Vision for Adult Social Care: Capable communities and active citizens	Set out the plans for a new direction for adult social care, putting personalised services and outcomes centre stage, based on six principles, personalisation being one such principle.
2012	The Health and Social Care Act	Requires the Clinical Commissioning Groups to promote the involvement of every patient.
2013	The Berwick Advisory Group	Greater involvement of patients and their carers at every level of the health service in order to deliver safe, meaningful and appropriate health care.
2014	The Care Act	Requires local authorities to involve adults in their assessment, care and support planning and review.

As we can see from the laws and guidance published since 2000, there has been a major revamp of adult social care law in England, all with the effect of seeking to transform care. The move to a single piece of legislation so people were clear about their rights had been called for and this was realised in the Care Act 2014.

Reflect on it

1.3 Legislation and your setting

Reflect on the ways in which the laws and papers in Table 12.1 have affected the way in which your setting delivers its care.

There may be other policies that are pertinent to your area of practice and these might include:

- **The National Service Framework and the Single Assessment Process (SAP)**. This was introduced in the Older People Framework and ensures that the elderly person in care receives appropriate care to meet their individual needs. The SAP calls for a holistic assessment to be made, with the emphasis on partnership working (see Unit M2c).
- **National Minimum Standards**, although not legal requirements, are guidelines which instruct the registered manager to 'develop and agree an individual plan' for all service users.

1.3 Legislation, policy and person-centred practice

What has been the effect of legislation and policy on person-centred practice in your setting?

- **The Care Programme Approach (CPA)** (1990) is similar to the SAP. This applies to the individual with mental health problems and ensures that they are fully involved in their own care plan.
- **The Personalisation Agenda (2008)** defines personalisation as 'the way in which services are tailored to the needs and preferences of citizens to empower citizens to shape their own lives and the services they receive'.
- **DOH (2012) 'Liberating the NHS; No decision without me about me'** outlines the need to increase opportunities for patients and their representatives to have more involvement in decisions about their care at all points in their care.

AC 1.4 Explain how person-centred practice informs the way in which consent is established with individuals

Person-centred care and verbal and written consent

Person-centred care demands that the individual requiring care is fully involved in the whole planning process and as such can be deemed to have consented to such arrangements in a verbal way as well as in a written document. Any discussion about treatment and care must be given in a sensitive and understandable way and the individual should be given enough time to think about the information and to ask questions if they need to. By engaging with the care worker, they have 'implied' that they consent to the process and this is an acceptable way of obtaining consent.

Key term

Consent means informed agreement to an action or decision; the process of establishing consent will vary according to an individual's assessed capacity to consent.

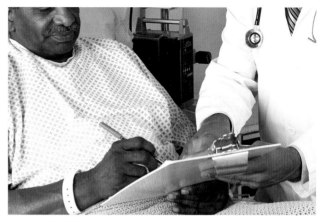

Figure 12.3 Written consent will remain in the individual's notes

In all cases dignity and respect must be considered and values and beliefs taken into account.

Often we ask for written consent and this is certainly true if the case involves any risk, such as with surgery. In this case, a written record will remain in the individual's notes recording the treatment and care agreed on. The actual process of writing up the notes of the consent must be rigorous, accurately recording all discussions and decisions made relating to obtaining consent.

Mental capacity

In approaching the care planning process, the assumption is that every adult must be presumed to have the mental capacity to consent or refuse treatment, unless they have undergone a capacity assessment and have been judged not to have the capacity to make a specific decision. If this is the case then with their best interests in mind that decision can be taken for them. If capacity is likely to diminish in the future then the MCA advises the appointment of a trusted person to make a decision on their behalf.

Source: Adapted from the http://www.nhs.uk/ Conditions/social-care-and-support-guide/Pages/ mental-capacity.aspx

The decision as to whether the individual lacks capacity must be made with the medical staff providing the treatment or care and in consultation with family and care staff. In an emergency situation when an individual requires treatment but is unconscious, treatment to preserve life may be given, as long as it is in the best interests of that individual. This is covered in the Mental Capacity Act.

Refusal of treatment by a person with capacity should be respected and a record made. If the person who has refused treatment or care is confused or mentally incapacitated in some way, care staff must make a full and frank assessment of their care and ensure that the individual is safeguarded.

If referral to court to obtain permission to treat is necessary, guidelines list the following circumstances:

- sterilisation for contraceptive purposes
- donation of regenerative tissue such as bone marrow
- withdrawal of nutrition and hydration from a patient in a persistent vegetative state
- where there is doubt as to the person's capacity or best interests.

Source: http://www.nhs.uk/conditions/consent-to-treatment/pages/capacity.aspx

Your knowledge of the Mental Capacity Act (MCA) 2005 (England and Wales) will be useful to enable you to manage decision-making for service users. It allows people over the age of 16 to appoint a proxy decision-maker who has the legal power to give consent to medical treatment when the patient loses the capacity to consent. In the case of a person who is detained under mental health legislation, the principles of consent continue to apply and care staff must ensure that the individual is aware of the circumstances and safeguards needed for providing treatment and care without consent.

If you are dealing with a child, then obtaining consent is complex as young people under the age of 16 are considered to lack the capacity to consent or to refuse treatment. Parents or those with parental responsibility must give consent. If the child is considered to have significant understanding and intelligence to make up his or her own mind about what is happening to them, that may be waived.

A child of 16 or 17 is considered to be able to consent for themselves, but good practice demands that parents or guardians are involved. Refusal of consent by a child of any age up to 18 years can be overridden by the parents or in exceptional circumstances an order from the court.

There are a couple of exceptions where a capable individual may be treated without first obtaining their consent. For example, a magistrate can order detention in hospital if a person has an infectious disease that presents a risk to public health –

such as rabies, cholera or anthrax (Public Health (Control of Disease) Act, 1984).

AC 1.5 Explain how person-centred practice can result in positive changes in individuals' lives

There can be little doubt that person-centred practice means that individuals feel more in control over their care and indeed their lives. They experience increased confidence and the benefits improve relationships the family and also the community. The traditional service-led approach was an easy way to deliver care for care workers but meant that people did not receive the help they really needed at the right time.

Personalisation gives more choice and control over lives and ensures that people have wider choice in how their needs are met. They are able to access universal services such as transport, leisure and education, housing, health and opportunities for employment regardless of age or disability (SCIE).

A campaign launched in 2006 entitled 'Dignity in Care' outlines the means by which intolerance of indignity in health care can be eliminated. The Dignity Challenge led by the Department of Health states that high-quality care services that respect people's dignity should (among other things):

- treat each person as an individual by offering personalised services
- enable people to maintain the maximum possible level of independence, choice and control.

In practice

1.4 Person-centred practice and consent
Explain to a new member of staff how consent is obtained.

Research it

LO1 Models underpinning person-centred practice
Research the models and principles that underpin person-centred practice and compare the Medical Model to the Social Model. How beneficial has the change to this approach been to care work?

235

LO2 Be able to lead a person-centred practice

In this section you need to undertake the activities in order to meet the outcomes and to supply your assessor with evidence-based practice. Each assessment criteria refers to working with and supporting others and in this context **'others' refers to family, friends, advocates, paid workers, as well as carers and other professionals.**

AC 2.1 Support others to work with individuals to establish their history, preferences, wishes and needs

In your role as manager your staff need to be supported and guided in obtaining information from service users which ensures that wishes and choices are all detailed. Taking a personal history may require a lengthy process in which the service user is encouraged to tell their life story. Telling their life story enables the individual to identify their needs and wishes in a more meaningful way, one which fits in with their life. Therefore, the value of communicating well can never be underestimated when developing good relationships. Drawbacks of this method include the potential for large parts of the story being missed due to memory loss, or for traumatic memories to emerge. For good quality care to be given, all biographical details need to be documented accurately.

AC 2.2 Support others to implement person-centred practice

Person-centred planning

In leading person-centred practice you and the others involved in the process need to keep in mind the following points:

- The central figure in the process is the client.
- Family and friends are partners in the care process.
- The care plan is a guide to what is important for the client and shows what support they need.
- A care plan helps the person to be a part of the community and is not merely about what services they need.
- The plan is a continuous process and does not stop when it has been written. The people involved continue to evaluate and act within the plan to help the client to achieve the best quality care (DOH, 2002).

AC 2.3 Support others to work with individuals to review approaches to meet individuals' needs and preferences

In reviewing care we need feedback about how the needs and preferences of the service user have been met and whether changes may be required. The supervision process is a good way in which to gain feedback from staff and time can be given to review which approaches worked well and which did not. Additionally, the team meeting can be a useful forum for discussing this. For others such as family members, friends, advocates and other professionals, reviews of care need to be planned and there should be regular meetings or perhaps forums to enable this.

The Action on Elder Abuse Toolkit provides us with a useful set of questions when undertaking the planning process. It states, in section 3.9 of the document:

Such an approach ties in with an emphasis on person centred approaches, and encourages engagement, time and patience. Key questions for a person centred approach include:

- *What is the person communicating about their views? How can we help them understand and communicate more?*
- *What is life like for this person? How do they experience the world?*
- *What would it be like to be in their shoes?*
- *What is important for them?*
- *What might their hopes and dreams be?*

Source: Action on Elder Abuse Toolkit

AC 2.4 Support others to work with individuals to adapt approaches in response to individuals' emerging needs or preferences

This section requires you to evaluate the whole process carried out in the above activities.

In adapting approaches to account for emerging needs, there needs to be an evaluation of the care process that has been undertaken. Sometimes emergencies happen and we need to review the care. A service user may deteriorate overnight, for example, and require a more hands-on approach to care. Person-centred practice recognises that needs change over time and plans for a change in the service provision. We may need to inform family, friends, advocates and other professionals as to the changes that may have occurred and which may affect the part they play in the care.

LO3 Be able to lead the implementation of active participation of individuals

AC 3.1 Evaluate how active participation enhances the well-being and quality of life of individuals

Langer and Rodin (1976) conducted a study to assess the effects of enhanced personal responsibility and choice on two groups of nursing home residents. In the experimental group, the residents were told they had responsibility for their own care. The second (control) group were informed that the staff were responsible for all care. Residents in the experimental group were free to make choices, had no decisions made for them and were also given a house plant to take care of. The opposite arrangements were in place for the control group. The results of the study showed a significant improvement for the experimental group over the control group in alertness, active participation and a general sense of well-being.

The expectation at the start of the study was that the debilitated condition of many of the aged individuals residing in institutional settings is the result of living in a virtually decision-free environment and consequently is potentially reversible.

Being unable to make a decision or to have a dialogue about their care and needs may inevitably lead to a major reduction in self-esteem, health and well-being.

Consider for a moment how you might feel if you were a patient in hospital and never consulted about your treatment. You merely had to accept the decisions made and do as you were told. It would not be very long before you were completely switched off and passive in whatever was being done to you. You might even feel that you were being undervalued with respect to any of your wishes.

The Nursing and Midwifery Council standards of conduct make it very clear that health care workers should listen to the people in their care and respond to their needs as individuals. They should be aware of their preferences and act in accordance with these. The General Social Care Council echoes this and the Code of Practice states that care workers must treat people as individuals and support their right to control their own lives and make informed choices.

In evaluating how active participation has enhanced the well-being and quality of life of our service users, we may ask for feedback via questionnaires, for example.

Research it

3.1 Active participation

Undertake a small-scale study of a group of individuals in your care and ask them to comment on how well active participation in their own care enhances their well-being and quality of life.

In practice

3.1 Active participation and well-being

How did the service users evaluate their involvement and their subsequent well-being in your setting?

AC 3.2 Implement systems and processes that promote active participation

A study commissioned by the Joseph Rowntree Foundation and carried out by Wilcox (1994) outlined ten key ideas about active participation and, in particular, community participation.

The publication, *The Guide to Effective Participation*, is worth looking at in more detail, but the key ideas are as follows.

1 Level of participation

A five-rung ladder of participation relating to the stance an organisation promoting participation may take:

- Information: telling people what is planned.
- Consultation: offering options, listening to feedback, but not allowing new ideas.
- Deciding together: encouraging additional options and ideas, and providing opportunities for joint decision making.
- Acting together: not only do different interests decide together on what is best, they form a partnership to carry it out.
- Supporting independent community interests: local groups or organisations are offered funds, advice or other support to develop their own agendas within guidelines.

Your policies and procedures which are in place will support this.

2 Initiation and process

Many problems in participation develop because of poor preparation within the promoting organisation – with the result that when community interest is engaged, the organisation cannot deliver on its promises. There needs to be a process or system in place to allow others to be involved and to allow the process to be controlled and monitored.

3 Control

The initiator or person in control can decide how much or how little control to allow to others – for example, just information, or a major say in what is to happen.

4 Power and purpose

Many organisations fear loss of control and may be unwilling to allow people to participate. However, working together allows everyone to achieve more than they could on their own. The guide emphasises the difference between power *to* and power *over*. People are empowered when they have the power to achieve what they want.

5 Role of the practitioner

Practitioners control much of what happens and the guide is written mainly for people who are planning or managing participation processes. It may be difficult for a practitioner both to control access to funds and other resources and to play a neutral role in facilitating a participation process.

6 Stakeholders and community

Anyone who has a stake in what happens is a stakeholder and some of these will have influence in the community.

7 Partnership

Partners must trust each other and share commitment.

8 Commitment

People are committed when they want to achieve something and apathetic when they do not. They care about what they are interested in. If people are apathetic about proposals, it may be that they do not share the interests or concerns of those putting forward the plans and that can be a starting point for dialogue.

9 Ownership of ideas

People are most likely to be interested and committed if they have a stake in the idea. Brainstorming workshops and helping people think through the practicality of ideas can be useful.

10 Confidence and capacity

Ideas and wish-lists are little use if they cannot be put into practice. Many participation processes involve breaking new ground – tackling difficult projects and setting up new forms of organisations. Training may be needed or the opportunity to learn formally and informally, to develop confidence and trust in each other.

The above is adapted from the findings of *Community Participation and Empowerment: Putting Theory into Practice*, published in 1994 by the John Rowntree Foundation. Reproduced by permission of the John Rowntree Foundation.

The process above is very much a social work model of practice and can be seen in initiatives such as the Sure Start programme. When arranging care packages for service users, it is important to involve as many partners in the community as possible in order to widen choice and options. By having an understanding of community developments, you are better able to refer service users to the right services.

Other systems and processes to support service users include policies and procedures. For example, risk assessment needs to form part of the systems and processes. You should also agree on how the care required is assessed in your workplace and how wishes, choices and preferences are agreed upon and met.

In practice

3.1, 3.2 Active participation

Show evidence of the systems and processes in your own work that promote active participation.

How effective are the systems and processes in ensuring active participation is working?

AC 3.3 Support the use of risk assessments to promote active participation in all aspects of the lives of individuals

The National Occupational Standards have identified six key roles for social work practitioners, one of which highlights risk assessment.

In key role 4, the social work practitioner is instructed to manage risk to individuals, families, carers, groups, communities, self and colleagues. The standard requires practitioners to manage and identify risk, balance rights and responsibilities, and monitor the risks to individuals, families, carers, groups, self and colleagues. It also demands that immediate action to deal with the behaviour that presents a risk is taken and strategies to help change behaviour are developed.

Helping individuals to make choices in their own care means that, occasionally, a choice may involve a risk at some level. Generally, we can view risk in two ways:

1 The risk a person poses to other people.
2 The risk a person may be subject to, whether by a chosen action or not.

In the first case, risk assessment focuses on how the person may pose a risk to others. For example, mental health workers and prison officers will have risk assessments in place, together with strategies and procedures which will protect them in the event of a situation developing.

Risk assessments and active participation

In the second case, the risk is not necessarily viewed as a negative and may in fact be positive. If the risk to be taken is life enhancing for the person, for example a young cared for person wishes to move away to attend university but is deemed as vulnerable, then the assessment needs to identify what the risks may be and whether they are acceptable to take or not.

In social work there are two types of risk assessment favoured and these are worth studying:

- actuarial assessment
- clinical assessment.

Actuarial assessment

This came from the insurance model of assessment and involves a statistical calculation of the risk whereby the risk is calculated according to the probability of something happening and then expressed in numerical form. You are predicting what might happen, together with the likelihood of that happening, and then making a judgement as to whether to take the risk or not.

Clinical assessment

This type fits better with the person-centred approach to care as it undertaken on a case-by-case basis and is therefore more individual in nature. It also proposes that there is a better understanding of the nature of the risk rather than merely a calculation of the probability.

Being based upon professional judgement, it is largely subjective and as such may be inaccurate – a risk to a service user may not register as a risk in your assessment.

Two forms of error have been cited with clinical assessment and these are false negatives and false positives. Walker and Beckett (2005) make the following points about this.

False negative is where a situation is identified as having a low risk and a harmful event occurs anyway. For example, if a person is left in the care of their family and comes to harm, the risk assessment is deemed to be 'wrong'.

False positives represent situations which are viewed as high risk, where a harmful event would not occur, even in the absence of intervention. For example, if the elderly person had remained in their own home, they would not have come to any harm, but moving them to a care setting causes distress and therefore harm has been caused.

These cases illustrate the uncertainty of risk assessment and Walker and Beckett conclude that it is imperative to review any situation in which a mistake has been made in the risk assessment and to determine whether there are any factors that should have been noted and were not. Alternatively, it may have been that the situation that emerged could not have been reasonably foreseen and prepared for because 'a bad outcome in and of itself does not constitute evidence that a decision was mistaken' (MacDonald and Macdonald, 1999).

In supporting the use of risk assessments to promote active participation we need to feel safe in the decisions made and one way is to ensure that you can defend each decision you make with respect to the assessment of the individual. You might think about the following questions to guide your assessment.

- Have you taken all reasonable steps in the process?
- Have you used reliable methods?
- Have you collected enough information and looked at it in an evaluative manner?
- Are you working within policy and law?
- Have you recorded all the decisions that were made?

In addition to the above, you might actually take a purely health and safety approach to risk:

- Step 1: Look for hazards.
- Step 2: Identify who could be harmed and how.
- Step 3: Evaluate the risk.
- Step 4: Record the findings.
- Step 5: Assess the effectiveness of the precautions in place.

Unit M1 on health and safety gives a more detailed account of this approach and you are advised to read this unit again.

Risk assessments may be viewed as onerous tasks in which a paper filling exercise is yet another additional job. However a more positive view is one in which we see risk assessing as a means to enabling our service users to actively participate in all aspects of their lives in a safe manner and in a way that will improve the quality of that life.

In practice

3.3 Risk assessments and active participation
Undertake a risk assessment for one of your clients and reflect on how you will ensure that active participation is promoted for that person.

Reflective exemplar

Geri's exemplar

An incident arose today at work which made me really think about how I was approaching personalised care. Mrs Casey, an 83 diabetic client, was keen to use her new scooter to attend an art group in the town. She had arranged to meet her friend at the centre and was going to leave at 8.30 for a 9.30 start. I usually ensured that she had her insulin at about 7.30 each morning to ensure she could eat breakfast at 8.30. On the day in question we would need to review that arrangement and change the times. I was not concerned about that at all and felt it was fine to do that, however, my real worry was allowing her to go at all. Mrs C is rather forgetful lately and has only just learned to use her scooter. My worry is that she will not be in full control of the appliance and may forget the key or lose her way. I am also worried about her diabetes and have a concern that should she need help when at the group, she may be unable to articulate what she wants. I feel that I will need to arrange for somebody to be with her when she goes and this is going to have staffing implications.

As I went through all these thoughts, it became clear to me that I had lost sight of the full picture. Mrs C is an individual with complete control over her own care and choice and I am merely there to ensure that she remains safe in the decision she makes. I spoke to my manager who said I needed to risk assess the event and then discuss with Mrs C anything she needed to help her to meet her goals.

Case study

LO3 Risk assessment and person-centred care

A care worker for a domiciliary care service was assisting an elderly client to get undressed so that she could be moved from her bed to her shower chair. Unfortunately the client fell to the ground. The carer, who was new to the role had not accessed the care plan so was unaware that the care plan assessment carried out a month earlier stated that two people were required to transfer the client safely from her bed into the shower chair. The elderly client was taken to the general hospital, where she was found to have sustained a broken back. She died the following day from the injury. An investigation carried out by the HSE found that although there had been a 'Safe System of Work Assessment' carried out on how to move Mrs X safely, it required updating after 12 months or sooner if there was any significant change in her mobility. Mrs X had recently had a chest infection and had become less mobile as a result of this and this should have alerted the care workers to carry out a further assessment. This was not done and additionally the carer who had been assisting the client on the morning of her fall had been given insufficient instructions and was not adequately supervised. She should also have been aware that two people were required to help with this task.

The care company therefore had to pay a fine of £60,000 for failing to review and update a risk assessment and to provide adequate instruction and supervision to its employees engaged in moving and handling residents.

Source: Adapted from a case on the HSE website: www.hse.gov.uk.htm

What can you learn from this tragic case study in relation to risk assessment and person-centred practice?

Legislation

All legislation pertaining to this unit is shown in Table 12.1 in section AC 1.3.

Assessment Methods

LO	Assessment criteria and accompanying activities	Assessment methods *To evidence coverage of the ACs, you could:*
LO1	1.1 In practice (p. 229)	Explain person-centred practice and describe its benefits to a member of your staff, or write a short piece to demonstrate your knowledge of this.
	1.2 Research it (p. 229)	Write a short account.
	1.2 Reflect on it (p. 232)	Write a short reflective account.
	1.2 In practice (p. 232)	Provide a written account or discuss this with your assessor.
	1.3 Reflect on it (p. 233)	Write a reflective account.
	1.3 In practice (p. 234)	Provide a written statement.
	1.4 In practice (p. 235)	Explain how consent is obtained to a new staff member or write a short piece about this.
	LO1 Research it (p. 235)	Prepare a short staff training session to complete the activity. Ask staff to comment upon how beneficial the change to this approach has been to care work and write a short statement of the findings.
	1.5 In practice (p. 236)	Give some examples or write a case study on one client.
LO2	2.1, 2.2 In practice (p. 236)	Write a case study to complete the activity.
	2.3 In practice (p. 237)	Complete the activity. You could discuss this with your assessor.

LO	Assessment criteria and accompanying activities	Assessment methods *To evidence coverage of the ACs, you could:*
	2.4 Reflect on it (p. 237)	Write a reflective account.
	LO2 Research it (p. 237)	Prepare a short questionnaire.
	2.4 In practice (p. 237)	Complete the activity. Provide a written account and discuss this with your assessor.
LO3	3.1 Research it (p. 238)	Undertake a small-scale study. Take your findings to the team at a meeting and write a report to evidence them.
	3.1 In practice (p. 238)	Discuss this with your assessor.
	3.1, 3.2 In practice (p. 239)	Complete the activity and discuss with your assessor.
	3.3 In practice (p. 241)	Complete the activity and discuss with your assessor.
	LO3 Case study (p. 242)	Discuss with your assessor what you have learned from this tragic case study in relation to risk assessment and person centred practice.

References

Action on Elder Abuse at http://lx.iriss.org.uk/sites/default/files/resources/Elderabuse.pdf.

Beresford, P., Shamash, M., Forrest, V., Turner, M. and Branfield, F. (2005) *Developing Social Care: Service users' vision for adult support*. London: SCIE.

Berwick, D. (2013) *A Promise to Learn – a Commitment to Act: Improving the safety of patients in England*. London: Williams Lea.

Darzi, A. (2008) *High Quality Care for All: NHS next stage review final report*. Norwich: TSO.

Department of Health (2000) *The NHS Plan: A plan for investment, a plan for reform. Cm 4818-I.* Norwich: HMSO.

Department of Health (2013) *The NHS Constitution for England*. www.gov.uk/government/publications/the-nhs-constitution-for-england.

DOH (2001) *Valuing People: A new strategy for learning disability for the 21st century; planning with people; towards person-centred approaches – accessible guide*. London: HMSO.

DOH (2005) *Improving the Life Chances of Disabled People*. London: HMSO.

DOH (2006) *Our Health, Our Care, Our Say: A new direction for community service*. London: HMSO.

DOH (2006) *Dignity in Care: Becoming a champion*. London: HMSO.

DOH (2009) *Personal Health Budgets: First steps*. London: HMSO.

DOH (2012) *Liberating the NHS: No decision without me about me*. London: The Health Foundation.

DOH (2008) *The Wanless Report: Securing good health for the whole population*. London: HMSO.

Francis, R. (2013) *Report of the Mid Staffordshire NHS Foundation Trust Public Inquiry*. London: TSO. www.midstaffspublicinquiry.com/report.

Health and Social Care Act 2012, section 13H.

Health Foundation (2014) *Person-centred Care Made Simple*. www.health.org.uk/sites/default/files/PersonCentredCareMadeSimple.pdf.

HM Government (2009) *Shaping the Future of Care Together*. Green Paper.

Langer, E. J. and Rodin, I. (1976) 'The effects of choice and enhanced personal responsibility for the aged: a field experiment in an institutional setting,' *Journal of Personality and Social Psychology*, 34(2), 191–8.

MacDonald, K. and Macdonald, G. (1999) 'Perceptions of risk' in Parsloe, P. (ed) *Risk Assessment in Social Work and Social Care*. London: Jessica Kingsley.

Putting People First: A shared vision and commitment to the transformation of Adult Social Care (2007). London: HMG.

Sanderson, H. (2000) *Critical Issues in the Implementation of Essential Lifestyle Planning Within a Complex Organization: An action research investigation within a learning disability service*. Manchester Metropolitan University. Unpublished Ph.D. thesis.

Sanderson, H. (2003) 'Implementing person-centred planning by developing person-centred teams,' *Journal of Integrated Care*, 11(3),18–25.

Stalker, K. and Campbell, V. (1998) 'Person-centred planning: an evaluation of a training programme,' *Health and Social Care in the Community*, 6(2), 130–42.

Walker, S. and Beckett, C. (2005) *Social Work Assessment and Intervention*. Dorset: Russell House Publishing.

Wanless, D. (2002) *Securing Our Future Health: Taking a long-term view*. London: HM Treasury, April.

Wilcox, D., Holmes, A., Kean, J., Ritchie, C. and Smith, J. (1994) *The Guide to Effective Participation*. York: Joseph Rowntree Foundation.

http://webarchive.nationalarchives.gov.uk/20130107105354/http://www.dh.gov.uk/en/Publicationsandstatistics/Publications/PublicationsPolicyAndGuidance/DH_081118

www.nmc-uk.org

'Person-centred planning – finding directions for change using person centred planning' (1992) http://www.helensandersonassociates.co.uk/readingroom/how/person-centred-planning.aspx

Useful resources and further reading

Innes, A., Macpherson, S. and McCabe, I. (2006) *Promoting Person-Centred Care at the Front Line*. York: Joseph Rowntree Foundation/SCIE.

Ladyman, S. (2004) 'Health and social care advisory service: new directions in direct payments for people who use mental health services,' speech, Department of Health, London, 18 May.

www.kingsfund.org.uk/projects/PFCC

www.health.org.uk/areas-of-work/programmes/family-patient-centred-care

www.nationalvoices.org.uk/what-care-and-support-planning

Unit SS 5.1

Assess the individual in a health and social care setting

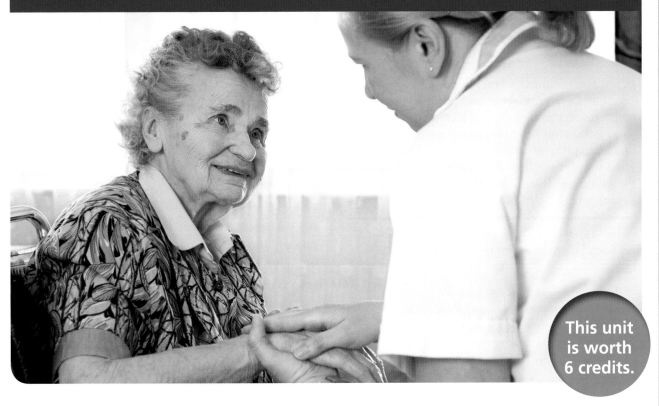

This unit is worth 6 credits.

Assessment is an important part of care as it involves collecting information about an individual and analysing it to enable us to understand what the service user needs for their safety and well-being. This unit addresses the different forms of assessment in the context of partnership working and looks at how you can manage the whole process of carrying out, reviewing and planning assessment for service users. Reference is made to several models of assessment and how partnership working can aid the process. Throughout the unit a series of activities will help you to build a portfolio of evidence to cover the learning outcomes of the unit.

This unit should be read in conjunction with Unit M3 'Manage health and social care practice

Learning outcomes

By the end of this unit you will:

1 Understand assessment processes.
2 Be able to lead and contribute to assessments.
3 Be able to manage the outcomes of assessments.
4 Be able to promote others' understanding of the role of assessment.
5 Review and evaluate the effectiveness of assessment.

to ensure positive outcomes for individuals' and Unit M2c 'Work in partnership in health and social care'.

LO1 Understand assessment processes

AC 1.1, 4.1 Compare and contrast the range and purpose of different forms of assessment and develop others' understanding of the functions of a range of assessment tools

> **Key term**
>
> **Care assessment** simply refers to collecting data and evidence about an individual's needs with respect to care. During a care assessment, you determine what care needs the individuals have, together with the level and type of care and support required to meet those needs. This is a fundamental role of the care worker and a manager.

The Social Care Institute for Excellence (2003) states:

'Although assessment has been recognised as a core skill in social work and should underpin all social work interventions, there is no singular theory or understanding as to what the purpose of assessment is and what the process should entail.'

With no one theory to support it, the process of assessment then becomes a huge subject and one which potentially might differ with each service in a partnership group. This is why when working with partners we bring together people who know the service user well and can contribute to the care positively. These people may be from other services but also include family, friends and informal carers. When this type of working is not done well this can lead to fragmentation of a service user's care, with many differing approaches to assessing their needs being used at the same time. It becomes imperative, then, to determine how we as care providers will assess the service user and to simplify the process.

Care planning

The care planning process is a good place to start. In any assessment of a client's needs the following 'basic helping cycle', as suggested by Taylor and Devine (1993), is useful.

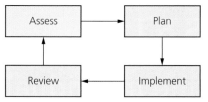

Figure 13.1 The basic care cycle (based on Taylor and Devine 1993)

In this basic cycle, the service user and the care professional work together to assess the needs, resources and potential risks for the service user. In doing this we are responding to the needs of the service user and are also working in conjunction with policy to ensure, for example, that we are providing individualised care and maintaining independence. The care to meet those needs is then planned and put into action at the third stage and finally evaluated or 'reviewed', starting the cycle again.

In 2005 Thompson described what he called the 'ASIRT' model of care planning:

AS – Assessment phase, which is the start of the process and the first part of an action plan leading onto the …

I ntervention stage when aims and objectives for the intervention are selected

R – Review when the evaluation of what has happened takes place, before finally

T – Termination, when the intervention is no longer needed and can be stopped.

Models of assessment and purpose

The care planning process, however we approach it, is just one part of assessment. Three different models of assessment have been suggested in research by Smale *et al.* (1993):

- **The Questioning Model** – in which the care worker leads the process and questions and listens, before processing the information. This means that the process is service led.
- **The Procedural Model** – in which information is gathered by the care professional who then makes a judgement as to 'best fit' for the service. This is criterion based and a range of checklists is used to determine which service is best for the service user.
- **The Exchange Model** – in which the care workers view the service users as the expert in their own care needs. This is really the most person-centred approach of the three. This model seems to describe the most holistic form of assessment, with the care professional managing a more client-centred approach.

The types of assessment we carry out will differ according to the setting we are in or according to the type of needs the person has. If the person living in their own home is having difficulty with their personal care, they might consider getting support by having a community care assessment of their needs. These assessments are carried out by social services and can vary, depending on the particular needs of the person being assessed.

Older people
Community care assessments for older people are carried out under the single assessment process.

People with mental health problems
Assessments for people in need of mental health services are carried out under the Care Programme Approach (CPA), which assesses:

- risk and safety
- psychiatric symptoms and experiences
- psychological thoughts and behaviours.

Mental health issues require the help of mental healthcare professionals and the community care assessment entitles the individual to a care plan that is regularly reviewed by the professional.

If the person has a range of needs and is considered to have severe mental health problems, their care may be coordinated under a CPA and a CPA care coordinator will be appointed to oversee the assessment and planning process. The coordinator is usually a nurse, social worker or occupational therapist.

People with learning disabilities
For service users with learning disabilities, assessment is governed by the principles set out by the 'Valuing People' plan, which aims to improve services for people with learning disabilities by treating them all as individuals. This 'person-centred approach' considers the client's ability to exercise choice and control over their lives.

Other types of assessment
- Needs-led Assessment: in this type of assessment the focus is on the individual's needs in a given situation.
- User-led assessment or self-assessment: the responsibility for decisions made about the care of an individual are shared between the care worker and the individual, but the person requiring the care is at the forefront in managing decisions. They assess their needs supported by a health professional and are proactive in determining issues surrounding their care, for example.

- Single assessment process (SAP): All care agencies need to work together so that assessment and the resultant care plan is effective and coordinated. The Single Assessment Process (SAP) was introduced in the National Service Framework for Older People (2001) in Standard 2: Person-centred care, the aim of which was to ensure that the NHS and social care services treat older people as individuals, enabling them to make choices about their own care.
  Many older people have wide ranging needs and in recognition of that, care must be holistic and centre on the whole person. The requirement to develop a Single Assessment Process was based on just this fact, to provide a person-centred health and social care framework, which includes entry into the system, holistic assessment, care planning, care delivery and review.
  In working with partners to deliver care there is always the potential for repetition of work and overlap of delivery. SAP aims to ensure that the individual's needs are assessed thoroughly and accurately, without duplication by different agencies. By sharing the information appropriately between all relevant agencies, SAP coordinates the assessment and ensures effective delivery care.
- Risk assessment: in undertaking an evaluation of risk it is important not to lose sight of person-centred approaches to care and service user choice. (See Unit M1 on risk assessment.) In this approach, risk is identified and assessed as to the possibility of danger, harm or accident happening.

Develop others' understanding of the functions of a range of assessment tools
Your understanding about the assessment process is crucial to delivering care that is of a high quality. As a manager of a service you are also responsible for ensuring that others, such as carers/family members, advocates and colleagues in your own service and other professionals outside your setting, understand the process. You therefore need to be able to develop others' understanding of assessment and why it is beneficial to the service user, as well as how they can contribute.

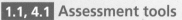

Research it

1.1, 4.1 Assessment tools
Research other types of assessment, including resource-led assessment.

There are a number of tools at our disposal which enable us to assess various functions and care activities. For example:

- Subjective Units of Distress Scale (SUDS) measures anxiety levels.
- Pain Assessment Scales to determine severity and types of pain.
- Scales which measure activities of daily living.
- Scales to measure pressure area risk.
- Patient Health Questionnaire – PHQ-9, which measures severity of depression.
- The Glasgow Coma Scale (GCS) used to rate the severity of coma.

In practice

1.1, 4.1 Assessment and others' understanding

Consider the different forms of assessment used in your care setting and determine how useful they are and what changes might be made to improve what you are doing.

Undertake a staff training session to ensure that 'others' have an understanding of the assessment tools in use.

Research it

1.1 Assessment tools

Research a couple of the assessment tools discussed and identify their use in your assessment process.

Reflect on it

1.1, 4.1 Assessment

Reflect on the staff training session you undertook on assessment. What have you learned from it? What were the strengths and limitations of the session?

AC 1.2 Explain how partnership work can positively support assessment processes

The 2010 to 2015 government policy: Health and Social Care Integration paper (May 2015) outlined the need for integrated care – 'services that work together to give the best care based on a person's personal circumstances'.

Additionally, the Health and Social Care Act 2012 sets out specific obligations for the health system and its relationship with care and support services. This is to make it easier for health and social care services to work together to improve the quality of services. It gives a duty to NHS England, clinical commissioning groups, monitor and health and well-being boards to make it easier for health and social care services to work together. (Source: www.gov.uk/government/publications/2010-to-2015-government-policy-health-and-social-care-integration/2010-to-2015-government-policy-health-and-social-care-integration)

With an increase in the number of people requiring both health and social care and the population becoming older, the likelihood of those with 'complex health needs' will be an issue in the near future. The need to address areas where services are not working well together or where people are not receiving 'joined-up services' is clearly being looked at.

In terms of the assessment process, the current government is keen to fund local councils to ensure that health and social care organisations work together to meet people's needs, and to allow individuals more choice with respect to the services that are right for them, giving them control over their own budgets for health and social care.

Working in partnership means that we have greater access to specialist services, but in working with partners such as other care professionals or family to deliver care, there is always the potential for repetition of work. The need to share information may also compromise confidentiality. However, by sharing the information appropriately between all relevant agencies, and ensuring that the individual remains at the centre of the assessment process, there is likely to be a more effective delivery of care.

In practice

1.2 Partnership work and assessment

How do all the partners you work with contribute to the assessment of care in your setting? Use a client as a case study to show the input.

LO2 Be able to lead and contribute to assessments

Leading on assessments necessitates you having knowledge about what is required and demonstrating that you know how to initiate an assessment and support a service user to participate in the process. The activities you carried out in the last section will help with this.

AC 2.1, 2.2 Initiate early assessment of the individual and support the active participation of the individual in shaping the assessment process

Early assessment

In recent years, there have been media articles about the need for early assessment with respect to memory loss in patients and signs of stroke. The National Institute for Health and Clinical Excellence (NIHCE) recommends that early assessment should take place, to enable planning for the future or, if treatment is to be given, to enable its institution at an early stage. In the case of stroke, the quicker the condition is assessed, the sooner the individual can access treatment and there is the possibility of full recovery. In these cases, then, early assessment is crucial to enable a better outcome for the client.

In all other cases of need, the assessment process should be initiated immediately or as soon as the care requirements of the client change. Early assessment enables the care plan to be implemented with speed and meet the needs of the clients as they arise.

When the assessment takes place, the client needs to be the central figure in the negotiation and this is recognised in legislation as being the optimum process for care planning. Others in the process, including other care workers, family or informal carers, should be clear about their roles and need to know how to record and report on the process.

Any delay that occurs in the assessment process will mean that risk and needs increase and this could lead to care not being given and the service user suffering as a result. The Care Act 2014 clearly states the obligations of the local authority to ensure that patients and carers have access to care services together with an assessment of their circumstances, needs and risks, and also early identification of needs and support.

Support active participation of the individual in shaping the assessment process

To aid the client in the assessment process the best way to proceed is to ask the questions, 'what would you like, what do you need, and how are you feeling at the moment?' By actively encouraging the client to voice their needs, concerns and how they would like their care needs met, a good rapport is developed and the client will feel actively involved in all decisions. Occasionally we may find that the service user is not fully able to engage with the process due to conditions that prevent understanding or sensory impairments which may make the process difficult. In this case an **advocate** needs to be called in to act on their behalf and to ensure they are fully represented.

The NHS recognises that the patient is an expert in their own care and thus developed the Expert Patients Programme (EPP) (2007), which is specifically designed for those with chronic conditions. People living with conditions that are long term know more about their condition and the way in which to manage it than health professionals, and as such are more than able to communicate their needs and what support they may require. (Go to www.nhs.uk/NHSEngland/AboutNHSservices/doctors/Pages/expert-patients-programme.aspx for more information).

Key terms

Active participation enables individuals to have a say in their care and how they live their life. The individual is regarded as an active partner in their own care rather than a passive recipient.

Advocates represent individuals or speak on their behalf to ensure that their rights are supported.

2.1, 2.2 Early assessment and active participation

Present a case study to show how you ensure that clients are assessed early and are a central part of the assessment process. Show the paperwork for one client, ensuring that confidentiality is maintained.

AC 2.3 Undertake assessments within the boundaries of own role

Boundaries for the way in which we practice are in place to keep us and service users safe. For example, some roles require additional training before we are deemed competent to undertake them and assessments are no different. As a health care professional and as a manager, your duty is to provide safe care and to ensure that the staff are equally competent. Staff may therefore need to undertake further training about how to carry out assessments or may require assistance to do so and your role as manager is to support them in this. Job descriptions which clearly outline roles in the position for which staff are employed are invaluable in ensuring boundaries are not breached.

AC 2.4 Make recommendations to support referral processes

Your role in the assessment process may be as a key worker undertaking the whole process and referring the client to various other services, or you may be a care professional who delivers care in another capacity. Whatever part you are playing, you need to ensure that you are able to successfully negotiate with others and refer clients on if you cannot fulfil their needs.

The Commission for Social Care Inspection, in its National Minimum Standards, publishes standards for your particular setting and as such you should make yourself and your staff aware of the regulations for assessment and the updating of clients' care plans. For example, Standard 6.9 states that:

'The service user is made aware of the respective roles and responsibilities of the care manager/CPA care co-ordinator, key worker and/or advocate and knows how to contact them.'

The client needs to be fully aware of the roles of each person involved in their care and you must ensure that you explain to them what your role is. You need to make sure that:

- as far as possible, the needs of the client are being met
- any information obtained from the client is relevant to meet their needs
- the information you provide is coherent and meets the individual needs of the client.

Referrals

At times you may be required to refer the client to another care professional and this can mean a delay in treatment or service delivery. It may be that the service required has a waiting list or it may be simply that the way in which the referral system works is cumbersome or confusing for the client. Clients are often told that a referral to another service will be made, only then to realise they have little or no influence over the process or any knowledge about who the client will be referred to or how long they can expect to wait. This inevitably leads to increased dissatisfaction with the care being given and you are likely to end up with a very unhappy client.

As a manager you can pre-empt this by implementing referral agreements. In the event that referrals need to be made between the partners delivering the client's care, you can undertake the following.

Develop referral guidelines which define the conditions that should be referred

The partnership group should work together to draw up a set of guidelines that outlines the conditions best managed by the setting and the conditions that need to be referred. With each group undertaking this work, there will be information about local practice habits, previous patterns of referral and availability of specialists, as well as current information on how each condition should be managed.

Any referrals to other services should be discussed with the client in advance and the client's consent obtained to disclosing information. You then need to ensure that the recipient of the referral is able to provide the required service and that any confidential information disclosed will be protected.

In practice

2.3, 2.4 Boundaries and referrals

Give evidence to show how referrals are made in your own setting and write a reflective piece about the boundaries within your role in the assessment process.

LO3 Be able to manage the outcomes of assessments

AC 3.1, 3.2 Develop a care or support plan in collaboration with the individual that meets their needs and implement interventions that contribute to positive outcomes for the individual

Developing care plans that meet service-user needs

The responsibility for organising the care planning meeting with the client may lie with you as the manager of the care setting and therefore you need to have gathered all the information for the meeting to take place. This needs to be done in advance of the actual meeting to enable people to read about and understand the services that may be on offer. Only then can informed choices and decisions be made. Personalised care is about focusing on what the service user would like from their care, looking at all their needs and not just medical ones. These may include factors such as personal circumstances, financial difficulties, cultural and ethnic differences, and also mental health needs to name a few. The service user should be encouraged to articulate what they need in respect of resources and support, and what they wish to achieve with the care plan. They should inform the care professional of their preferences for care.

Key term

A care or support plan is a written document or something recorded in patient notes which is an agreement between a service user and health professional to help manage their day-to-day health and care needs.

In practice

3.1, 3.2 Care plans and interventions

Provide evidence that you have developed a care or support plan in collaboration with a client in your care that meets their needs. Describe and analyse the interventions that were implemented, detailing how they contributed to positive outcomes for the client.

Interventions that contribute to positive outcomes for the individual

Before the meeting you need to ensure that contact is made with all who should attend and you also need to be aware of the professional with whom you will be working in order to support this client. For the client, the meeting may be quite a daunting process. They may lack the confidence to be part of a meeting where there are GPs, health visitors and housing officers present and as such, may not participate fully. It is good practice to meet with the client and the family before the meeting to help them through the process and to discuss what will happen and who will be there. You might also help them to prepare what they wish to say and perhaps they might make some notes to help them.

It is possible that you may need to act as an advocate for the client or you might enlist the help of an independent person to do this job, particularly if you are chairing the meeting. This is a difficult situation since it is quite easy to make suggestions as to what you or the advocate thinks is best for the client and yet may be far from what they actually want and would be the best outcome for them. Care must be taken to listen to what the client is saying and to put forward their views, not your own. To ignore a service user's wishes or preferences will lead to lowered self-esteem and demoralisation, so steps need to be taken to ensure this does not happen. Planned interventions must promote positive outcomes and a well-planned care package will build the service user's confidence. If this is not the case then the process has not served its purpose.

Reflect on it

3.1, 3.2 Care plans and interventions

Having completed the above activity, reflect on what you have learned from it.

Research it

3.1, 3.2 Positive outcomes

Using the care plans and assessments in your setting, prepare a short report which shows how the plans developed have led to positive outcomes for the service users.

LO4 Be able to promote others' understanding of the role of assessment

AC 4.2 Develop others' understanding that assessment may have a positive and/or negative impact on an individual and their families

The main aim of any assessment has to be to improve the client's quality of life, but so often, care workers focus merely on the *needs* of the client and fail to recognise their strengths. If we continually focus on what the client is unable to do, we negate the fact that they have strengths in certain areas and they can miss out on optimising their well-being.

In helping others such as other professionals, carers/family members, advocates and colleagues in the care process to understand this, we remind them of the positive and negative impact of assessment on individuals. For example, social dynamics for the family may change when an individual opts to stay at home as this will impact the way family members live their lives. Adjustments made to the fabric of the building may impact on social events that previously took place at home. Perhaps a person being cared for in the home means children have to share bedrooms which may also impact family life. Others in the care process therefore need to understand the impact the assessment is likely to have on their living arrangements and other areas of their lives.

AC 4.3 Develop others' understanding of their contribution to the assessment process

As a manager, you will need to ensure that others understand what their contribution to the assessment process is. Everyone around the service user has the responsibility of being involved in and contributing to assessment – this includes other professionals, informal carers, family members, advocates and colleagues. Colleagues may help by simply listening to what the service user needs and wants and ensuring that their voice is heard. An advocate can contribute by giving the service user information and helping them to understand what they can expect as well as a voice for the individual. The contribution of health professionals will be the application of their specialist knowledge to a situation, but family and informal carers can support the process by supplying much-needed personal information, history and knowledge about the service user's needs and wishes for care as well as emotional support. Everyone involved in care has a contribution to make, which should be encouraged and applauded.

Look at case study 4.3 and answer the questions.

In practice

4.2, 4.3 Developing others' understanding

Using case study 4.3, prepare a staff training session to address Mrs Jones's needs in a more positive manner and encourage the staff to undertake a further assessment which results in a positive outcome for Mrs Jones.

Reflect on it

What have you learned as a result of the training session and your completion of the activities in the unit? How have you ensured that staff have an understanding of the positive and/or negative impact that assessment may have on an individual and their families? How do staff feel they are contributing to the assessment process?

Key term

Others in this learning outcome refer to other professionals, carers/family members, advocates and colleagues.

Case study

4.3 Mrs Jones

Mrs Jones is 75 years old and has recently lost her husband. She is feeling lonely and has problems with her mobility following a stoke four years ago. She is able to cook and clean her house with no problems and manages to go to a local lunch club once a week as the bus stops outside her house every Tuesday. Shopping is difficult and her children and their families all live over 100 miles away and cannot offer any support. She has caring neighbours who pop in from time to time and help with the garden.

Mrs Jones enjoys baking and as an active member of the WI regularly bakes for sales. She also likes to swim but has found it difficult to get to the pool as she doesn't drive. Bathing at home is also a bit of a problem and she does not have a fitted shower so is 'strip washing' every day.

As a manager, you assign a care worker to assess Mrs Jones and ask her about her needs. The care worker notices that Mrs Jones has a mobility problem. Mrs Jones says she has trouble with getting to the shops and is a little lonely.

The care worker puts into place home help to aid Mrs Jones with her housework and arranges a regular supermarket delivery for her main food needs. A care worker also comes in once a week to help Mrs Jones with her bath.

As the manager of the service:

1 What are your views on this outcome for Mrs Jones?
2 How do you think she will be feeling about the services that have been put into place?
3 How might you assist the care worker to revise the care plan?
4 How might you engage with colleagues to determine their contribution to the assessment process?
5 What might you ask them about the plan that has been put into place?

It is possible that you have noticed that although Mrs Jones's needs may be met in this scenario and with these services, there are major limitations in the outcomes.

LO5 Review and evaluate the effectiveness of assessment

AC 5.1, 5.2 Review the assessment process based on feedback from the individual and/or others and evaluate the outcomes of assessment based on feedback from the individual and/or others

Review the assessment process based on feedback

Once the care plan is in place and being implemented, it is most important to monitor its effectiveness, to check whether it is meeting the needs of the individual and to make changes as and when necessary.

At the outset you will have agreed on the following:

- How often should we monitor the plan?
- What methods will we use to monitor the plan?
- Who will be expected to contribute to the evaluation?

How often? This largely depends upon the complexity of the plan and the needs of the client. If the client has severe needs to be met, then changes are likely to happen with more regularity, in which case a weekly meeting may need to be planned to monitor how the plan is working. If, however, the client needs very little support, the need to monitor the plan may become necessary only when a change occurs.

Methods? This can be in written form or at case meetings, but whatever method is used, it is wise to document what has been said, so a verbal report would not be best practice since there is no record.

Who? The more people involved in the care of the client, the more evidence there will be to check the outcomes. There is a danger that too much information may be forthcoming, so you may limit the evaluation to key people. It is also not good practice to overload a lay carer with forms to fill out on a regular basis since they may already feel overwhelmed with the care they are giving.

Once you have the information on how the plan is working, you need to collate the evidence and respond to the changes that are identified.

In reviewing the process you may have asked such questions as whether there was active participation of the services and if this was useful, whether the assessment process was clear for the service user and others, for example.

Evaluate the outcomes of assessment based on feedback

In evaluating outcomes we need to weigh up the positives and negatives within the process. We need to get the services users' views and the views of other professionals, informal carers, family members, advocates and colleagues. Some examples of the sorts of things that might become evident from your monitoring are:

- deterioration or improvement of the client's physical condition
- deterioration or improvement of the client's mental condition
- change in support from neighbours, friends or family
- change in housing
- change in finances
- change in local services on offer
- change in staff in agencies being used.

Whatever changes have been noted for your client need to be recorded and then acted on. The information about the changes must be shared with all involved in the care and action taken as to how the changes will impact on the care and the client.

In reviewing the process there should be a planned meeting in order for all involved in the process to be present to discuss the changes and how they can be dealt with. As the care manager, it is likely that you will be responsible for organising the meeting and drawing up an agenda or a checklist of things that need to be discussed.

In practice

5.1, 5.2 Feedback and assessment

Using the care plan of the client you have recently assessed, provide evidence of the assessment process and show the feedback from the individual and/or others. From the feedback gained, how would you evaluate the outcomes for the individual?.

Research it

5.1, 5.2 Assessment

How effective is assessment? Interview a couple of staff members to as certain their views on the assessment process, in your setting.

AC 5.3 Develop an action plan to address the findings

At the end of the review meeting, you will need to ensure that the care plan is revised and updated with respect to the changes that have been discussed. The client needs to understand how the changes will impact on their care and the significance of the changes.

Revisions to the plan can be as follows:

- **Outcome achieved**: in this case, the client's condition has changed and they no longer require an intervention to help. For example, perhaps they had been suffering from bronchitis which necessitated additional care being put into place. Their recovery means this care is no longer needed.
- **Reduction in support**: this links in with the first outcome and as the client becomes more independent, they may need a reduced level of support and this can be planned for here.
- **Increase in support**: sometimes the client may require more care in certain areas, for example a change in the client's family circumstances. Perhaps a family member moving from the area may mean that they need other care put into place to fill this void.
- **Increase in the type of support needed**: in this case, if the client has become more disorientated or forgetful, they may need a different type of service put into place. The onset of a physical disability may also require a change in care.
- **Changing the method of support**: occasionally, a service provider may go out of business or be unable to offer the service due to resource limitations. In this instance, a new service provider needs to be provided and the change noted in the action plan.

The care planning process is an important one and every step of the way needs to be documented, reviewed and accurately recorded. Good practice demands that confidentiality is respected and that records are maintained in good order. Written reports must be included in the care package. Minutes of meetings with staff in attendance must also be kept and a record of the pre-review meeting should also be available to show how the client was prepared for the meetings.

Changes to the package should be identified clearly and the revised plan made available to all involved in the care to be delivered.

In practice

5.3 Action plan to address findings

Using the care plan and the recent review notes of the client, develop an action plan to address the findings.

Legislation

The Care Act 2014 highlights the obligations of the local authority to ensure that patients and carers have access to care services and can ask for an assessment of their circumstances, needs and risks. It also stresses that the early identification of needs and support helps to stop needs increasing, something that delays in care can cause. You should also look at:

- The Freedom of Information Act 2000
- The Data Protection Act 1998.

Assessment methods

LO	Assessment criteria and accompanying activities	Assessment methods *To evidence coverage of the ACs you could:*
LO1	1.1, 4.1 Research it (p. 247)	Write a short account about other types of assessment.
	1.1, 4.1 In practice (p. 248)	You could consider the questions, and undertake a staff training session and provide a written account to complete the activity.
	1.1 Research it (p. 248)	Provide a written account and document the activity.
	1.1, 4.1 Reflect on it (p. 248)	Provide a reflective account. Ask your assessor to comment on your work.
	1.2 In practice (p. 248)	Conduct an interview, prepare a client case study. Provide a written account.
LO2	2.1, 2.2 In practice (p. 250)	Present a case study and document the paperwork.
	2.3, 2.4 In practice (p. 251)	Provide a (reflective) written piece.
LO3	3.1, 3.2 In practice (p. 251)	Provide evidence through a case study. Write a short report as suggested in the activity.
	3.1, 3.2 Reflect on it (p. 252)	Write a small piece detailing your thoughts.
	3.1, 3.2 Research it (p. 252)	Prepare a short report.
LO4	4.2, 4.3 In practice (p. 252)	Complete the activity and provide a written account.
	Reflect on it (p. 252)	Complete the activity. Discuss this with your assessor.
	4.3 Case study (p. 253)	Read the case study and answer the questions.
LO5	5.1, 5.2 In practice (p. 254)	Complete the activity and provide a written account.
	5.1, 5.2 Research it (p. 254)	Conduct an interview and provide a written account.
	5.3 In practice (p. 255)	Develop an action plan.

References

DOH (2015) *2010 to 2015 Government Policy: Health and social care integration paper. London. Crown copyright.* Also to be found at www.gov.uk/government/publications/2010-to-2015-government-policy-health-and-social-care-integration/.

SCIE (2004) *Leading Practice: A development programme for first line managers* (www.scie.org.uk/publications/guides/guide27/files/lp-participants.pdf).

Smale, G., Tuson, G., Biehal, N. and Marsh, P. (1993) *Empowerment, Assessment, Care Management and the Skilled Worker.* London: HMSO.

Taylor, B. and Devine, D. (1993) *Assessing Needs and Planning Care in Social Work.* London: Arena Press.

Thompson, N. (2005) *Understanding Social Work: Preparing for practice.* Basingstoke: Palgrave Macmillan.

Useful resources and further reading

http://www.local.gov.uk/web/guest/care-support-reform/-/journal_content/56/10180/6522308/ARTICLE

http://www.scie.org.uk/care-act-2014/safeguarding-adults/

Unit CCLD OP 5.25

Undertake a research project within services for health and social care

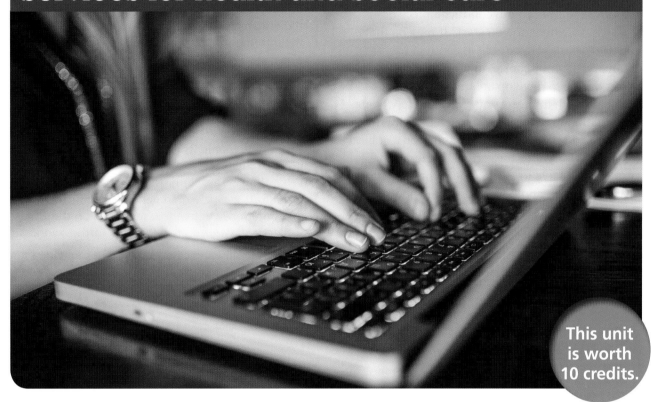

This unit is worth 10 credits.

The purpose of this unit is to assess your knowledge and understanding of the skills that are required to undertake a research project within services for health and social care. Evidence-based practice is now a common expectation for all health and social care practitioners, and to meet these expectations you are required to participate in research initiatives as part of everyday practice. All care practitioners are duty bound to perform care in a safe way. You may also be asked to account for why you undertake a particular practice, and therefore the skills and knowledge for doing so need to be up to date. To 'do no harm' then is the essential premise of evidence-based practice, and the need to be able to demonstrate that the care provided is safe and effective is a reasonable expectation.

Learning outcomes

By the end of this unit you will:

1 Be able to justify a topic for research within services for health and social care.
2 Understand how the components of research are used.
3 Be able to conduct a research project within services for health and social care.
4 Be able to analyse research findings.

LO1 Be able to justify a topic for research within services for health and social care

AC 1.1 Identify the area for the research project

This unit requires you to conduct a piece of research, so where do you start? It may be that you are fortunate to be able to conduct research on an area of your choice, in which case you might decide to develop an area of your own practice which interests you. Alternatively, your organisation may wish to advance their own agenda and ask you to conduct work on a subject they have chosen for the setting. Either way you will still have to think about what you are proposing to do and how you will go about it. Essentially you need to define your starting point and eventually develop a research proposal.

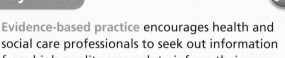

Key terms

Evidence-based practice encourages health and social care professionals to seek out information from high-quality research to inform their own clinical practice and decision making.

Research proposal provides an outline description of the research to be carried out. It summarises the research process and gives information about the information to be discussed in the project.

In practice

1.1 Identify areas for research

Take a few moments to think about an area of practice that you would like to study further. What is an area of interest for you or for your organisation that would benefit from further investigation? Write a few sentences on the subject and why you feel it merits further work.

Read the following case study to get some idea about how you might start to identify areas for research.

Case study

1.1 Julie

Part One

Julie, a care manager in a nursing home, was particularly good at staff training and enjoyed this aspect of her work. Her opportunity to capitalise on this came when she was asked to conduct research into the training needs of newly appointed staff to the care home. She used her 'people skills' to find out as much as she could about the training needs of the staff in order to understand the problem further, and she started interviewing staff in her organisation and comparing this with information from another similar care home. Her love of reading was also useful here, and she started to look at published work on training in health and social care and comparing this with what she had learned in her exploratory work.

She soon realised, however, that this was a huge area and the more she read the more she realised that she had to refine her study to just a small topic area. She decided to focus on induction training and so started the process of limiting her topic and developing just one question she felt needed to be answered.

1 How might she be helped to limit her topic?
2 What questions might you suggest she start with?

AC 1.2 Develop the aims and objectives of the research project

In AC 1.1 and the In practice activity you completed, you will have identified an area of practice that you have an interest in and wish to study further. The case study highlighted the need to refine the area of interest, limiting the range of the topic, and this can be done by clearly stating a question you wish to answer or a problem you wish to solve by the end of the project. This will help to guide your thinking and to keep you focused on the work. It is all too easy at this stage to gather huge amounts of data and to undertake lots of reading, thus losing sight of the actual problem you are trying to solve. Stating the aim of your research will give structure to it which can then guide your reading at the outset. At this point you should also give thought to the reason you are carrying out this piece of work, and the aims and objectives should include this together with an understanding of the sorts of methods that would be useful to use.

Case study

1.1 Julie

Part Two

Julie decided to focus her work on one of the challenges that her setting faces. This is providing good-quality induction training. She refined her aim to:

This project aims to develop a response to the challenges currently faced by organisations in meeting the requirements of the principles underpinning the induction standards for care staff. It is intended that the research findings will contribute to a better understanding of staff needs and the development of a model of induction training.

The objectives to meet this aim are to:

- identify aspects of the induction standards that organisations currently find challenging by auditing the current process by using a questionnaire
- evaluate current practice in my setting and two others
- propose ways in which these may be addressed
- develop a model of training.

In practice

1.2 Aims and objectives

In the case study, Julie gives the reasons for her study ('to respond to current challenges'), together with methods (questionnaire, audit and evaluation of current practice), intention to develop a model of training, as well as to provide a better understanding about the challenges with respect to training.

What is the aim of your project and how do you envisage accomplishing that aim? Describe your understanding of the problem briefly and the reason for your interest. Identify some methods for collecting the information you need in conducting your research.

AC 1.3 Explain ethical considerations that apply to the area of the research project (include confidentiality, sensitivity of data, seeking agreements with participants)

Key terms

Aims are the broad statements of intent of your research project. They highlight what is to be accomplished and seek to address the expectations of the research.

Objectives are the steps you will be taking to answer your research questions. They show how the aims will be accomplished. Aims and objectives include the reasons, understanding and methods for conducting the research project.

Ethics refers to the standards of right and wrong that describe how we ought to behave and that distinguish between acceptable and unacceptable behaviour. This, for example, includes the obligations we have as humans to refrain from murder, assault and causing harm to others, etc. Ethical standards relate to human rights, such as the right to life, or the right to privacy or to freedom. These are the ethical considerations we need to be aware of and examine to ensure that they are reasonable and morally sound.

Historical background and ethical considerations

The key ethical principles that underlie the conduct of research have come about as a result of various historic events in which questionable practice with respect to research was undertaken. Notably, the Nuremburg War Crimes Trial brought attention to the way in which German scientists had conducted experiments on human captives which were often humiliating but more so led to disfigurement and death. (For a report about the Nuremburg Code, see www.cirp.org/library/ethics/nuremberg/)

The Helsinki Declaration (1975) Guidelines required researchers conducting clinical trial procedures, on human subjects to ensure patient safety, by obtaining consent and applying to ethics committees for permissions.

Additionally, the Tuskegee Syphilis Study in the 1950s and 1960 involved African-American participants who were infected with syphilis and had known effective treatments withheld in order to continue the research study and not jeopardize the results. In the light of these particular events, ethical standards had to be re-examined and human subjects protected by the implementation of ethical principles. These principles include:

- **voluntary participation**
- informed consent/seeking agreements with participation
- confidentiality
- anonymity
- sensitivity to data.

There are, however, many more depending upon the research guidelines of the settings in which you are working.

If participants in research are misled in any way, then deception is said to have occurred. This can be the withholding of information or misleading participants in some way.

- **Seeking agreements with participation/informed consent**: any participants in research have the right to be fully informed about the procedures and risks involved and must give their consent to participate. Additionally, participants must not be put at risk of harm, either psychologically or physically as a result of their participation. It is up to the researcher to fully brief participants on the objectives of the study and to explain all aspects of the study, including any interventions that might be carried out.
- **Confidentiality**: participants in research have a right to privacy, and any information they provide during the course of research must be treated confidentially. Any publication of material gained during the study will be anonymised and not be identifiable as theirs. If confidentiality and/or anonymity cannot be guaranteed, then the participant must be warned of this in advance and is then at liberty to refuse to participate. Researchers need to be aware of the Data Protection Act 1998 and to understand what their responsibilities are with regard to confidentiality.
- **Anonymity**: this guarantees that the identity of the participant will remain unknown to others and even to the researcher. It is sometimes difficult to accomplish, especially in situations where the research study is small and the researcher has contact with each participant.
- **Sensitivity of data**: any information or data collected in the course of the research study must be respectfully treated and used honestly. Researchers need to respect the information and avoid any bias at all in the publication of data, and above all publish honestly without deception. Sensitive information collected about participants must be dealt with in a manner that is confidential, and should in no way link to the names of the participant so as to identify them.

Research governance and ethics

The Health Research Authority (HRA) is responsible for publishing guidance on principles of good practice in the management and conduct of health and social care research in England, and in 2015 issued their UK draft policy framework for health and social care research for consultation. It sets out the principles and responsibilities that underpin high-quality research in all health and social care settings.

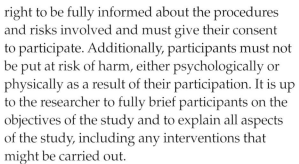

Key term

Voluntary participation refers to the rights of participants to refuse to be part of research if they so choose. People must not be coerced into participating in research.

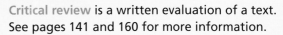

In practice

1.3 Ethical considerations

Explain the ethical considerations that apply to the area of your research project.

Previous to this, responsibility for issuing guidance for research in England was the domain of the Research Governance Framework (RGF).

This framework ensures that there is:

- a quality framework in place
- public confidence in quality research
- principles of good practice
- monitoring and regulation, e.g. through funding bodies; National Patient Safety Agency (for reporting adverse effects).

Department of Health (2005) *Research Governance Framework for Health and Social Care.* London. Department of Health.

Following the analysis of comments from the consultation, a revised version of the guidance will replace the Research Governance Frameworks previously issued by each of the UK Health Departments.

You can find out more by going to www.hra.nhs. uk/documents/2015/02/uk-policy-framework-health-social-care-research-v-1-0-feb-2015.pdf.

In addition to the above, the Economic and Social Research Council have developed a framework for Research Ethics to ensure that all research is carried out to a high ethical standard.

AC 1.4 Complete a literature review of chosen area of research

Undertaking a review of literature ensures that what we are reading is appropriate and of good quality, and also gives structure to our thoughts about the study in question. You may already have undertaken some reading and have conducted some searches for literature.

Reviewing literature has a number of purposes. It helps you to:

- define the subject you wish to work on
- gain a historical perspective of your subject
- make a judgement about the research methods used in the studies
- enables you to suggest further research on the basis of previous knowledge in the area.

Key terms

Critical review is a written evaluation of a text. See pages 141 and 160 for more information.

Critique is similar to evaluation and refers to an analysis. It has both positive and negative connotations as it involves recognising merit but also passing judgement or finding fault.

Reading critically

A 'critical' eye is needed in reading new material. This will help you to get the best out of the review. When we use the word 'critical' or 'critique' we often attach a negative connotation to it. We may feel uncomfortable 'criticising' another's work, but we need to put this into some perspective. The study you read may well be a really good one – you are still undergoing a 'critique' of it, but will be showing it in a positive light. Critical appraisal, then, is not always negative.

Here are some pointers to help you to read in a critical way:

- Keep your purpose in mind when you read. Ask yourself why you are reading this particular study.
- Don't let any extraneous or superfluous arguments in the book or article distract you from your reading.
- Think first about what you are expecting from the article or chapter.
- Skim the headings and the abstract of the piece.
- Look at the first line of each paragraph and the conclusion.

In getting the most out of your reading you should start developing good habits now. For example, make notes about each article or source read and ensure that you include details of the reference. Author, date, title, publisher, place and any page numbers if relevant. It is soul destroying to get to the end of a good piece of work to find you now need to access all the references again! Keep your reading and notes organised and your bibliography up to date as you go along. It is also a good idea now to jot down some topic headings for your literature review.

When you have finished reading your texts, summarise what you have read and write a draft section commenting on it. Ensure that you make the links between what you have read and your own research. Is there anything else you now need to look at which may not have been covered in the review so far?

Sometimes it is difficult to know when to stop reading and to start the actual study, but this will depend on the requirements of your course. If you are undertaking an undergraduate piece of research and are required to submit a 2,000-word literature review, then reading hundreds of articles is likely to make your job a little difficult! Try to stick to the major pieces of work submitted for your research subject and the most up-to-date references.

The next step is to group what you have read into different themes which can then become headings as you write your review. It is wise to be selective here and to only include relevant material that is related to your area of study.

Structure of the literature review

Your literature review should be a coherent piece of work, and so the writing-up of your review must be planned and structured well.

The first task is to make sense of the notes you have made, and organise and arrange them. It is important that the ideas from your reading of articles and books are presented in an order that makes sense in the context of your research project.

Tips

A number of reviews I have read contain a common error – they tend to present material from one author, followed by another, and so on. You can avoid this by organising your review into ideas. You will need to identify common themes and categorise the work you have read into groups of ideas. You could group authors who draw similar conclusions and other authors who disagree. Try not to just describe the work you have read but make comments as to how the work has been used in the field and what it means for you in your own work. By linking what you have read to your study, you are ensuring that the literature review is related to the hypothesis and methodology to follow. A summary of what the

Key terms

Hypothesis is an 'educated guess' which attempts to explain a set of facts. For example, we may guess that smoking causes lung cancer and pose such a hypothesis. We would then go on to devise an experiment to either prove or disprove our hypothesis.

Methodology is an analysis of the ways in which we examine or research phenomena or hypotheses. If we apply the term to a research study, we are referring to the methods or principles we use to study the topic.

literature means and implies will clearly show you have thought about your reading in the light of what is to follow.

Writing your literature review

A literature review has an introduction, main body and conclusion, not dissimilar to an essay. The introduction describes what your research is about and the main topics you are interested in looking at. It will also highlight the background to the study and will describe the focus of your interest.

In the main body there will be an analysis of the literature and it may be structured with headings.

The main body of the review will show how your research develops what has been done before and provides justifications and rationales for what you are doing and why. It will give some indication as to how you intend to carry out the research.

The conclusion provides a summary of where the research you are interested in lies currently, and should highlight any gaps or problems with the existing research. You can then fully address how your research will move the subject forward and address those gaps in knowledge.

The following checklist may prove useful to you in your assessment and any research you may undertake in the future. It should be completed after you have completed your literature review as it will help you to structure the rest of the study.

Selection of sources	Tick
What is the purpose of the review and have you identified it?	
How did you go about it and have you justified your choices?	
Have you justified your choice of materials and stated why you discarded others?	
Have you rationalised what years you excluded?	
Have you emphasised recent developments in the subject under study?	
Have you focused on primary sources with only selective use of secondary sources?	
Is the literature you have selected relevant? How do you know?	
Is your reference data complete?	
Have you critically evaluated the literature?	
Have you organised your material according to issues?	
Have you organised the material in a logical way?	
Does the amount of detail included on an issue relate to its importance?	
Have you critically evaluated design and methodology?	
Have you shown results which were conflicting or inconclusive and suggested possible reasons?	
Have you shown the relevance of each reference to your research?	
Have any interpretations been applied to the topic from what you have read?	
Can you say that the reader's understanding has been enhanced by your summary of the current literature?	
Has your literature review affected the choice of research design and the method for your study?	

Source: Adapted from Worcester University checklist

In practice

1.4 Literature review

Undertake and complete a literature review of chosen area of research.

Using the above checklist, does your review have any gaps which may need to be addressed?

How will you now proceed?

LO2 Understand how the components of research are used

AC 2.1 Critically compare different types of research

Research methods can be divided into two types, primary and secondary:

- **Primary research** focuses on original research which you yourself originate and carry out. Examples include surveys, interviews and observations.
- **Secondary research** is the presentation of other writers' 'primary' research. You will have carried out secondary research in much of your course work. You are accessing secondary sources when engaging in any research for a project or an essay.

When talking about research methodology we also use the terms quantitative and qualitative. These two terms refer to the way in which the research is carried out and the methods used. The data presented at the end of the research is also different.

Quantitative research

If your research is focusing on questions such as 'How many' and 'How often', then you are likely to present your data in terms of numbers and statistics and it will therefore be quantitative in nature.

Originally developed to study natural phenomena, this was the method of choice of natural scientists but is now widely used in education and health care. The methods include surveys, experiments and statistical data.

Strengths of the quantitative approach

- Subject to rigorous controls and checks throughout the process.
- An objective approach to data collection is favoured, and therefore the results are often thought to be more accurate.
- Large numbers of participants (samples) are used in this type of research, therefore a large amount of information can be obtained.
- The findings can be **generalised** to the wider population.
- Studies can be replicated or repeated, and therefore the results obtained can be more readily compared with similar studies.
- In this type of work it is also possible to reduce personal bias, simply because researchers are able to keep their 'distance' from participating subjects.
- This type of research is well controlled, and the methods and instruments used, such as questionnaires, are standardised.

Weakness of the quantitative approach

- Some of the methods involve the use of laboratory conditions, and this is not entirely appropriate when studying human subjects.
- The validity of the study is questionable.
- The way in which questionnaires or survey methods are written may not elicit responses that are useful or real.
- Misunderstanding about the questions can occur.
- The relationship between what somebody says and actually does cannot always be truly tested.
- We all have own unique experiences and this can certainly change the manner in which we behave. In other words, we may all bring a different way to behave to an experiment which is not useful for quantitative research.
- Gathering primary data can result in data unreliability.

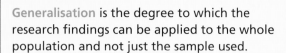

Key term

Generalisation is the degree to which the research findings can be applied to the whole population and not just the sample used.

Ethnography refers to the observation of other people's cultures and customs.

Qualitative research

Qualitative research methods were developed in the social sciences when it was felt that the study of social and cultural phenomenon required a different means of inquiry. This approach seeks to gain insight into people's lives. Their attitudes, behaviours and value systems are the areas of interest for the qualitative researcher who wants to seek out the 'why' of a particular topic. Rather than merely trying to describe a certain phenomenon, this approach attempts to gain a greater understanding and depth about what is happening in a given circumstance.

Using the *phenomenological* approach, as posited by sociologists in an attempt to study the experience of the subjects and how they interpret their world, the researcher becomes an interpreter and attempts to reveal concealed meaning. The four major qualitative approaches are ethnography, phenomenology, field research and grounded theory.

Source: Tilmouth, T., Davies-Ward, E., Williams, B.,(2011) *Foundation Degree in Health and Social care*, London, Hodder Education.

Ethnography

This approach comes from the field of anthropology and is mainly associated with studying culture. Although in the past such research usually concentrated upon culture in terms of ethnicity and geographical location, it now accepts a wider definition and includes studies of any group or organisation. So it is as perfectly acceptable to study the culture associated with a business or health and social care setting, as it is to study the behaviour of a tribe in another part of the world.

The participant–observer method from field research is the method of choice in the ethnographic approach. In this respect the researcher becomes a participant in the culture and observes and records extensive notes. This approach is sometimes known as 'going native'.

Phenomenology

Phenomenology focuses on an individual's subjective experiences and interpretations of the world and how it appears to others. Sometimes considered a philosophical and sociological perspective, it is used in social research disciplines including psychology, sociology and social work.

Field research

Field research is the means of gathering qualitative data in ethnographic research where the researcher goes 'into the field' to make his/her observations of the phenomenon in its natural state. Extensive field notes are generated which are coded and analysed in a variety of ways. Ethnography refers to the way in which the data gathered from participant observation is written into a more meaningful report.

Grounded theory

Grounded theory is an approach that was originally developed by Glaser and Strauss in the 1960s. The purpose of it is to develop theory about phenomena of interest that is grounded in observation.

Strengths of the qualitative approach

- Produces some very in-depth work and rich data about phenomena which is impossible to collect from sets of statistics.
- Enables the researcher to look far more closely at the meanings within behaviour and to understand what is happening in settings, and to question participants' responses to certain issues.
- Enables the study of people in their own settings where there are naturally occurring events that provide rich data for study.
- Enables collection of information in areas where there has been little knowledge in existence in the past, and where the issues under study may be sensitive.
- Enables the researcher to get close to the material under study and to gain in-depth data which can later be subjected to quantitative research.

Weakness of the qualitative approach

- It can be very time consuming to conduct this type of research to gain a valid response.
- Collecting and analysing the material which is often unstructured in nature can also be time consuming.
- Finding themes in reams of notes can at the very least be a little daunting, and trying to find meaning in the materials can also take time.
- The sample size is usually quite small with just a few participants taking part.
- Some critics are concerned that the type of study lacks rigour since variables cannot be controlled.
- Results produced cannot be readily generalised to the population as a whole.

This type of research lends itself to small-scale study and therefore data obtained, while rich, is too small to allow valid conclusions.

Table 14.1 Comparison of quantitative and qualitative research

Quantitative	Qualitative
Quantitative analysis is thought to be objective.	Qualitative data is generally thought to be more subjective.
Thought to have little human bias attached to it.	As it is dependent on people's opinions, and assumptions, there are biases present.
Lack of bias is seen as the data collected relies on the comparison of numbers according to mathematical tests.	Bias is thought to occur because the researcher interprets people's statements or other communication, and this might be influenced by the way the researcher sees the world or approaches the work.

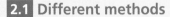
AC 2.2 Evaluate a range of methods that can be used to collect data

Methods for gathering quantitative data

Checklists/scales

A checklist is a tool for identifying the presence or absence of knowledge, skills or behaviours, and is used for identifying whether key tasks have been completed. A good example is the NHS Continuing Healthcare Needs Checklist, which can be found at www.gov.uk/government/uploads/system/uploads/attachment_data/file/213138/NHS-CHC-Checklist-FINAL.pdf.

A rating scale is a tool used for assessing the performance of tasks and skill levels as well as processes and qualities. It is similar to checklists, except that it demands more than a yes or no response; it requires an indication of the level at which something has been accomplished and usually comprises a list of performance statements in one column, and the range of accomplishment stated in descriptive words in another column. This column can indicate a range of achievement, such as from *poor* to *excellent*, *never* to *always*, or simply *strongly disagree* to *strongly agree*. For example, the care worker is honest; *strongly disagree*, disagree, neither agree nor disagree, agree, *strongly agree*.

Both these methods can only tell us that something happens and the extent to which it happens, but they cannot answer questions such as why they happen or how, and therefore have their limitations.

Surveys

Surveys are useful if you want to learn what a larger sample of the population thinks and you need to keep the costs of research down. Surveys tend to have a different way of questioning than interviews and are most useful for gathering data through a wide variety of methods such as emails, post or face-to-face interviews and provide useful statistical data. The disadvantages of using this type of method is that poorly written questions can limit the types of responses you get and may also affect reliability and validity of the study if the questions are biased in any way. Types of surveys include: interview, postal, telephone, internet or online surveys.

(Adapted from Sincero 2012).

Source: Explorable.com: https://explorable.com/advantages-and-disadvantages-of-surveys

The types of survey include:

- **Interview surveys**
  - These may be face-to-face.
  - Can be conducted either 'in-street', 'on-the-doorstep' or 'in-house'.
  - Participants may be randomly selected from a list/database, or specifically chosen.
- **Postal surveys**
  - These are commonly used in lifestyle research.
  - Sample of names and addresses are drawn from a database of the population such as the national census.
- **Telephone surveys**
  - These offer an opportunity for good coverage of the population.
  - They can require a team of interviewers, preferably using a computer-assisted telephone interviewing (CATI) system.
  - Can be costly due to the specialist equipment needed.
- **Internet/online surveys**
  - Individuals are invited to visit (or are sent a link) to a website to complete the questionnaire.
  - The questionnaires may also be attached in an email.

Questionnaires

These are a useful way of engaging large number of people and can be of the 'paper-pencil' variety or may be web based. They can save time and money, and people may well respond in a more truthful way due to anonymity. Unfortunately, the response rate can be very low. Think about the number of questionnaires you may have received in the post and how many went straight into the bin!

Experiments

An experiment generally involves two or more groups: a test group and a control group to which an intervention is applied and then the results observed and measured. This type of study involves the control and observation of variables, with the researcher affecting (controlling) what happens to the subjects and then investigating the effects of the intervention. Experiments are conducted to make comparisons between groups and to examine causal relationships. Experiments are invariably associated with laboratories where there is an assumption that more control can be applied.

It is referred to as the 'Scientific Method' and you may come across this term in your further reading.

One of the major drives for this type of method is the desire to minimise the influences of personal or cultural beliefs on a phenomenon. Therefore this method is concerned with eliminating bias or prejudice in testing a theory. In a health and social care setting it is unlikely that you would choose this type of method, although it is used in medical research and in drug testing.

Experiments usually have three types of variables:

● Independent variable (IV): This is the variable the experimenter manipulates or changes and may have a direct effect on the dependent variable. It is a variable that is not changed by the other

variables you are trying to measure. For example age is an independent variable as is eye colour.

● Dependent variable (DV): This is the variable the experimenter measures, after making changes to the independent variable (or the variable which is changed). It depends upon other factors. For example, the way you deliver care depends upon other factors such as how much sleep you had the night before or even how you are feeling during the shift. So we could say that the Independent Variable (IV) causes a change in the Dependent Variable (DV) but the Dependent Variable cannot cause a change in the Independent Variable. Here is an example to clarify this: perhaps we have a hypothesis that carers with blue eyes are more likely to give better care. The IV is the eye colour of the carer (IV) and we are hypothesising that this will cause a change in care being given (DV). It is, however, not possible to say that the care being given (DV) could cause a change in eye colour of the carer (IV).

● Controlled variables: These are quantities within an experiment that the researcher wishes to remain constant, and he must observe them as carefully as the dependent variables.

Observation

In quantitative research observational methods are more direct and structured and may be undertaken in a laboratory-contrived situation. The downside to using observation as a method is the time it takes and also that behaviour changes when there is another person in the room which may affect the results. It differs from the qualitative type of observation we cover later on pages 268-269.

Interviews

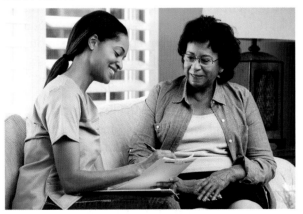

Figure 14.1 Face-to-face interviews allow you to create a rapport with the participants

Research it

2.2 Methods

Look at the methods discussed and carry out some secondary research which identifies the advantages and disadvantages of experiments, the different types of interviews and observational methods.

In quantitative research, interviews are more structured than in qualitative research with standard sets of questions and little else.

Face-to-face interviews enable the establishment of rapport between participants and researcher, allowing the researcher to clarify any answers given. They can be quite time consuming and this is a disadvantage of this type of approach. These are also a qualitative good way to gain qualitative data.

Telephone interviews are quicker and more affordable and give access to many more participants. However, not being able to see the person means that non-verbal cues may be missed which may affect results.

Computer Assisted Personal Interviewing (CAPI) is almost like an online survey where the researcher brings in computers with questions already set up. Although this is a quick way to get information, it is a more expensive approach.

Physiological measurement

This type of research is useful if we want to know how frequently something happens or to test whether a cause and effect relationship is occurring. Pre-test post-test designs measure a variable before and after a procedure, e.g. heart rate before and after exercise to measure recovery rates. A disadvantage of this type is that the equipment used in research may differ. For example, if you are weighing people you need to ensure that the scales being used are giving true readings every time.

Methods for gathering qualitative data

There are a number of ways in which qualitative data can be gathered. These include:

- individual and face-to-face interviews
- focus groups
- observations and ethnography
- action research
- case study.

Individual interviews

This is a good way to gain detailed information from a single individual or small number of individuals, or if you need to gain an expert's view or want more in-depth knowledge of a certain phenomenon.

Face-to-face interviews

These provide the means by which you can adapt your questioning to the answers of the person and you can record the interview. The strengths of these methods are that you can interview people from a wide population, gaining direct feedback. There is also the opportunity to allow the person to clarify their answers. Rich data can be gained using this method in that more sensitive and emotive subjects can be addressed due to the personal interaction involved. There are different kinds of interviews you can conduct, and there is the added advantage of being able to interview people from around the world by phone, email and even online messaging boards, including pages on Facebook. They are, however, less personal ways to collect information, and may limit the amount of information you gain. They may also prevent follow-up questions.

Focus groups

These constitute a group of people being asked about their attitudes towards a product, service, an idea or even the packaging on a brand. The pros and cons for this type of work are similar to interviews, in that you can gain a deep understanding of complex issues due to the more personal contact you will have with the group. The downside is that effort is needed to get people together, and the small numbers involved mean the data will be limited.

Observations and ethnography

Observations involve watching people or animals interact with each other and the setting around them. As a means of gathering information this type of primary research is excellent, since observations do not need to be structured around a hypothesis. Before undertaking more structured research, a researcher might choose to go into a setting and merely observe what is going on. In this way he/she can more readily form a research question. There are different types of observation and each will affect the results obtained, and whichever way observation is done consideration should be given to how the observer may change the event. Have you ever been in a situation where you are aware of a person with a clipboard jotting down notes? The chances are this event in itself will make you change what you are doing.

For example, if Julie (in our case study in this unit) were to observe the induction training in a setting, she may not get a true picture of what is really going on. Her presence may change the outcome. However, becoming a participant in the induction training may mean she is able to gain a lot of information. But in doing her work in this way there is a question of the ethics involved. For example, does Julie tell the other participants that she is a researcher and risk their behaviour changing? If she chooses not to then she risks losing the trust of the participants but also her research may be deemed unethical.

There are ways to address these issues in order to maintain an objective stance, but Julie would need to be very focused and sometimes make several visits to the setting. If she were to attend the training once a week for four weeks, it is likely that she may start to blend into the background and her presence would be forgotten, thus enabling clients and staff in the setting to act in a more normal manner. This is what anthropologists and ethnographers do in studies of different cultures. By becoming part of the culture or community for a period of time, they can blend in and observe from the stance of a participant. We call the types of participation in observation as covert and overt.

Covert observation

- People being studied are unaware of the researcher's presence or the purpose of their being there.
- The researcher needs to assume a false identity, so this immediately raises ethical concerns.
- Although the data collected contributes to the greater understanding of behaviour, critics are concerned with the ethical issues this creates.
- This presents the main drawback to covert observation, and the issues involving informed consent and privacy are most important.

Overt observation

- The researcher reveals him/herself to the group and then carries out observations.
- It may change the manner in which those under study may act and therefore may not give a true picture of what is happening.
- The behaviour may be contrived.
- It reveals something of how they feel about being watched or about showing their feelings.
- Behaviour is often difficult to maintain over a long period, so if the study is long term then natural behaviour can be seen at some point.
- Ethical issues are minimal since the participants know the researcher is there and potentially have the ability to stop the proceedings if they feel it is necessary.

Action research

As the term implies, this is research which is active in nature and is firmly grounded in practice. It is a form of self-reflective inquiry in that it encourages the participants to improve their practice by addressing their understanding about what they are doing and making changes for the better (Tilmouth *et al.*, 2011). This is a practical method used to solve problematic situations in a work setting, and takes the form of completing a number of steps shown below:

- analysing qualitative data/generating hypotheses
- planning action steps
- implementing action steps
- collecting data to monitor change.

The research cannot be generalised or seen to be representative of wider society, and the findings are applicable only to the setting in which the research is carried out. However, this does in no way invalidate the results. Cohen and Manion's (1980, p. 178) definition of this type of research is still valid:

'an on the spot procedure designed to deal with a concrete problem located in an immediate situation … the step by step process is constantly monitored … over varying periods of time and by a variety of mechanisms … so that the … feedback may be translated into modifications, adjustments, directional changes … so as to bring about lasting benefits to the ongoing process.'

This definition implies an ongoing cycle of events, and can be described as a 'cyclical process of change' or a series of planning actions initiated within the setting to address a problem or issue which needs to be explored. The researcher takes on the role of a change agent and works with the clients in the setting.

Case study

A case study usually takes a group and provides an in-depth study of a certain aspect of their lives or setting. The strength of this approach lies in the researcher being able to concentrate on one issue in depth. For example, you may be interested in finding out how a setting is implementing the Safeguarding Agenda, and decide to spend time gathering data about how this particular institution is addressing this issue. You will be able to question, observe, listen and access documentation and then write a report on your findings. Critics of this type of research identify the lack of generalisability of the findings.

You may have recalled that this term is used to describe how representative of the greater population the findings are. In other words, can we safely assume that the setting we are conducting the case study in is similar and contains staff who are similar to other settings in another part of the country? Probably not, and as such we cannot therefore use the findings to suggest that all settings are at the same level of operation as the one we have studied. To apply findings in studies to the wider population we would need to conduct research which involves a bigger sample and more widespread data gathering. The case study does have limitations.

> ### In practice
>
> **2.2** **Methods to collect data**
>
> Which methods to collect data do you favour and why? Evaluate them in the light of your own study and say how they might be used.

> ### Research it
>
> **2.2** **Methods**
>
> Research and look at two qualitative and two quantitative methods that can be used to collect data and information from other sources. Make an evaluation of the four methods and determine which you find the most valuable for your own study.

AC 2.3 Identify a range of tools that can be used to analyse data

There are a number of tools which you can use to analyse and present your data, including:

- tables
- charts
- lists
- maps
- wordclouds (the method by which frequently occurring themes and words are shown on a radiagram in specific colours – see Figure 14.2).

Written reports

Having identified the manner in which you wish to collect your data, you should put it into action and implement your plan. You will then need to organise the data.

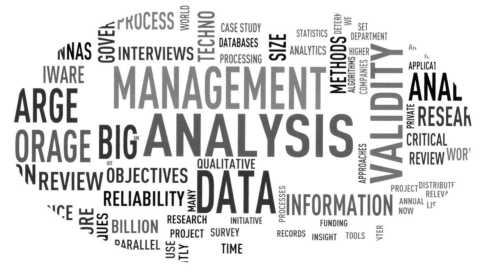

Figure 14.2 Wordclouds

When this part of the work is complete you then need to analyse the data, and this involves examining it. You are now trying to answer your research question and trying to find out whether there are any relationships in what you have seen or if patterns or trends have emerged within the work you have done.

If you have used **quantitative methods** then the data collected might be translated into numbers, which can then be displayed and analysed mathematically. You may need to apply statistical tests to analyse this type of data. Some examples are given below:

- the frequency rate and duration of specific behaviour or conditions
- compilation of test scores from scales, etc.
- survey results of reported behaviour, or ratings of satisfaction, stress, etc.
- numbers or percentages of people with certain characteristics in a population
- statistical procedures such as calculating the mean, median or mode (average) number of times an event or behaviour occurs.

Qualitative data is often written as descriptions of something or opinions given in response to questioning, and is likely to result in huge amounts of written material making analysis an ongoing process rather than a task undertaken at the end of the research.

You may find you have a lot of quotes and there may be many interpretations of an event or phenomenon. However this information is collected, in this form it is unlikely to be able to be analysed using a numerical format.

Unlike numbers, **qualitative information** cannot always be reduced to something definite. While a numerical value placed on an event or situation may tell us how much or how many times something is done or favoured, it cannot possibly inform us as to how an individual *feels* about that event or situation.

Qualitative data is useful to show patterns in behaviour that the numbers in quantitative data cannot, but in good research the use of both quantitative and qualitative information is encouraged.

There are a number of steps the qualitative researcher is likely to take to analyse their results.

- **Step One:** The material from interviews and observations is read and recurring themes are identified. Make a record of this information by constructing a hard copy of transcripts of audio/visual recordings and comprehensive notes of any conversations you have had.
- **Step Two:** Themes are sorted into categories which involves the use of coding which is simply the means by which themes or words are labelled in the text for easy identification later. We might use a simple highlighter pen to do this or a number system. Coding enables the researcher to search the data and to compare it and identify patterns that might be of interest or require further investigation.
- **Step Three:** Links between categories are identified, and charts, thought maps, matrices, flow charts, or time lines may be used to group data.
- **Step Four:** The data is validated (triangulation) using group discussions, and perhaps statistics to investigate how often themes occur. This helps to maintain accuracy. By involving the participants in checking the work you have done you can help improve the accuracy and credibility of the research. Group discussions with peers can also be used to check findings, and questioning can help to validate findings.

Research it

2.3 Quantitative research

In quantitative research, descriptive statistics are used to provide a summary of the data. These include ordinal data, nominal data, interval measurement, ratio measurement, frequency distribution. Conduct some research into these. It will also be useful for you to find out about terms such as central tendency, mean, mode and median, standard deviation, and hypotheses testing.

Key term

Triangulation refers to the use of several methods to test the results in a data set. In order to ensure the work being carried out is valid, the researcher is wise to use multiple methods to compare findings in the data. If the researcher relies on one method only there is no external check to test the result. By using three methods to get at the answer to one question, it is hoped that two of the methods will give similar results thereby validating the study. If the three methods all come up with conflicting results, at the very least the researcher knows that they need to refine the question and readdress the data.

Reflect on it

2.3 Tools

Think of the tools you might use for your own study and reflect on the ones you feel are the best to analyse the data for your own planned project.

In practice

2.3 Tools to analyse data

Identify the tools that you will use within your study to analyse data.

- **Step Five:** Thematic pieces are integrated into a whole – a theory may be posited or an integrated description of the findings made. In this final stage the researcher presents the findings.

AC 2.4 Explain the importance of validity and reliability of data used within research

Validity

This refers to whether a study measures or examines what it claims to measure or examine. A researcher who is trying to measure people's attitudes to pregnant women and smoking, for example, needs to construct a tool that he/she knows is measuring that specific attitude. In this way the results can be accurately applied and interpreted for a test to be valid.

For example, in constructing the tool, attention must be paid to the selection of participants, which should be random, and to the experimental design and methods which must be structured and controlled. Any inconsistency in this or if there is poor use of the methods will compromise the research and it will be deemed to be invalid.

Reliability

Reliability refers to the extent to which an experiment, test or other measuring procedure gives the same results on repeated experiments. Other researchers must be able to perform exactly the same experiment under the same conditions and generate the same results in order to reinforce the findings. This is called replicating findings.

For example, if you are performing a test involving the measurement of a client's blood pressure, you will be using some type of sphygmomanometer (blood pressure monitor). We would hope that the monitors used are calibrated or regulated well enough to give the same results in a reliable fashion, and that a true assessment of the client's blood pressure is recorded each time. However, in order to maintain accuracy, the researcher may decide to take recordings a number of times to minimise the chances of malfunction and maintain validity and reliability.

In qualitative research, however, human judgement may be a concern. For example, if researchers are being asked to rate a certain skill or observe behaviours, their judgement of what they are seeing may vary and this can compromise reliability.

Reliability and validity exit side by side and cannot be mutually exclusive of each other. For example, a measuring tool that is not reliable cannot at the same time be valid. How so? There is no validity if the instrument being used to measure a test is doing so in an inaccurate way. How can your measures of weight be valid if the scales do not operate accurately and reliably?

On the other hand, a measuring tool can be reliable without being valid.

Consider your scales again. Although they are accurate and reliable they cannot be used as a valid measure of blood pressure however reliable they are!

Any tool or test used in research to measure data must be reliable, and by this we are referring to how consistent a measuring device is. The quality of the research itself will be measured by these criteria. This term also refers to its accuracy. For example, if we use a set of scales to measure the weight of our service users, then we would expect that scale to provide consistent and reliable results and the tools we use in research are similar.

LO3 Be able to conduct a research project within services for health and social care

It is now time to conduct your own research and for the remainder of this section you will undertake activities to help you do this.

AC 3.1 Identify sources of support whilst conducting a research project

Your primary source of information and support will be your line manager or the person who will supervise your work. You could also access the library either locally or perhaps at a partner university or college and the internet. If you are undertaking a piece of research for your organisation then you will need to ensure that management is informed about what it is you are doing. For support on a day-to-day basis you might approach your tutor or assessor to see if they are willing to be a mentor to you. A mentor is somebody who has experience in a subject and who can provide you with information about the research process or the subject you are studying.

AC 3.2, 3.3, 3.4 Formulate a detailed plan for a research project; select research methods for the project and develop research questions to be used within project

You may wish to use the following list of steps to plan your research:

- **Step 1** – Choosing the project: In this part you need to identify the things which interest you. Then ask yourself questions such as what are the interesting topics within those themes and what are the key things you want to know about those topics. This is likely to engender a question you wish to answer and you will need to check that it is a reasonable question. This may sound a little obvious, but you should consider whether it is a question that can be answered in your size of project and if it is worth answering. In developing your question, make sure that it is one that you are interested in because this makes the whole process much more enjoyable. Start by listing all the questions you have about the subject and then choose one that stands out. Make sure the question is not too broad and possible to study. This is covered in-depth in LO1.
- **Step 2** – Initial literature review: Now it is time to research and review the literature to enable you to find out what research has already been completed on your subject. This is covered in-depth in AC 1.4.
- **Step 3 (AC 3.3)** – Choose your methods: At this stage you need to choose the best approach to enable you to answer your research question. This is covered in LO2.
- **Step 4 (AC 3.4)** – Finalise your research questions: Having finished the literature review, you may now find that your question has changed as you now have a clearer grasp of what is already known and what may need to be looked at in more detail.

Pilot study is a small-scale preliminary study which is conducted before the main study to check whether it is feasible, how much time it is likely to take and at what cost; and whether there might be any problems. It is designed to predict any issues that might arise before the full study is carried out and to improve on the study design; essentially it is a practice run.

- **Step 5** – Pilot the methods: Whatever method you use, you should check that you can use it correctly and that it will work.
- **Step 6** – Organising the data collection: Think about how you will collect and then organise the evidence you will use to arrive at your conclusions.
- **Step 7** – Data collection: Collecting the data is time limited so make sure you work back from the date the research study is due to be completed.
- **Step 8** – Data analysis: You now need to think about the methods you will use in order to analyses and interpret the information you have gained.
- **Step 9** – Drawing conclusions and interpretations: This is where the detailed interpretations are pulled together to find answers to the research question. It is here you will be reflecting on the conclusions you have drawn and talking about the methods you have used. Finally, you will probably make recommendations for future research in the field.
- **Step 10** – Preparing the final thesis: At this stage you make sure that the work is clear and you start the process of:
  - writing and editing
  - drawing diagrams, tables or charts

In practice

3.2, 3.3, 3.4 Detailed plan, research methods and questions

Produce a detailed plan for a research project and check it with your supervisor.

Consider the research methods you have selected and provide a rationale for the choice.

What other questions may emerge as you undertake the study?

- completing and checking the bibliography and appendices
- preparing the contents and the abstract
- printing and binding the work.

AC 3.5, 3.6 Conduct the research using identified research methods and record and collate data

See LO2 for the information you require in conducting research and recording and collecting data.

In practice

3.5, 3.6 Identified research methods and recording and collating data

Conduct the research using identified research methods and record and collate data.

Is your research method appropriate to the study or do you now feel you should have used a different one? In collating the data what methods will you use and why?

LO4 Be able to analyse research findings

AC 4.1, 4.2 Use data analysis methods to analyse the data and draw conclusions from findings

See AC 2.3 for more information on using data analysis methods to analyse data.

Drawing conclusions from the research study is the final part of the process and probably the most important, because it is here you can determine the success or failure of the study. As part of your conclusion, you will need to state what you found and what you determine the findings to mean. You will also need to remind the reader of the introduction to your research and say what has been achieved.

If you write a weak conclusion to a study that is otherwise really well planned and executed, then there is a chance the findings will not be taken seriously.

In practice

4.1, 4.2 **Analyse data and draw conclusions**

Analyse the data you have collected through your research and summarise the findings. What conclusions have you drawn?

AC 4.3 Reflect how own research findings substantiate initial literature review

In this part of the research you need to ask yourself how your findings link to the original literature review. Do they substantiate what you found in the original literature, or has the research highlighted some new learning on the subject?

AC 4.4 Make recommendations related to area of research

When undertaking this part of the research you must ensure that your results support the recommendations. If, for example, you have researched and developed a new policy, your recommendation may show the steps required to implement the policy, and the resources needed. You might also make recommendations for further research to continue what you have started.

In practice

4.3, 4.4 **Literature findings, review and recommendations**

How have your research findings substantiated the initial literature review, and what recommendations related to the area of research will you make?

AC 4.5 Identify potential uses for the research findings within practice

Here is where you can justify the research carried out and put the findings to practical use. The recommendation section in your study will be useful here, and a short report on what has been accomplished can show how you intend to put the findings into practice.

As part of everyday practice, you are required to participate in research initiatives and provide evidence-based practice, and this is now a common expectation for all health and social care practitioners. One possible use for research findings in practice might be to change care or improve resourcing of an area.

It might even show that an increase in budget is required if certain areas of the service are to remain viable. In carrying out a research study you will have increased your own and others' knowledge about a particular practice, and in so doing will have demonstrated that the care provided is safe and effective.

Reflect on it

4.5 **Findings and practice**

How might you use the findings from your study in practice?

In practice

4.5 **Potential uses for research findings**

Write a report for your staff to show how the research undertaken may be used in practice.

Legislation
- Data Protection Act 1998
- The Equality Act 2010

Assessment methods

LO	Assessment criteria and accompanying activities	Assessment methods *To evidence coverage of the ACs you could:*
LO1	1.1 In practice (p. 258)	You could provide a written account. You could also discuss this with your manager. Justify the choice. Study the 1.1 Case study.
	1.1 and 1.2 Case studies (p. 258 and 259)	Answer the questions and provide written accounts.

➔

LO	Assessment criteria and accompanying activities	Assessment methods *To evidence coverage of the ACs you could:*
	1.2 In practice (p. 259)	Verbally describe the aim of your own project to your assessor before you embark upon the research. Make sure you are fully aware of the problem you are interested in solving and then discuss some of the methods you might use to collect information. Alternatively you could complete a small piece of writing which would become part of the research later which answers the tasks in the activity.
	1.3 In practice (p. 261)	Undertake a professional discussion with your assessor.
	1.4 In practice (p. 263)	You could simply use the checklist to identify any gaps which may need to be addressed or you might first discuss with your assessor the type of literature you need to access and then complete a literature review of chosen area of research.
LO2	2.1 Research it (p. 266)	You need to show your understanding of qualitative and quantitative research. You can do this by defining the two terms and then identifying the different methods of research. Or you could compile a table which show the pros and cons of each type. Finally write a short paragraph to say which you favour and why?
	2.1 In practice (p. 266)	Choose four methods of research and critically compare them in a written piece.
	2.2 Research it (p. 268)	With your assessor discuss the different types of methods and the advantages and disadvantages. Alternatively you could produce a mind map which shows the methods, the pros and cons of each and notes about which you feel are most valuable for your own study.
	2.2 In practice (p. 270)	Provide a written account.
	2.2 Research it (p. 270)	Complete the activity. Prepare a written evaluation.
	2.3 Research it (p. 271)	Produce a diagram that summarises the different types of quantitative data.
	2.3 Reflect on it (p. 272)	Discuss the points in the activity with your assessor.
	2.3 In practice (p. 272)	Provide a short written piece.
	2.4 Reflect on it (p. 273)	Write a short piece or use a spider diagram to show what the two terms mean and where they fit into research.
	2.4 In practice (p. 273)	Explain this to your assessor or you could write a short piece to show your understanding.
LO3	3.1 In practice (p. 273)	Provide a written piece.
	3.2, 3.3, 3.4 In practice (p. 274)	Produce a detailed plan for a research project and check it with your assessor. Use the checklist in the text.
	3.5, 3.6 In practice (p. 274)	Answer the following questions. You might like to discuss these with your assessor.
LO4	4.1, 4.2 In practice (p. 275)	This requires you to take a detailed look at your work so far and make a judgement about the data you have collected through your research and summarise the findings. Discuss your conclusions with your assessor.
	4.3, 4.4 In practice (p. 275)	Write a short account.
	4.5 Reflect on it (p. 275)	Discuss this with your staff at a team meeting. You could write a short piece.
	4.5 In practice (p. 275)	Write a report.

References

Cohen, L., Manion, L. and Morrison, K. (2000) *Research Methods in Education*. London: Routledge.

Department of Health (2005) Research Governance Framework for Health and Social Care (DOH).

Katz, J. (1972) *Experimentation with Human Subjects*. New York: Russell Sage, pp. 305–6.

Nuremburg code, www.cirp.org/library/ethics/nuremberg/.

Tuskegee study, www.cdc.gov/tuskegee/timeline.htm.

Useful resources and further reading

Atkinson, R.L., Atkinson, R. G., Smith, E. E. and Bem, D. J. (2002) *Introduction to Psychology*. San Diego, CA: Harcourt Brace.

Becker, S. and Bryman, A. (2004) *Understanding Research for Social Policy and Practice* (1e). Bristol: The Policy Press.

Bowling, A. (2002) *Research Methods in Health: Investigating health and health services* (2e). Milton Keynes: Open University Press.

Burns, N. and Grove, S. K. (1987) *The Practice of Nursing Research. Conduct, critique and utilisation*. Philadelphia, PA: W. B. Saunders.

Carnwell, R. (2000) 'Essential difference between research and evidence-based practice,' *Nurse Researcher*, 8(2), 55–68.

Clarke, A. M. (1998) 'The qualitative–quantitative debate: moving from positivism and confrontation to post-positivism and reconciliation,' *Journal of Advanced Nursing*, 27, 1242–9.

Coolican, H. (1999) *Research Methods and Statistics in Psychology*. London: Hodder & Stoughton.

Cormack, D. (2000) *The Research Process in Nursing* (4e). London, Edinburgh: Blackwell Science.

Denscombe, M. (2002) *Ground Rules for Good Research: A 10 point guide for social researchers*. Milton Keynes: Open University Press.

Denscombe, M. (2003) *The Good Research Guide for Small-scale Social Research Projects* (2e). Milton Keynes: Open University Press.

Department of Health (1993) *Research for Health*. London: Department of Health.

Dey, J. (1993) *Qualitative Data Analysis: A user friendly guide for social scientists*. London: Routledge.

Economic and Social Research Council (2002) *Research Ethics Framework*. London: HMSO.

Gomm, R. and Davies, C. (2000) *Using Evidence in Health & Social Care*. London: Sage Publications.

Health Research Authority (2015) *Draft UK Policy Framework for Health and Social Care Research*,

www.hra.nhs.uk/documents/2015/02/uk-policy-framework-health-social-care-research-v-1-0-feb-2015.pdf

Holliday, A. (2001) *Doing and Writing Qualitative Research*. London: Sage Publications.

Kerr, A. W., Hall, H. K. and Kozub, S. A. (2005) *Doing Statistics With SPSS* (2e). London: Sage Publications.

Knight, P. T. (2001) *Small Scale Research: Pragmatic inquiry in social science and the caring professions*. London: Sage Publications.

Lincoln, Y. and Guba, E. G. (1985) *Naturalist Inquiry*. Newbury Park, CA: Sage Publications.

Lincoln, Y. S. and Guba, E. G. (2000) 'Paradigmatic controversies, contradictions, and emerging confluences' in Denzin, N. K. and Lincoln, Y. S. (eds) *The Handbook of Qualitative Research*. Thousand Oaks, CA: Sage Publications, pp. 163–88.

Oppenheim, A. N. (1992) *Questionnaire Design, Interviewing and Attitude Measurement*. London: Pinter Publishers.

Robson, C. (2002) *Real World Research: Resources for social scientists and practitioner-researchers*. Oxford: Blackwell Publishing.

Sallah, D. and Clark, C. (2005) *Research and Development in Mental Health Theory, Framework and Models*. London: Churchill Livingstone.

Sincero, S. M. (2012) *Advantages and Disadvantages of Surveys*, Explorable.com: https://explorable.com/advantages-and-disadvantages-of-surveys.

Tesch, R. (1990) *Qualitative Research: Analysis types and software tools*. Basingstoke: The Falmer Press.

➡

Thompson, C., McCaughan, D., Cullum, N., Sheldon, T., Thompson, D. and Mulhall, A. (2001) *Nurses' Use of Research Information in Clinical Decision Making: A descriptive and analytical study: final report.* London: NCC SDO.

Walliman, N. S. R. (2000) *Your Research Project: A step-by-step guide for the first-time researcher.* London: Sage Publications.

www.elsc.org.uk

http://gateway.uk.ovid.com/athens/ (requires ATHENS username and password)

www.pubmed.com

http://bmj.com

www.medicine.ac.uk/bandolier/

www.dh.gov.uk

www.dh.gov.uk/en/Publicationsandstatistics/ Publications/PublicationsPolicyAndGuidance/ DH_4108962

www3.interscience.wiley.com/cgi

Data Protection Act 1998 – Governance Arrangements for Research Ethics Committees (GAfREC), 2011 – see more at www.hra.nhs.uk/ resources/research-legislation-and-governance/ governance-arrangements-for-research-ethics- committees/#sthash.kSJ6x6Nx.dpuf

The Equality Act 2010 – Health Service (Control of Patient Information) Regulations 2002 – see more at www.hra.nhs.uk/resources/before-you-apply/ types-of-ethical-review/ethical-review-of-research- using-confidential-patient-information/#sthash. O1zhhHPv.dpuf

Unit O30c

Facilitate coaching and mentoring of practitioners in health and social care

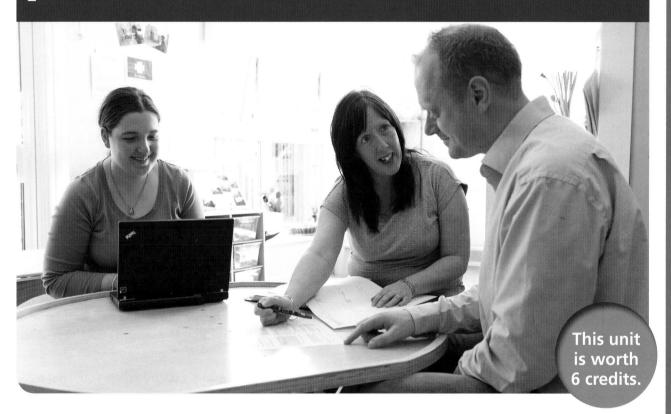

This unit is worth 6 credits.

Continuing Professional Development and lifelong learning are particular requirements for any care professional and are essential for the development and improvement of safe and effective care services, leading to better staff retention as well as contributing to good management practice. Coaching and mentoring are fast becoming an important part of staff development in the support of health care staff.

In this unit you will be introduced to the benefits of coaching and mentoring practitioners in health and social care settings, and look at ways in which you will be able to promote this. Using the activities provided you will be encouraged to identify practitioners' coaching and mentoring needs, implement coaching and mentoring activities and review the outcomes of coaching and mentoring.

Learning outcomes

By the end of this unit you will:

1 Understand the benefits of coaching and mentoring practitioners in health and social care settings.
2 Be able to promote coaching and mentoring of practitioners in health and social care settings.
3 Be able to identify the coaching and mentoring needs of practitioners in health and social care settings.
4 Be able to implement coaching and mentoring activities in health and social care settings.
5 Be able to review the outcomes of coaching and mentoring in health and social care.

LO1 Understand the benefits of coaching and mentoring practitioners in health and social care settings

AC 1.1 Analyse the differences between coaching and mentoring

Coaching and mentoring are similar in nature so we should be clear about what they refer to. Both roles are in place to enable individuals to flourish in their work and also their personal lives.

Gallwey defined coaching as unlocking a person's potential to maximise their performance. It is helping them to learn rather than teaching them (Gallwey 1986, Whitmore 2002)

Successful coaches, according to Parsloe (1999), require knowledge and understanding of process and have at their disposal a variety of styles, skills and techniques. A coach therefore may not have direct experience of a client's formal occupational role, but will be able to use a process to help them to make the changes they desire.

On the other hand, mentoring is a proffesional relationship and is about following in the route of a colleague who can pass on knowledge and experience of a role.

Research it

1.1 Coaching and mentoring

Search definitions of the two terms and prepare a short account of how they differ.

AC 1.2, 1.3 Explain circumstances when coaching would be an appropriate method of supporting learning at work and when mentoring would be an appropriate method of supporting learning at work

In the setting, you may be approached by a member of staff who feels they need to develop new skills in order to enable them in their current work issues. In this situation a coach would be a good option. For example, a coach will assist and challenge the individual to help them work out what they need to do to improve. The coach will ask them to articulate what motivates them and what gets in the way in their work. Rather than direct or teach the individual, a coach will help them to gain confidence and increased awareness about what they need to do to improve their work.

Coaching will be the most useful option when new skills in the workplace are needed and will offer learning opportunities which are geared to individual needs.

On the other hand, the relationship between a mentor and 'mentee' is different and mentors can be more directive in their approach and provide specific advice where appropriate – a coach would not offer their own advice or opinion, but help the individual find their own solution. Mentoring might be a more appropriate route to follow when a supportive role is required. For example, mentoring is about a more experienced colleague supporting the development of those less experienced. Using their greater knowledge and understanding of the work setting, this role is less formal with the mentor acting as a facilitator enabling the individual to perform effectively in a new role.

Mentoring will be most useful when you need to increase team commitment to the workplace and its goals, or you want to improve communication or change the organisational culture in some way.

By engaging with a mentorship system you are more able to help the workforce gain a greater insight into how organisation functions.

In practice

1.1, 1.2, 1.3 Coaching and mentoring

1 What do you understand to be the differences between the two terms?
2 Analyse the differences and say which you feel is more appropriate in your setting. Perhaps you might give examples of the uses.
3 Give an account of when you have used coaching and mentoring as methods of supporting learning at work.

AC 1.4, 1.7 Explain how coaching and mentoring complement other methods of supporting learning, and explain how coaching and mentoring in the work setting can contribute to a learning culture

Continuing Professional Development and lifelong learning are particular requirements for any care professional, and are essential for the development and improvement of safe and effective care services, improving staff retention and contributing to good management practice.

However, Skills for Care in its 'Keeping Up The Good Work – a practical guide to implementing continuing professional development in the adult social care workforce' document (2010) highlights the fact that traditionally the formal training offered to staff ignored a range of other activities such as coaching and mentoring. It writes:

'CPD for the social care workforce ought also to include any development opportunity which contributes directly to improving the quality of service and improved outcomes for people who use services. This may include work-based learning through supervision and other opportunities supported and provided by employers, such as in-house courses, job-shadowing, secondment, mentoring, coaching' (2010, p. 1).

There is much to commend coaching and mentoring in the workplace and this has become a major way in which learning takes place.

As methods of developing staff, coaching and mentoring should be seen to complement traditional training. While attendance at training courses is necessary and a useful way in which to develop staff, the use of one-to-one support through coaching and mentoring relationships can help to focus on developing specific new skills that benefit the individual and the work setting.

Clutterbuck (2011), an authority on coaching and mentoring, argues that significant studies of effective managers revealed that those managers who spend a high proportion of their time and energy coaching or mentoring others get the best results from their teams.

Norman and Roche's (2015) article shows how mentoring is fast becoming an important part of staff development in the support of health care staff.

Research it

1.7 A learning culture

Go to this link, https://www.networks.nhs.uk/nhs-networks/nwas-library-and-information-service/documents/Coaching%20and%20Mentoring%20V2.3%20Word%20EDITED.pdf and download a copy of Coaching and Mentoring: a Quick Guide (2013). This gives you a list of articles about coaching and mentoring.

Look at two articles and give an overview of how coaching and mentoring could become part of your setting to improve the learning within it. Give examples from the articles you have read.

In practice

1.4, 1.7 Coaching and mentoring

Show evidence of your use of coaching and mentoring to support your staff's CPD and comment about how it contributes to a learning culture.

Coaching and mentoring in the workplace means that every opportunity where learning may be required can become an informal learning opportunity and, unlike conventional training, means the focus is on individual and organisational goals or sharing experiences to help a staff member develop new skills while working. This type of activity contributes to the learning culture of the workplace.

AC 1.5 Analyse how coaching and mentoring at work can promote the business objectives of the work setting

Key term

Talent management and development is about using all types of learning, planned and unplanned, to achieve and maintain changes in an organisation in order to gain a competitive edge.

Coaching and mentoring programmes are activities which are part of the spectrum known as 'talent management'. When we spend time developing specific new skills that benefit staff and the workplace (coaching), or we work with a staff member to help them to think through a problem situation or help them to progress their career (mentoring), we are investing time and energy into managing and developing the workforce or the **'talent'** we have in our staff. We should never take for granted the fact that our work setting is only as good as the people who work within it. (Serrat, 2009; CIPD, 2012)

The Institute of Leadership and Management (ILM) research shows that:

> '95% of learning and development managers say that coaching has delivered tangible benefits to their business. 90% of organisations with over 2,000 employees use business coaching.'

Source: https://www.i-l-m.com/Learning-and-Development/Qualifications-explained/coaching-and-mentoring-qualifications/what-is-coaching

The National Skills Academy programmes (www.nsasocialcare.co.uk/programmes/coaching-and-mentoring) also promote coaching and mentoring as a key driver to improved care delivery. With coaching or mentoring schemes in place, staff can be assisted to deal with challenging situations with increased confidence. Additionally, mentoring conversations with the staff can help to promote the objectives of the organisation, and by giving coaching in certain skills objectives can be met more readily.

Reflect on it

1.5 Talent management

Think about the term talent management and development. How do you think staff would feel if they were to be viewed in this way, i.e. as 'talent'? Do you think this is a positive way in which to develop your staff?

In practice

1.5 Coaching, mentoring and business objectives

Write a short piece showing how coaching and mentoring in your workplace might be used to promote the business objectives.

AC 1.6 Evaluate the management implications of supporting coaching and mentoring in the work setting

In practice

1.6 Implications

What do you think are the implications on your role as manager of supporting coaching and mentoring? What do you think are the pros and cons of supporting coaching and mentoring in your role as a manager? Do you think the practice is worth the time and effort?

There is much to commend the use of coaching and mentoring in your workplace. It can empower employees to develop their careers and also helps to build commitment to the setting and the service users. Putting energy into developing the staff will increase the success of the setting. The benefits of such schemes within the workplace are well documented, and the implications for you as a manager will be the development of a committed and skilful team. One downside to the use of coaching and mentoring is the time needed to meet with staff on a one-to-one basis.

AC 1.8 Explain the importance of meeting the learning needs of coaches and mentors

Numerous courses are available for coaches and mentors, and you need to bear this in mind if you are going to ask staff to fill these roles.

Coaching, in essence, requires a person to have high **emotional intelligence** and to be able to relate to people. Not only do they need to understand people but they also need to show interest in them.

Key terms

Emotional intelligence is the capacity some people have to recognise not only their own but others' emotions, and to be able to discriminate between different feelings and labels and deal with them properly. It is about being sufficiently self-aware about our reactions to situations and dealing with the emotions appropriately.

Empathy is the ability to share and understand the feelings of another person.

Some people have a natural ability to show **empathy** and can build rapport quickly, and it is this sort of person who would make a good coach. Additionally, they will have good communication skills, including listening skills. A coach needs to be able to gather information about what the coachee requires, and reflect and clarify that information using good questioning skills to guide the person. Someone who is able to maintain a calm atmosphere during the process is more likely to get better results for the person being coached.

Coaches do not have to have experience of the role they are coaching in, so in your workplace you might use the skills of a person who is from the wider multi-disciplinary team.

With respect to mentoring this is normally a person who is experienced in the job and one who acts as a support for the worker. As with coaching, the skills are similar, although often a friendship might develop.

It is important that those chosen for the coaching and mentoring roles feel that they are able to carry out the role and also are trained in certain techniques. Training coaches and mentors will give them more confidence in their role and will ensure that staff under their tutorship will be given the best opportunities to improve their practice. They should also be people who display the sorts of qualities that one would expect would help them to develop a good relationship with another member of staff. External training courses are in abundance, but just as much can be gained through supervision and learning through others in the workplace.

Reflect on it

1.8 Qualities and characteristics

Have you ever met somebody you instantly warmed to? What was it about them or what they did that made you feel so comfortable?

In practice

1.8 Importance of meeting learning needs of coaches and mentors

Explain how you will meet the learning needs of coaches and mentors in your workplace.

LO2 Be able to promote coaching and mentoring of practitioners in health and social care settings

AC 2.1 Be able to promote the benefits of coaching and mentoring in health and social care

In LO1, we read about some of the benefits of coaching and mentoring. Effective managers are able to motivate and move their teams to action. Clutterbuck (2011) highlighted the benefits of coaching and mentoring for managers, saying that it enabled them to delegate more therefore freeing up time to focus on the most important tasks. He also noted the changes that occurred in the way that people communicate, as well as the quality of personal and organisational decisions and levels of employee retention.

To promote the benefits of this way of working, you need to evaluate the changes that you have noted in the way in which the service runs. For example, you may have seen an improvement in the way in which the team communicate with each other, and you may be reaping the benefits of a more cohesive workforce. These changes promote the on-going practice and development of coaching and mentoring.

In practice

2.1 Promote benefits of coaching and mentoring

Prepare a presentation to staff promoting the benefits of coaching and mentoring for the staff.

AC 2.2, 2.3 Support practitioners to identify learning needs where it would be appropriate to use coaching and where it would be appropriate to use mentoring

Coaching in the setting is a useful option when the learning needs of the staff require confidence to use new skills or to develop areas of practice. For example you may notice that a member of staff is struggling with a clinical skill such as moving and handling of a service user. You notice they take a long time which is not good for the service user who is getting a little frustrated. Coaching in this case would be useful as the coach could offer some suggestions as to how they might carry out the task and how they could improve their technique. They might also suggest completing a further training course or a refresher course to enable them to really grasp the principles they need.

Mentoring, on the other hand, is a less formal approach and in this instance a mentor will work with the care worker and support them in the role they are trying to undertake by giving them advice. They may show them how to carry out the task and be with them as they complete it. It is a more nurturing approach.

There are similarities with both roles but sometimes one is more appropriate to use over the other.

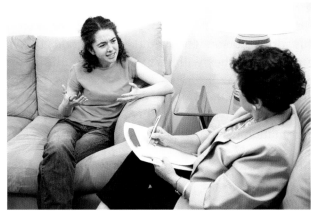

Figure 15.1 Mentoring on a one-to-one basis

In practice

2.2, 2.3 Learning needs

With your staff members, identify learning needs where it would be appropriate to use coaching and then learning needs where it would be appropriate to use mentoring.

AC 2.4 Explain the different types of information, advice and guidance that can support learning in the work setting

Information, Advice and Guidance (IAG) help organisations to develop the work skills and qualifications staff need to do a good job. The Skills for Health website is a useful aid and identifies specialist resources to help you offer such guidance to your staff. Look at the website now.

With high-quality IAG you and your staff can plan the training more effectively and improve the recruitment and retention of staff in the workplace.

Case study

2.2, 2.3 Identifying learning needs for coaching and mentoring

You notice that Jamie, your care supervisor, has a rather difficult relationship with the staff on his shift. They seem to find him a little difficult to work with due to the exacting nature of his style and his somewhat overbearing nature. Often the staff leave the shift feeling worn out and unhappy. In supervision you discuss this with Jamie and he is agreeable to having some help to change his behaviour.

How would you organise help for Jamie and what is more appropriate here – coaching or mentoring?

Jamie is clearly in need of some help and has some learning to do with respect to how he approaches the staff. He clearly needs to learn how to deal with the staff in a more empathetic way so a coach may be able to help him here.

A coach might be a person from another workplace who can come in and observe Jamie at work and then provide feedback as to how he dealt with certain situations. Jamie might be encouraged to look at how his non-verbal communication is impacting the problem, or the way he verbally addresses the staff, and could then be guided as to how this could change. The coach may ask Jamie to undertake some reading work or to collect data on how certain interventions put into place have worked. He/she may also have arranged to see Jamie on a weekly basis and given homework to undertake in between visits.

The mentor on the other hand is likely to work on a one-to-one basis with Jamie in the workplace and is likely to be a colleague Jamie trusts. As a 'critical' friend the mentor is on hand to support Jamie when the going gets tough and can guide him.

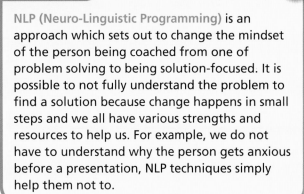

In practice

2.4 Information, advice, guidance

What information, advice and guidance arrangements do you have in place in your work setting? Can you improve their effectiveness?

Key term

NLP (Neuro-Linguistic Programming) is an approach which sets out to change the mindset of the person being coached from one of problem solving to being solution-focused. It is possible to not fully understand the problem to find a solution because change happens in small steps and we all have various strengths and resources to help us. For example, we do not have to understand why the person gets anxious before a presentation, NLP techniques simply help them not to.

Additionally, the Matrix Standard is a nationally recognised quality standard for any organisation that delivers information, advice and guidance (IAG) on learning or work. It helps organisations to demonstrate the quality of their IAG by showing what they are doing and communicating it in a clear way. It is a tool that provides a framework for development and improvement in the workplace, and achieving the standard gives national recognition that the organisation provides high-quality IAG practices and procedures. Health employers that have already been accredited and are planning a future review.

More information about current arrangements and how to arrange for assessment can be found on the EMQC website.

It is also possible that you will have links with local further education colleges and universities, all of which have dedicated teams dealing with IAG. These may be approached for help with respect to learning in the workplace.

AC 2.5 Demonstrate a solution-focused approach to promoting coaching and mentoring in the work setting

In solution-focused coaching and mentoring, the focus is on finding solutions instead of seeking answers to and finding reasons for the problems. It differs from other coaching models and approaches which tend to be more problem focused.

This approach highlights what works well and then makes plans to replicate that work, rather than repeating strategies that are not working well. The Neuro-Linguistic Programming (NLP) adage of 'if you always do the same thing you always get the same results' comes to mind here.

By focusing on the existing skills of the person being coached or mentored, the goals that the person has set for themselves can be reached more

In practice

2.5 Solution-focused approach

Write a short account of what a solution-focused approach to coaching and mentoring is and then give an example of its use from your workplace.

---

readily since they recognise they have the ability and skills to achieve them.

An example of this type of work can be seen in Solution-Focused Brief Therapy which originated as a method of counselling. Since its use in this type of work it has been applied to many other areas such as in schools, supervision sessions, meetings with colleagues, and with professionals in all walks of life.

In coaching and mentoring a solution-focused approach will not focus on the problem that is occurring but the solution that is needed. The coach will elicit information about what might happen if the goal was achieved, if the problem was eradicated, and then discusses with staff how this might have happened. So in this type of work the focus is on the signs that the results are starting to happen. For example, a member of staff may experience anxiety when giving a presentation to managers. Rather than looking at the problem, the coach will look at how the person wants to be during the presentation. They will then discuss the means to achieving this. They look at the steps to completing the presentation successfully.

LO3 Be able to identify the coaching and mentoring needs of practitioners in health and social care settings

AC 3.1 Use different information sources to determine the coaching and mentoring needs of practitioners in the work setting

The different information sources you might use are:

- **Strategic/business plans** – these may well highlight areas of practice that need to change, and coaching and mentoring can then be used to develop this.
- **New legislation/regulation** – if new policies are being brought into practice then there is a need for training and development. Coaching and mentoring is a useful way to ensure the policies are available to staff.
- **Supervision agreements/professional development plans** – staff agree at supervision their developmental needs, and while they may opt to attend lengthy courses, coaching and mentoring can also be a useful addition to the learning and may even provide an alternative way to learn.
- **Availability and expertise of coaches and mentors in the work setting** – staff may require training in the roles of coaching and mentoring.
- **Service users who have different needs** – coaching and mentoring can be a valuable tool, and coaches from different settings can be brought in to help staff develop skills needed to work with these service users.

AC 3.2 Plan coaching and mentoring activities

There are a number of activities for coaching and mentoring and we have covered a few. You will recall the GROW model and the SMART targets in units SHC 52 and LM2c, and these are a couple of ways in which you can work with a mentee or coachee. You might simply start by setting goals and then highlighting steps to reach the outcome and build an action plan. You could also take the time to identify top priorities, challenges and barriers.

For example, a new member of the staff may require help in their role. They may have a mentor who will work alongside them during a shift supporting them in the day-to-day work and to whom they can turn should they feel concerned about the role. Coaching may come in the form of working with other members, for example the multidisciplinary team. They may, for example, be coached by the physiotherapist in moving and handling techniques.

LO4 Be able to implement coaching and mentoring activities in health and social care settings

AC 4.1, 4.2 Support the implementation of coaching and mentoring activities, and select the most appropriate person to act as coach or mentor

One of your main tasks as a manager is to be clear about what the staff need to know in order to carry out their work efficiently and safely. You will have a range of training activities that must be carried

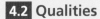

Reflect on it

4.2 Qualities

Reflect on the skills and qualities of the ideal coach or mentor. Think about how to select the most appropriate person to act as mentor.

In practice

4.1, 4.2 Implementing activities and selecting the appropriate person

Using a suitable person (this may be you or another staff member) implement a coaching and mentoring activity.

State the issue. Clearly show the coaching and or mentoring activity and document it. Say why the person was the most appropriate person for this task.

out over the course of the year, but staff will also have identified their own needs with respect to further skills and knowledge they wish to gain. In implementing coaching and mentoring in your workplace you should know your staff well and be able to identify people who have the sorts of qualities we discussed in AC 1.8. In AC 4.3 and 4.4, we explore further how you can select the most appropriate coach to act as coach or mentor. In supporting coaching and mentoring activities, you will need to identify on your CPD plan, the sorts of training and development that might be undertaken during the course of the year for the staff and then determine how best it can be delivered. It might be that some of the sessions can be undertaken by coaches already working in the service.

AC 4.3, 4.4, 4.5 Explain the support needs of those who are working with peers as coaches or mentors, provide coaching in a work setting according to the agreed plan, and provide mentoring according to the agreed plan

Successful mentors and coaches are those who are masters of their craft. They are the people in your organisation who are able to plan and carry out their work using excellent organisational skills, creating a positive climate for care. They are also staff members and peers of the people they are helping, and they will be committed to their own professional growth because they realise this will have a positive benefit for their colleagues and service users. These are the staff who are people oriented, have good interpersonal skills and are well liked by their peers. They should also be willing to share their expertise with others. Having coaches and mentors who are from the same peer group means they are usually at a similar level to those they are working with and they understand the work context and role. As this might well be an additional role for staff members, the support system in place must include training and supervision. A regular meeting may be all that is needed to check in with the coaches and mentors, or they may discuss their experiences during supervision.

Provide coaching and mentoring according to the agreed plan

Your CPD plan for the year identifies what it is that staff need to do in order to practise safely and to develop in their roles. In identifying potential mentors and coaches among the staff, a plan needs to be put into place, and those approached should feel that the role is one which demonstrates their expertise and person-centred skills. You might meet the potential coaches and mentors and identify with them what they can offer to the role and what training needs they may have. This can become part of the overall plan for providing coaching and mentoring, and will include coverage of the skills of the coaches and mentors and how they might be able to provide these skills to others. They should recognise just how important it is to be asked to carry out this task, but should not be made to feel obligated to accept the role.

In practice

4.3, 4.3, 4.5 Supports needs and agreed plans

Show the plan for coaching and mentoring and demonstrate how the choice of staff was made and how they have been prepared for this role. Using your CPD plan, identify the additional training needed for the coaches and mentors. How have the coaches and mentors in your setting been prepared for their roles and how does this fit into the overall CPD plan?

LO5 Be able to review the outcomes of coaching and mentoring in health and social care settings

AC 5.1, 5.2 Review how the use of coaching and mentoring in the work setting has supported business objectives, and evaluate the impact of coaching and mentoring on practice

In evaluating just how well the coaching and mentoring has impacted on the workplace, you will need to discuss the positives and the negatives of the venture. For example, can you show any tangible improvement in staff delivery of certain aspects of care, or is there a concern about the way in which the whole project has been used? Perhaps you have found that a particular project in the workplace has moved on at a great pace and there has been positive feedback from service users to suggest a change in care has had a positive effect. Alternatively, you may find the opposite, and in reviewing what has happened you will need to talk to staff involved and get feedback from both parties to ascertain what has happened. You may discover that personality issues between those involved in mentoring and coaching programmes have emerged and these need to be discussed. Perhaps you have poorly matched staff with mentors and coaches and some resentment has built up. It might even be that the goals set have been unrealistic, leading to the member of staff being overwhelmed by what they have had to do.

See AC 1.5 for more information on how coaching and mentoring can promote business objectives.

AC 5.3 Develop plans to support the future development of coaching and mentoring in the work setting

The plans for your coaching and mentoring programme in your work setting need to link into the strategic plan of the organisation. You will already have identified the training needs of staff and should now be able to see where the coaches and mentors may fit into the plan. In developing the plan further you should be looking at the changes to care work and identifying training to ensure the

In practice

5.1, 5.2, 5.3 Outcomes of coaching and mentoring

Prepare a report which:

a) shows how coaching and mentoring in the work setting has supported business objectives
b) evaluates the impact the plan has had on practice in your setting
c) provides a list of recommendations for the future development of coaching and mentoring in the work setting.

staff remain skilled in what they are doing. For example, the new Associate Practitioner role may appeal to some of your senior health care staff who express a wish to undertake further training.

In your plan there will need to be some reference to how this might be accomplished. This is a positive move and enables your service to keep up to date with developments. On the down side, there will be implications for the budget and also for staff skill mix which will change.

In highlighting exactly what your organisation needs for future care, you clarify how your coaches and mentors will work and what they need to do to develop their roles. Plans need to show what training is mandatory and what is developmental. It also needs to show what can be delivered in-house by coaches and that which needs to be completed off site.

Legislation

Currently there is little by means of legislation that affects coaching and mentoring. A recommendation from the Francis report (2013) to regulate health care assistants, while not taken up by the government, led to plans to introduce a set of mandatory minimum training standards and a code of conduct applicable to all HCAs who report to nurses, midwives and adult social care workers in England (Skills for Care and Skills for Health, 2013). This includes recommendations for personal development to be undertaken. While not specifically mentioning coaching and mentoring, this type of approach is now becoming an attractive way to develop staff.

Assessment methods

LO	Assessment criteria and accompanying activities	Assessment methods *To evidence coverage of the ACs you could:*
LO1	1.1 Research it (p. 280)	Demonstrate to your assessor the difference between coaching and mentoring or undertake a search of the two terms and prepare a short account of how they differ. Be sure to reference your sources.
	1.1, 1.2, 1.3 In practice (p. 280)	Have a professional discussion with your assessor about the points in the activity giving an account of when you have used coaching and mentoring as methods of supporting learning at work, showing an understanding of the differences. Alternatively provide a written account of the answers to the questions.
	1.7 Research it (p. 281)	Complete the activity. You could provide a written piece.
	1.4, 1.7 In practice (p. 281)	Provide a written piece to show evidence of your use of coaching and mentoring to support your staff's CPD and comment about how it contributes to a learning culture.
	1.5 Reflect on it (p. 282)	Interview staff to find out what their views are on the term 'Talent Management'. Ask them how they feel about this term and whether it is a positive one? Alternatively you might discuss this with your assessor.
	1.5 In practice (p. 282)	Obtain a copy of the business objectives for your setting and with the team identify how coaching and mentoring in your workplace might be used to promote these. You could write a short piece.
	1.6 In practice (p. 282)	Write a (reflective) piece about the implications on your role as manager of supporting coaching and mentoring and with your assessor answer the following questions.
	1.8 Reflect on it (p. 283)	Consider making a short journal entry.
	1.8 In practice (p. 283)	Write a short report which explains how you will meet the learning needs of coaches and mentors in your workplace. Or discuss with your assessor ways in which the learning needs can be met.
LO2	2.1 In practice (p. 283)	Prepare a presentation to staff promoting the benefits of coaching and mentoring for the staff.
	2.2, 2.3 In practice (p. 284)	Complete the activity. You could also compile a table showing the differences of each with examples of learning needs.
	2.2, 2.3 Case study (p. 284)	Using the case study, write a reflection about what Jamie needs and the most appropriate manner in which you might help him.
	2.4 In practice (p. 285)	Put a copy of the policy which mentions information , advice and guidance into your portfolio or show some of the documentation. Alternatively you could write a short report about the IAG arrangements in place in your work setting, and then say how you might improve their effectiveness.
	2.5 In practice (p. 285)	Write a short account.
	2.5 Research it (p. 286)	Complete the activity and provide a written account.
	2.5 Reflect on it (p. 286)	Discuss with your assessor the coaching and mentoring that occurs in your setting and demonstrate how effective is it and how might you encourage more practitioners to promote its use?

→

LO	Assessment criteria and accompanying activities	Assessment methods *To evidence coverage of the ACs you could:*
LO3	3.1, 3.2 In practice (p. 286)	Complete the activity. Or you could prepare a table using the headings in the text to identify and plan the coaching and mentoring needs of practitioners in the work setting.
LO4	4.2 Reflect on it (p. 287)	You could write a reflective piece addressing points in the activity. Or you could undertake a real situation and appoint one of the staff to be a coach or mentor. Write a short account of how you selected the person
	4.1, 4.2 In practice (p. 287)	Ask your assessor to observe a coaching and mentoring activity and provide a witness testimony of the observation. Ask the assessor to comment upon the issue being coached or mentored as well as the progress of the session Discuss with the assessor why the person conducting the session was the most appropriate person for this task.
	4.3, 4.4, 4.5 In practice (p. 287)	Place a copy of the plan for coaching and mentoring into your portfolio and write a short report to show how the choice of staff was made and how they have been prepared for this role. Using your CPD plan, identify the additional training needed for the coaches and mentors. Discuss with your assessor how the coaches and mentors in your setting have been prepared for their roles and how this fits into the overall CPD plan?
LO5	5.1, 5.2, 5.3 In practice (p. 288)	Present a mind map or write a short report which addresses the points on the activity.

References

Clutterbuck D (2011) Creating a coaching and mentoring culture, accessed from www.gpstrategiesltd.com/downloads/Creating-a-coaching-and-mentoring-culture-v2.0-June-2011[23].pdf

Gallwey, T. (1986) *The Inner Game of Tennis*, London: Pan.

Gov. (2013) Report of the Mid Staffordshire NHS Foundation Trust Public Inquiry accessed from http://webarchive.nationalarchives.gov.uk/20150407084003/http://www.midstaffspublicinquiry.com/report

NWAS LIS (2013) Coaching and Mentoring: A Quick Guide, accessed from https://www.networks.nhs.uk/nhs-networks/nwas-library-and-information-service/documents/Coaching%20and%20Mentoring%203.0%20pdf.pdf

www.i-l-m.com/About-ILM/Work-with-us/coaching-and-mentoring/coaching-in-organisations

www.nsasocialcare.co.uk/programmes/coaching-and-mentoring

Parsloe, E. (1999) *The Manager as Coach and Mentor*. London: Chartered Institute of Personnel & Development p. 8.

Serrat, O. (2009) *Coaching and Mentoring*. Available at: www.adb.org/publications/coaching-and-mentoring

Skills for Care (2010) *Keeping Up The Good Work – A practical guide to implementing continuing professional development in the adult social care workforce*. Leeds: West Gate,

www.skillsforcare.org.uk

www.management-mentors.com

Skills for Care and Skills for Health (2013) *National Minimum Training Standards for Healthcare Support Workers and Adult Social Care Workers in England*. Bristol: Skills for Care and Skills for Health.

Useful resources and further reading

Davidson, K. (2011) 'Solution focused approaches.' Chapter in Northamptonshire TaMHS Project – Evaluation of Interventions.

Norman, K. and Roche, K. (2015) 'Mentors: Supporting Learning to Improve Patient Care,' *British Journal of Healthcare Assistants*, 9(3), 132–7.

Whitmore, J. (2002) *Coaching for Performance*. London: Nicholas Brealey.

Unit EOL 501

Lead and manage end-of-life care services

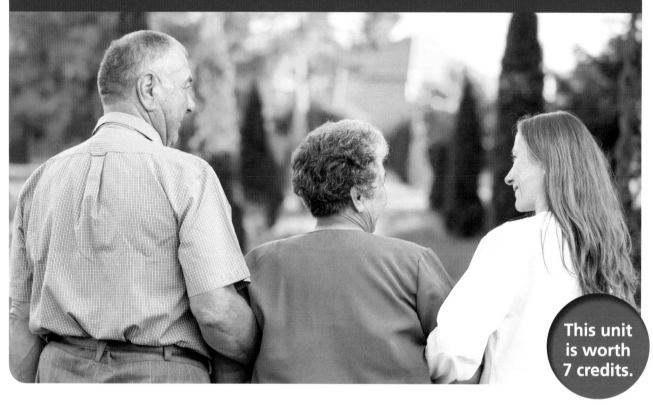

This unit is worth 7 credits.

Good end-of-life care (EOLC) enables individuals to make choices about how they choose to live at the end of their lives and to live as comfortably as possible until they die. The purpose of this unit is to assess your knowledge about EOLC as well as your skills and to help you to gain an understanding about leading and managing end-of-life care services. It will provide an overview of the main points with respect to caring for individuals at the end stage in their lives, as well as managing a service where staff will require more support in this area.

Learning outcomes

By the end of this unit you will:

1 Be able to apply current legislation and policy in end-of-life care in order to develop end-of-life services.
2 Understand current theory and practice underpinning end-of-life care.
3 Be able to lead and manage effective end-of-life care services.
4 Be able to establish and maintain key relationships to lead and manage end-of-life care.
5 Be able to support staff and others in the delivery of excellence in the end-of-life care service.
6 Be able to continuously improve the quality of the end-of-life care service.

LO1 Be able to apply current legislation and policy in end-of-life care in order to develop end-of-life services

AC 1.1, 5.4 Summarise current legislation relating to the provision of best-practice end-of-life care services, and support staff and others to comply with legislation, policies and procedures

> ### Key term
>
> **End-of-life care** is for individuals who are considered to be in the last year of their life or who are receiving palliative care. It refers to enabling people to live as well as possible at this time and to die with dignity. End-of-life care continues for as long as it is needed, and may include those services provided at diagnosis, during treatment or palliative care, including the dying phase, or following death.

Findings that inform legislation

The Department of Health launched the End of Life Care Strategy in 2008, and in 2010 the National End of Life Care Programme's Social Care Framework was proposed. This went a long way to raising awareness and confidence among the social care workforce to support people at the end of life. A 'care pathway' approach to providing end-of-life care has been the means for planning and providing the right kind of care at every stage.

In 2012, the government published the first NHS Mandate in response to a survey carried out in 2011. The survey revealed that although 43 per cent of bereaved people said they thought that care for their loved ones in the last three months of life was excellent or outstanding, 24 per cent had said it was fair or poor. The fact that a large percentage of people were not benefiting from high-quality care at the end of their life led to a government response. The mandate sets out what the NHS must achieve for older people and those people at the end of life. The responsibility for planning for end-of-life care was given to NHS England, an organisation leading and prioritising the care in the National Health Service (NHS) in England.

Legislation

The Human Rights Act 1998* came into force across the UK in 2000 and brought together the UK domestic laws and the rights set out in the European Convention on Human Rights (ECHR). This is currently under review.

(At time of writing, the Conservative Government has proposed to replace the Human Rights Act 1998 with the British Bill of Rights so it will be important to keep up to date with any changes.)

Under this act all 'public authorities', including the NHS, must act in accordance with the rights and duties set out in the act, and health professionals are required to observe the act in reaching decisions about individual patients.

The ECHR rights that are most relevant to decisions about treatment and care towards the end of a patient's life are:

- Article 2: The right to life and positive duty on public authorities to protect life.
- Article 3: The right to be free from inhuman and degrading treatment.
- Article 5: The right to security of the person.
- Article 8: The right to respect for private and family life.
- Article 9: The right to freedom of thought, conscience and religion.
- Article 14: The right to be free from discrimination in the enjoyment of these other rights.

These rights have been open to interpretation and much debate with respect to some challenges to medical decisions, in particular to ethical decisions with respect to withdrawing and withholding treatment and ending life. In addition to the above the NICE quality standard provides specific, concise quality statements and measures which provide the public, health and social care professionals, commissioners and service providers with definitions of high-quality care expected at the end of life.

Staff will need to be well supported if they are engaged in any decision making which may be open to interpretation and may draw them into ethical debates about care and withholding treatment. You can support them by ensuring they are well versed in the legal side of things so they are able to make rational decisions based on facts.

Other legislation relating to the provision of best-practice end-of-life care services that you will need to be aware of includes:

- Data Protection Act 1998
- Access to Health Records Act 1990
- The National End of Life Care Strategy 2008
- The National End of Life Care Programme 2010
- The Nursing and Midwifery Council Standards of conduct, performance and ethics for nurses and midwives 2015
- DH 2013 Code of Conduct for Heathcare Support Workers and Adult Social Care Workers in England, (London, Skills for Care)
- Medicines Act 1968
- Mental Capacity Act 2005
- Registration of Births and Deaths Act 1953

AC 1.2 Apply local and national policy guidance for end-of-life care to the setting in which you work

NHS England in its *Actions for End of Life Care: 2014–16* set out its commitment to developing a vision for end-of-life care beyond 2015, and the need to work with social care providers across the country to ensure the plan is devolved to local level. Your local commissioning group and health authority will have in place guidelines for end-of-life care in your area so it will be useful to ensure you have knowledge of these plans.

AC 1.3 Analyse legal and ethical issues relating to decision making at end of life

Legal issues

The legal position on end-of-life issues is clear and it remains illegal, despite several attempts to put bills through parliament to the contrary, to actively bring about someone's death, with or without the person's consent. However, the ethical considerations for some patients have brought about numerous legal cases in which individuals seek permission to die or to be helped to die.

In one case in 2012, Tony Nicklinson suffered a stroke which left him paralysed from the neck down. He fought for the right to allow doctors to end his life but lost a High Court battle. His response to this ruling was to refuse food. He contracted pneumonia and died aged 58 at his home.

Other cases include the Dianne Pretty 2002 case as well as the Airedale NHS Trust v Bland case. They highlight the ethical implications and difficulties with respect to assisted suicide and withholding treatment. In the Trust v Bland case, the court ruled that where it is not in the patient's interests to continue treatment (in this case Anthony Bland was in a Permanent Vegetative State), omission to act that (intentionally) results in the patient's death is permissible and that in future court approval should be sought in all cases where treatment is proposed to be withheld or withdrawn from a patient. Withholding and withdrawing treatment are both considered omissions to act.

If a person who is deemed competent to act refuses treatment which results in their death, the clinician in charge of the case would not be deemed to be assisting a suicide. It would be unlawful, however, for a competent patient to request that a positive act is taken to end life.

Ethical issues

Other ethical theories and principles are relevant when considering treatment decisions at the end of life. One such debate is the Sanctity of Life Doctrine. This argues that all human life has worth and therefore it is wrong to take steps to end a person's life, either directly or indirectly. Ethical dilemmas arise when individuals question the quality of their lives and request to die (see the Dianne Pretty case). The problems here lie with the definition of quality of life, as our objective view of an individual's life may be very different to the view of the person who is living it.

Health care professionals are expected to act in the patient's best interest (this is called beneficence) or in ways which benefit the patient. Person-centred care demands that the patient, the family and others such as lay carers or ministers and religious guides are part of the decision making in the care pathway. At the end of life, the dilemma often revolves around what course of action will be in the patient's best interests, and while it may be difficult to see how death can be a benefit, if existing quality of life is poor then there needs to be a discussion with respect to the balance of harms and benefits.

Finally, the concept of non-maleficence or doing no harm is sometimes difficult to comply with, particularly in end-of-life care. Many medical treatments may have harmful side effects but may actually save or improve lives. In such cases it is the question of how much harm is caused by the treatment which needs to be considered.

Reflect on it

1.3 Legal and ethical issues

Consider the legal and ethical issues relating to decision making at end of life and justify where you stand on the ethical principles outlined above.

In practice

1.3 Legal and ethical issues

Talk to the staff in your area and check and examine their understanding about the legal and ethical issues surrounding end-of-life care. How might you help them to gain more information about this?

AC 1.4, 5.5 Explain how issues of mental capacity could affect end-of-life care, and support staff and others to recognise when mental capacity has reduced to the extent that others will determine care and treatment for the person at the end of life

The Mental Capacity Act 2005 (England and Wales) and its Code of Practice, and the Adults with Incapacity (Scotland) Act 2000 and its Code of Practice make clear the legal aspects of the decision-making process for adults who lack capacity to make their own decisions.

Additionally, they guide adults to make provision for future decisions by appointing attorneys and by recording statements of their preferences. Adults can also make advance decisions or directives about refusing treatment.

The acts provide statutory safeguards to protect vulnerable individuals in helping them to make judgements about what course of action would be beneficial. Any adult who lacks capacity to make decisions, because of poor communication or mental or physical conditions that make it difficult for them to do so, is fully safeguarded.

End-of-life care becomes more difficult when the patient cannot communicate their wishes or is unable to make decisions due to failing health. These acts and codes therefore protect the person by ensuring that decisions are made in their best interests. Additionally, advocates can be called upon to assist in the decision making by ensuring that the person has as much information as possible to enable an informed decision to be made. Assessment of needs and advanced care planning is also useful here. Also, a member of the family may have lasting power of attorney directive which can help in this.

Staff need to be able to recognise when mental capacity is failing and ensure that the relevant people around the service user can be called upon to help with the decision making. Good advanced care planning will anticipate this happening and will allow you to plan accordingly, but staff must be aware of the importance of thinking ahead to ensure the best care can continue even when the mental capacity of the person is failing.

In practice

1.4, 5.5 Mental capacity and end of life care

1 What do you understand by the term mental capacity and how it might affect end-of-life care?
2 What support do your staff require with respect to recognising when mental capacity has reduced? How do you know they understand what they need to do and who they need to contact?

LO2 Understand current theory and practice underpinning end-of-life care

AC 2.1 Describe the theoretical models of grief, loss and bereavement

People react to grief in a variety of ways. There are many theories about grieving, loss and bereavement and here we mention but a small sample.

Bowlby, attachment theory (1958) and Parkes (1975)

Bowlby (1907–1990) pioneered the theory of attachment in children. His work focused upon troubled young people whose family circumstances separated them from primary care givers. In 1968 he published *Attachment and Loss* in which he asserted a new way of understanding the bonds between child and parent together with the implications of breaking these bonds and the effects this would have on the development of the child. He took these findings and applied them to the loss and separation felt in grief and bereavement. Bowlby suggested that the attachment bond being broken by the death of a loved one led to a normal adaptive response resulting in grief. This work was later developed in collaboration with Colin Murray Parkes, who broke down this natural adaptive grief response into four phases or stages of grief. Murray Parkes' (1975) work proposed four phases of mourning with associated feelings:

1 Numbness: the bereaved person feels a sense of unreality and denial of the event. Emotions become frozen, or cut off.
2 Yearning and Searching: the grieving person tries to relieve the pain of the loss by attempting to recover the lost person. This is associated with feelings of anger, guilt, tension and restlessness as the bereaved person searches potential places for their loss. Dreaming about the lost person and reliving the events surrounding the death is also common.
3 Disorganisation and Despair: described by Parkes as 'a period of uncertainty, aimlessness, and apathy' – this is when the individual experiences depression, anxiety, loneliness and fear.
4 Reorganisation: the individual starts to realise that while they may never really get over the death, they are able to get through it. With an increase in energy and a growth in self-confidence the person can now move forward in a life without the loved one.

Kubler-Ross and the five stages model (1969)

Elisabeth Kubler-Ross published her theory *On Death and Dying* (1969) as a result of work with terminally ill patients facing their deaths and going through various stages of what later became identified as grief. She introduced five stages of grief – denial, anger, bargaining, depression, acceptance. They supply us with a simple explanation of the emotions associated with grief.

William Worden and Tasks of Mourning (1991)

J. William Worden's (1991) model broke the grieving process down into four main tasks or 'flexible phases', some of which could be addressed at the same time or individually. He moved away from the fixed stages that other theorists suggested, with the suggestion that stages might well be revisited even if they felt 'completed'. The tasks were as follows:

1 To accept the reality of the loss and to support the grieving person to move from denying the death when they cannot come to terms with the event to fully realising the person has gone and will not return. Rituals surrounding death are helpful here.
2 To process the pain of grief and support them rather than distract them from it.
3 To adjust to a world without the deceased and enable the person to move forward to make the necessary adjustments to life without the loved one.
4 To find an enduring connection with the deceased in the midst of embarking on a new life, and helping the grieving person to stay connected to the one lost but moving on to a new life.

Stroebe and Schut's Dual Process Model (1999)

This model proposes a revised model of coping which identifies two types of stressors – loss and restoration. Loss-oriented stress results from being focussed upon the person who has been lost and we do this in a number of ways. We may visit places they liked to visit, or reminisce by talking at length about them. Playing music they liked and looking at photos are also loss-orientated activities.

Restoration-oriented stressors refer to the stress that comes to the bereaved person from having to carry out tasks the loved one used to do and the isolation that may come from this. Daily tasks such as cooking and cleaning or fixing the car all take on new meanings for the bereaved person and this can be very stressful. There is a constant movement between loss-oriented and restoration-oriented coping which in this model is referred to as is the concept of oscillation. Healthy grieving means the bereaved person will move constantly between engaging in a dynamic of moving between confronting the death and at other times avoiding it. Stroebe and Schut suggest, unlike other models, that it is healthy to avoid the loss at times and at other times confront it! http://www.whatsyourgrief.com/ offers some useful advice.

In practice

2.1 Models of grief, loss and bereavement
Compare and contrast the models of grief, loss and bereavement you are aware of.

AC 2.2 Explain how grief and loss manifest in the emotions of individuals who are dying and others

Individuals who are at the end of their lives or those around them such as carers, colleagues and other health professionals will inevitably experience emotions of loss and grief, and these manifest in a number of ways which will be unique to each individual involved.

For the individual, there is likely to be a change in their emotions. They may behave in a different way, or the shock of acknowledging the death or impending death may be such that at first it could be difficult to accept. They may exhibit such responses as crying, or in others a numbness may ensue with the person feeling nothing and or/showing no distress.

- Emotions such as anger and resentment are also common and these may happen suddenly, with the person feeling them exhibiting shame at such an outburst.
- Some individuals report a feeling of guilt which may be because of their anger or because of something they had said or done that they regret. There may also be thoughts about what they could have done to prevent the death, and these thoughts may be expressed as 'if only I had said this or done that' or 'what if'.
- Routine is disturbed at this time and this can often result in confusion or feelings of uncertainty about the future. The normal activities of everyday life may seem unimportant.
- The loss and loneliness experienced is also most painful and some people will feel depressed and withdraw from activities they had previously enjoyed.

For those around the person the emotions are likely to run just as high and will need to be acknowledged and managed. Stress levels may well increase and occasionally conflicts may arise. As the manager you need to be aware of the change in behaviour with the staff which might indicate they are finding it difficult to cope.

Those affected may also include care or support staff, colleagues, managers, non-direct care or support staff, carers, families, visitors, volunteers, health professionals, other organisations, social workers, occupational therapists, GPs, speech and language therapists, physiotherapists, pharmacists, nurses, Macmillan Nurses, independent mental capacity advocates, and clinical nurse specialists. We need to be aware of how they may be affected. For example, the family are likely to be greatly affected by the potential loss of a loved one but we should also be aware of those who have dealt with the person in a professional manner over the years and how they might be feeling at this time. The GP for example or the nursing and care staff who have been coming into see the person and delivering care may well have built up a relationship and are also likely to feel the effects of the potential loss. Due to their professional role they will approach this in a different way to the family but it may well have an effect on their emotions at this time.

Research it

2.2 How grief and loss manifest in others

'Others' in this AC may refer to care or support staff, colleagues, manager, non-direct care, or support staff, carers, families, visitors, volunteers, health professionals, other organisations, social worker, occupational therapist, GP, speech and language therapist, physiotherapist, pharmacist, nurse, Macmillan Nurse, independent mental capacity advocate, clinical nurse, specialists.

Choose three of the above, and explain how grief and loss may manifest in their emotions.

In practice

2.2 Grief, loss and emotions

As a care professional you may have experienced such loss when patients or clients are facing the end of life. Think for a moment about the emotions you have observed in yourself and others including health professionals, families and the patient themselves and write about this.

AC 2.3 Analyse how a range of tools for end-of-life care can support the individual and others

The range of tools for end-of-life care include the following.

The Liverpool Care Pathway

The Liverpool Care Pathway for the Dying Patient (LCP) developed by Royal Liverpool University Hospital and Liverpool's Marie Curie Hospice in the 1990s was hailed as a tool for the care of terminally ill cancer patients and was later extended to include all dying patients. It was initially developed to enable multi-disciplinary care teams to make decisions on continuing or discontinuing medical treatment, and putting into place comfort measures during the last days and hours of an individual's life. It became controversial and was largely discredited when a number of cases came to light alleging that people had been placed on the LCP without consent or their family's knowledge. This resulted in the Department of Health initiating an inquiry, the results of which advised that NHS hospitals should phase out the use of the LCP (2013). A review of this has also been carried out. It would be useful for you to research the 'More Care, Less Pathway: A Review of the Liverpool Care Pathway' further.

Gold Standards Framework (GSF)

The GSF provides an evidence-based approach to care for all patients approaching the end of life. It is designed to be applied to individuals with any condition or diagnosis, at any stage in the final years of life in any setting, and may be provided by anyone in health or social care. It represents a complete package of care to improve end of life (Department of Health, *End of Life Care Strategy*, 2008).

Preferred Priorities for Care (PPC) and advance care plan approaches

The Preferred Priorities for Care (2007) is a document in which the patient's wishes and preferences for the last year or months of their life are written down. (You can find this at www.nhsiq. nhs.uk/resource-search/publications/eolc-ppc. aspx.) This activity can help the patient and their carers to plan the care they need and want, and it means that everyone involved in that care knows exactly what the patient needs. It is also called an advanced care plan.

We all wish to provide care which is dignified and allows the patient to have the best care at times of needs. An advanced care plan when used in care homes and residential care allows older people to express their wishes and preferences about the way they want to be supported, particularly at the end of their lives. It also enables staff to care for people in the way they want. By keeping a record of these wishes and preferences, individuals can be supported by staff even if they are unable to express themselves, and their dignity can be maintained.

Welsh integrated care pathway

An Integrated Care Pathway or ICP is a document that records the processes within health and social care to ensure that guidelines and protocols used for end-of-life care are locally agreed and patient centred. Similar to the GSF, it aims to ensure that the care of the patient includes the correct people when they are needed, delivering care in the right place and giving the best attention to the patient experience.

In December 2015, NICE published guidelines on caring for adults at the end of their lives. These guidelines for the NHS are about improving care for people who are in their last days of life, putting the dying person at the heart of decisions about their care. See www.nice.org.uk/guidance/NG31/chapter/Recommendations-for-research

AC 2.4 Explain the pathway used by your local health authority

In your own area there is likely to be a preferred way of caring for people at the end of their lives, and as such a pathway or one of the tools above may have been chosen for use. Alternatively, you may have developed your own way of dealing with EOLC. One of the recommendations of More Care, Less Pathway (the review of the Liverpool Care Pathway) was that the Care Quality Commission (CQC) should review end-of-life care provision across sectors. As such the CQC and the Leadership

Alliance for the Care of Dying People are now implementing an approach to caring for dying people across England which will ensure that everyone who is receiving EOLC has access to high-quality care which meets their needs and wishes.

AC 2.5 Critically reflect on how the outcomes of national research can affect your workplace practices

Research-based evidence contributes to the development of policies and practices that affect the care we give to our patients. Everything we do in care should have a firm foundation in research.

With respect to end-of-life care, new approaches for care have been launched as a result of reviews into the LCP. At a health care conference in September 2014 (Improving End of Life Care – Implementing the New Priority Areas, Outcomes and Guiding Principles for Care at the End of Life), a new focus on giving compassionate care was published.

It recognised that enabling an individual to plan for death needed to start well before a person reaches the end of their life and should be an integral part of personalised and proactive care.

The publication of five new Priorities for Care aimed to promote a stronger foundation for good care and a culture of compassion in the NHS and social care, putting the individual and their families at the centre of decisions about treatment (DOH, 2014).

LO3 Be able to lead and manage effective end-of-life care services

AC 3.1 Explain the qualities of an effective leader in end-of-life care

One of the main areas in which you can set yourself apart as a good leader is to support and facilitate your team. Giving care at the end of life requires staff to provide the most exemplary work for the families and the patient involved, and to do this they need to know that they are in an organisational environment that keeps them safe and gives them support.

As a leader you need to ensure that supervision is available to address the care worker's emotional and development needs, and that staff have manageable workloads. You will also need to train staff so they have the correct skills to deal with the difficult emotions that can arise when working in end-of-life care. The team need to understand their roles in supporting people and be fully aware of issues around mental capacity, advance decisions and Safeguarding of Vulnerable Adults (SOVA), and this can be ensured by establishing systems and procedures that encourage information sharing and good communication.

At this time, staff may feel vulnerable and emotional and so a compassionate attitude is required to support them. Having empathy for how they are feeling and being aware of how this may affect performance at this time are useful qualities to exhibit.

In practice

3.1 Qualities of an effective leader in end-of-life care

Talk to your team and ascertain what they need from you as a leader in supporting them in caring for people at end of life. Write a short piece and then evaluate your skills.

AC 3.2, 5.3 Manage own feelings and emotions in relation to end-of-life care, using a range of resources, and support others to use a range of resources as appropriate to manage own feelings when working in end-of-life care

In the course of your work and in dealing with individuals who are at the end of their life, feelings and emotions run high. You are not only managing the last days or hours of somebody's life but will also be in contact with relatives and friends who are grieving and bereaved. Staff may also be struggling with their own emotions and you will therefore be helping them through this time. Your own emotions are not to be ignored here and one way in which you can help yourself is to debrief.

Debriefing is a process which allows you to discuss any emotions you may have surrounding a case or a particular event to enable you to let go of emotions. In doing so you are able to share experiences with a peer or your mentor and talk through what you are feeling at this time.

Mentoring another staff member in this type of work can be a crucial role. As somebody who is more experienced or knowledgeable about the work you are doing, you can be a valuable guide to the staff member and can provide much needed support in a trying time.

Supervision may also be sought and can help with any guidance, or you can give advice as required. If your supervisor is somebody who has experience in your field of work then they may be able to help you discuss problems and difficulties. They may also suggest counselling services if they feel you might benefit.

Counselling services is a therapy that allows a person to talk about their problems and feelings in a confidential environment. At times we may feel overwhelmed by the emotions we have and may need to talk to somebody impartial about what we are going through. It is not always appropriate to speak to the manager or the mentor, so a counsellor will be a useful contact. The counsellor is trained to listen with empathy and can help the person deal with any negative thoughts and feelings they may be having.

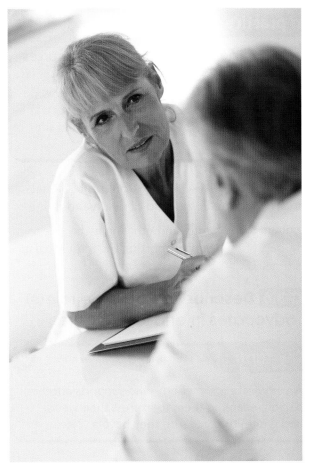

Figure 16.1 Supervision can help a person to deal with their feelings

Others involved in the care of the person at the end of their life will also require your support and you need to be prepared to discuss ways of coping. You could ensure that they know about sources of support and can access such things as counselling if they need it and supervision if available. They may also need to be debriefed following a particularly difficult task and you need to be aware that it may fall to you as the manager in the setting to arrange this or carry this out. A kind word or recognition of their feelings at this time may be all that is required to assure the person or member of staff that you understand how difficult this time may be for them and are there to provide support.

In practice

3.2, 5.3 Managing feelings

Put together a resource pack for staff which identifies where they might seek help to manage their emotions at this time. In dealing with your own emotions which ones do you find useful and why?

Reflect on it

3.2, 5.3 Managing feelings and emotions

Write a short journal piece to show how you have managed your own feelings with a recent end-of-life care case. What have you learned from this case? How would you support a member of staff who is struggling with their emotions?

AC 3.3, 3.4 Use effective communication to support individuals at end-of-life and others, and use effective mediation and negotiation skills on behalf of the individual who is dying

Effective communication

We know how important good communication is to any care situation, but when feelings and emotions are running high more sensitivity to the emotions that individuals are feeling is necessary. The NICE quality standard states that:

> 'People approaching the end of life and their families and carers are communicated with, and offered information, in an accessible and sensitive way in response to their needs and preferences'

Source: NICE quality standard [QS13], 2011

Any information about care must be culturally appropriate and be accessible to individuals with additional needs and to those who do not speak or read English. Access to an interpreter or advocate may be needed. Good communication requires that we need to be sensitive to personal preferences and take approaches that accept patient choice, regardless of our own views in the matter.

Mediating and negotiating

You may also experience difference in opinions about the care being offered. Families may want things done in a certain way, whereas the individual involved may have a different view. In this case you may find yourself acting as a mediator.

In a negotiation of this type the mediator tries to moderate the power imbalances between the family and the individual but does not take sides. It is essential that everybody is able to say what they feel and want. You, however, need to take a neutral stance and steer both parties towards a compromise they are happy with.

AC 3.5 Ensure there are sufficient and appropriate resources to support the delivery of end-of-life care services

Hospice teams are well resourced, but you may find that in your setting palliative care is not a major part of your work. Should you decide that it is in the best interests for a patient to stay in your setting at the end of their life, the resources required may need to be reviewed to enable this to happen. To support this process a coordinated input from the wider multi-professional team needs to be sought. This may, for example, include working in partnership with faith and non-religious communities, charities and volunteers,

and you might also seek help from professionals who are working in the field of death and dying.

Members of the family and others may be able to form part of the team supporting the individual at this time.

AC 3.6 Describe the possible role(s) of advocates in end-of-life care

At end-of-life, however, there may come a point when capacity to make decisions is difficult, and this might mean that the individual is at risk of not being offered all the opportunities and choices they might like. This is when an advocate becomes helpful, as they can listen to the person and help them to explore their options and express their views. By giving them the information they need they can help them to make informed decisions and support them in meeting medical staff. Some charity organisations can provide advocates. For example, MENCAP's Empower Me service is for people with learning disabilities. People who lack capacity due to severe ill health may also require the service of an advocate.

AC 3.7 Manage palliative care emergencies according to the wishes and preferences of the individual

An emergency is generally a condition which if left untreated may result in death. In palliative care dying is an expected outcome, so an emergency in this respect is one in which the quality of life remaining is compromised and prolonging life becomes unrealistic.

In managing such emergencies certain issues must be considered, and you need to be aware of the wishes of the patient and their family, the stage of the condition as well as the nature of the emergency situation.

The most common emergencies are:

- pain crisis or unrelieved symptoms
- spinal cord compression
- haemorrhage
- superior vena cava obstruction
- hypercalcaemia
- airway obstruction or severe shortness of breath
- seizures.

If one of your patients or clients does deteriorate as a result of an emergency, then certain questions need to be answered. Decisions about whether the problem can be treated for the benefit of the patient or whether it should be treated need to be made. Also, if a treatment to be performed is likely to cause more pain, then the appropriateness of such a course of action must be questioned.

Such decisions need to be made with the individual's family, if possible the patient themselves, and other health care professionals.

As some emergencies are expected, an advanced care directive to cover such an eventuality would be a useful way forward. Some people will have provided statements in their end-of-life care plans which clearly state 'Do not attempt cardiopulmonary resuscitation (DNA CPR)', or will expressly state that further treatment to sustain life be withheld at such a time.

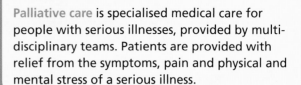

Key term

Palliative care is specialised medical care for people with serious illnesses, provided by multi-disciplinary teams. Patients are provided with relief from the symptoms, pain and physical and mental stress of a serious illness.

Equally they may request that attempts at resuscitation are always tried.

In managing care planning, these types of directives are the best way forward so that the care given at this time can be in the patient's best interest. Person-centred care means that the wishes and choices of the patient are paramount, and must always be foremost in our decision making. Records must be clearly kept which leave us in no doubt of the patient's wishes at crucial times.

In practice

3.7 Managing palliative care emergencies

Describe how you manage emergency situations such as these in your care setting. Can they be improved?

AC 3.8, 6.2 Use a range of tools for end-of-life care to measure standards through audit and after death, and critically reflect on methods for measuring the end-of-life care service against national indicators of quality

The Department of Health published its End of Life Care Strategy: Quality Markers and Measures for End of Life Care in 2009 in which it recommended ten top-quality markers:

1 Have an action plan for the delivery of high-quality end-of-life care, which encompasses patients with all diagnoses, and is reviewed for impact and progress.

2 Institute effective mechanisms to identify those who are approaching the end of life.

3 Ensure that people approaching the end of life are offered a care plan.

4 Ensure that individuals' preferences and choices, when they wish to express them, are documented and communicated to appropriate professionals.

5 Ensure that the needs of carers are appropriately assessed and recorded through a carer's assessment.

6 Have mechanisms in place to ensure that care for individuals is coordinated across organisational boundaries 24/7.

7 Have essential services available and accessible 24/7 to all those approaching the end of life who need them.

8 Be aware of end-of-life care training opportunities and enable relevant workers to access or attend appropriate programmes dependent on their needs.

9 Adopt a standardised approach to care for people in the last days of life.

10 Monitor the quality and outputs of end-of-life care and submit relevant information for local and national audits.

Source: DOH (2009) End of Life Care Strategy: Quality Markers and Measures for End of Life Care. London NSO)

This might be a useful tool to use to audit the end-of-life care your setting provides. In addition, the End of Life Care Quality Assessment (ELCQuA) Tool (http://www.endoflifecare-intelligence.org.uk/home) is an online self-assessment tool which was developed by the National End of Life Care Intelligence Network to help providers of end-of-life care to monitor the quality of services. A set of core measures structured around the NICE Quality Standard for end-of-life care for adults (2011), and other regulations and guidance and progress in care, is assessed against these. However, it was withdrawn in March 2016. (For more information go to www.nice.org.uk/guidance/qs13/chapter/quality-statement-/-identification)

End of life care does not finish when the person dies. In fact this can be a time fraught with all sorts of issues that require other service involvement. For example, the death must be certificated and there may be a need to contact the coroner. Additionally, the patient may have expressed a wish for organ donation so the team concerned with this will need to be contacted.

The way in which the body is handled and prepared for burial or cremation also requires sensitive handling and the staff dealing with this must be aware of cultural and religious differences. All of these factors must be considered and be a part of the care planning process and discussions before the patient dies. You can gain more information at https://www.gov.uk/government/publications/2010-to-2015-government-policy-end-of-life-care/2010-to-2015-government-policy-end-of-life-care.

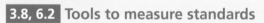

Research it

3.8, 6.2 Tools to measure standards

Go to the websites cited and look at the tools that are available to measure standards for end of life care. Compare two tools and make some recommendations as to how you might use what you have learned in your own setting. How do you think the use of such measures improves the care given to service users?

In practice

3.8, 6.2, 6.3 Tools, standards and improvements

Which tool to measure standards at end of life care is used in your setting?

How effective is the tool used in your setting and how does it fit with national quality indicators? What might you recommend your setting does to improve aspects of the end of life care service?

Research it

LO3, LO6 Tools and standards

The NICE Quality Standards on Caring for Adults at the End of their Lives (2015) outline the methods for measuring the outcomes. These can be found at the ELCQuA which are to be updated in 2016. Go to www.nice.org.uk/guidance/NG31/chapter/Recommendations-for-research

As a manager in a setting that deals with end of life care, you need to have a good understanding and have evaluated the methods you use for measuring the service against quality standards.

Look at how these standards are measured and examine how they might be used in your own care setting.

In practice

4.1, 4.3 Key relationships and decision making

With one patient who is nearing the end of their life, identify the key relationships they have in the form of a mind map and show how the decision making is being shared.

AC 6.3 Use outcomes of reflective practice to improve aspects of the end-of-life care services

Reflection requires practitioners to think deeply about their own practice and by studying the experiences that happen in the course of the working day to improve practice. For example, an incident at work may make you question the way in which you reacted and by reflecting upon it and linking in your current knowledge, you may gain further insight into how you might deal with a similar situation in the future. End of life care can be quite demanding emotionally and you may find reflective practice is a useful way in which to deal with these demands in the best way possible.

LO4 Be able to establish and maintain key relationships to lead and manage end-of-life care

AC 4.1, 4.3 Identify key relationships essential to effective end-of-life care, and implement shared decision making strategies in working with individuals at end of life and others

End-of-life care begins in the 6–12 months before death and ends 6–12 months after death. During this time you will develop a number of relationships with the patient, their family, friends and other care professionals from the multi-disciplinary team. The way in which these relationships develop and function is important to the kind of care the patient can expect and the support for the family following the death, and requires effective coordination and communication across all teams.

The development of the relationships at this time will revolve around the shared decision making that takes place in the months of planning the care. The End of Life Strategy (2008) highlighted the need for people to have choice over where and how they die. Decision making about such things will involve many people who have some sort of relationship with the patient both as family or in a caring role. Key stages put forward in the strategy involve:

1 Discussion on end of life.
2 Assessment and care planning.
3 Coordination of care.
4 Delivery of high-quality care in different settings.
5 Last days of life.
6 Care after death (DOH, 2008).

AC 4.2, 4.4, 4.6 Analyse the features of effective partnership working within your work setting, analyse how partnership working delivers positive outcomes for individuals and others, and explain how to overcome barriers to partnership working

Partnership working is all about sharing, with each partner having something to contribute in terms of skills, knowledge and resources. The partnership should be equal in power and decisions should be made jointly. In Unit M2c we cover partnership working and the essence of it extensively. See ACs 1.1, 1.3 and 1.4 in that unit.

In practice

4.2, 4.4, 4.6 Partnership working

What are the effective features of your own care setting? Why do you think they work so well?

How does your partnership mean your service users get positive outcomes in their care? What is it that you do well? Give some examples to show you have examined this.

What are the barriers you have noticed in your own partnership working and how have you overcome these?

Research it

4.2, 4.6 Outcomes and barriers

Go back to the sections in the unit above and refamiliarise yourself with the outcomes of positive partnerships and barriers to partnership working. What might be a barrier in the case of end-of-life care?

AC 4.5, 4.7 Initiate and contribute to multi-disciplinary assessments, and access specialist multi-disciplinary advice to manage complex situations

In some cases the care becomes very complex and you will need to liaise with other members of the wider multi-disciplinary team. In cases where further help or specialist care is needed, staff should be aware of how to refer the service user to such services.

Any patient who has continuing health care needs or is at the end of life must have a multi-disciplinary assessment. This will involve specified key professionals relevant to the care and treatment they need and might include staff, from nursing, medicine, occupational therapy, physiotherapy as well as relatives/carers.

In Unit SS 5.1 we cover the assessment process (AC 1.2 may be of particular use).

In practice

4.5, 4.7 Multi-disciplinary assessments and advice

In your own setting draw a flow chart of all the people in the multi-disciplinary team you will need to involve in the care of the patient you identified in the 'In practice' activity previously. What is the process of referral to other specialists in the wider team?

LO5 Be able to support staff and others in the delivery of excellence in the end-of-life care service

AC 5.1 Describe how a shared vision for excellent end-of-life care services can be supported

Staff must feel that they are supported in all aspects of their work, and as a manager it is your responsibility to ensure that there is a shared vision for excellence. This needs to be a part of ongoing team meetings in which the strategy for EOLC can be discussed and reviewed. Feedback from staff and other care professionals and families also provides useful information, and can inform you as to the progress of care being given.

AC 5.2, 5.6 Implement strategies to empower staff to ensure positive outcomes for individuals and others, and access appropriate learning and development opportunities to equip staff and others

We have talked at length in other units (including SHC 52, HSCM1 and M3) about how training and development empower staff to develop in their work. There are courses in EOLC that staff may be interested in undertaking in order to further their career, and also to enable them to give excellent quality care for this type of patient. Additionally, coaching and mentoring are useful in this type of care, and it can be very uplifting for staff to have a mentor at their side.

AC 5.7 Explain the importance of formal and informal supervision practice to support staff and volunteers at the end-of-life care

Supervision can be both formal and informal. You may meet regularly with staff at set times and keep records of what has been discussed and planned. This is a formal session and is a time when staff can be praised for their work and also when they can offload and talk about how they have coped with difficult care work. Even though we are busy, supervision should be available at the times arranged and should not be cancelled.

Informal supervision may occur at any time and occurs when the staff member feels they need advice or guidance and seek out their supervisor for support. For example, something may have happened on shift that the staff member feels they need additional help with, and contact with the supervisor will be valuable here. This sort of meeting is unplanned and delivered in response to the supervisees' immediate needs.

It is wise to record the situations (and things discussed in both formal and informal sessions) and then revisit them at the regular planned meeting.

In practice

5.1, 5.2, 5.6, 5.7 Shared vision, empowerment, opportunities and supervision

What is your shared vision for excellent end-of-life care services and how can it be supported?

What strategies do you employ to empower staff involved in the delivery of end-of-life care to ensure positive outcomes for individuals and others?

What learning and development opportunities do you use to allow your staff to equip themselves in this type of work? Are there any others you could suggest or will use in future?

Talk to a member of your staff about the supervision provision within your work setting. Evaluate how well it is managed and how supported staff feel.

Give an account of the formal and informal supervision carried out within your own setting?

How much of each type do you see happening in your setting and which do you value the most?

AC 5.3 Support others to use a range of resources as appropriate to manage own feelings when working in end-of-life care

In practice

5.3 Support others

What resources are available in your setting to support staff in managing their feelings?

How can you as a manager ensure that staff are aware of these resources and feel able to access them?

In end-of-life care the emotional support required by staff is likely to require a more sensitive approach. In SCIE's Effective Supervision Guide (2013) it reports on research into the emotional support of supervisors as being highly effective in dealing with anxiety and stress. By providing and undertaking supervision in a safe, confidential, quiet space with supervisors who are respectful and empathetic, staff could be offered debriefing sessions which deal with the emotional impact of specific cases.

Supervision can help staff to reflect on their feelings and areas of work where they feel vulnerable in a non-threatening way. It is essential that in any supervision work staff are able to feel safe in the relationship and can have trust and confidence in the process. Resources such as these may require appointments to be made and may also incur cost if they are privately obtained. Staff need to be aware that these will be available to them if and when they require them, Alternatively you as the manager may also offer support on an ad hoc basis for staff who are struggling to cope.

AC 5.8 Provide feedback to staff on their practices in relation to end-of-life care

Staff need to know that the work they have done and are doing with respect to EOLC is valued and of excellent quality, and they can be assured of this only if they have feedback. This may simply be a matter of thanking them for their help and hard work at the end of a shift, or may be a more formal form of recognition. Giving negative feedback can be trickier and needs to be delicately handled particularly when emotions are running high. In this case, it would be better to take the member of staff aside and identify what the issue is. They can then be supported to change their practice if that is what is needed. See Unit HSCM1 ACs 5.1 and 5.2 for more information on feedback.

LO6 Be able to continuously improve the quality of the end-of-life care service

AC 6.1, 6.3 Analyse how reflective practice approaches can improve the quality of end-of-life care services, and use outcomes of reflective practice to improve aspects of the end-of-life care service

In EOLC we are often faced with decisions about care that may impact upon our values and beliefs. For example, we may be challenged from time to

time with moral or ethical dilemmas that can make us feel uncomfortable. Reflective practice can help us look at those experiences and the actions we took and help us to really understand ourselves a little better. One method for reflection might be the use of a learning journal in which we think about an incident or experience and question it in the light of what we know we now need to know. We can ask ourselves questions that focus our thoughts and ideas. We can talk about how we felt in the situation and what it was like to feel like that. We might ask ourselves questions about how we could have done things differently and consider whether that might have been better. If we understand the effect our care is having and can have honest appraisals about our work (both positive and negative), we can start to determine how our actions and behaviours impact upon the service user and this will have an effect on care we provide.

Legislation

See AC 1.1 for a list of the legislation that is relevant to your understanding of this unit.

Assessment methods

LO	Assessment criteria and accompanying activities	Assessment methods *To evidence coverage of the ACs you could:*
LO1 (and LO5)	1.1, 5.4 In practice (p. 294)	Write a short essay which summarises the current legislation relating to the provision of best-practice end-of-life care services, and say how you will help staff to become familiar with their roles under this legislation. Or you could prepare a hand-out for staff detailing the current legislation relating to the provision of best-practice end-of-life care services
	1.2 Research it (p. 294)	Complete the activity. Alternatively you could look at the local policy for end-of-life care used by the setting in which you work and write a short piece to show your understanding of it.
	1.2 In practice (p. 294)	Write a short piece to show your understanding.

LO	Assessment criteria and accompanying activities	Assessment methods *To evidence coverage of the ACs you could:*
	1.3 Reflect on it (p. 295)	Write a reflective piece or prepare a training session for staff in which you ask the team to consider the legal and ethical issues relating to decision making at end of life and justify where they stand on the ethical principles outlined.
	1.3 In practice (p. 295)	Complete the activity. Discuss with your assessor how you might help them to gain more information about this?
	1.4, 5.5 Research it (p. 296)	Complete the activity. Make short notes on these and then have a discussion with your assessor about your findings. Deliver a training session for staff to ensure that your team are aware of the codes of practice.
	1.4, 5.5 In practice (p. 296)	Complete the activity, explaining the answers to you assessor.
LO2	2.1 In practice (p. 297)	Compile a table or a mind map which compares and contrasts the models of grief, loss and bereavement you are aware of.
	2.2 Research it (p. 298)	Provide a written piece or you might try to interview individuals for their accounts of how they feel.
	2.2 In practice (p. 298)	Complete the activity. Discuss this with your team and write short notes on their responses.
	2.3 In practice (p. 299)	Provide a written piece addressing the points in the activity.
	2.4 Research it (p. 299)	Complete the activity. Alternatively make notes on the pathway and determine its usefulness by discussing it with your staff.
	2.5 Reflect on it (p. 299)	Write a short reflective piece. Ensure that you put the notes into your portfolio for future reference.
	2.4, 2.5 In practice (p. 299)	Have a discussion with somebody from the wider multi-disciplinary team who has specialist knowledge in end of life care. Ask them the questions in the activity.
LO3 (and LO6)	3.1 In practice (p. 300)	Complete the activity. Write a short piece and then evaluate your skills.
	3.2, 5.3 In practice (p. 301)	Write a short journal piece to show how you have managed your own feelings with a recent end-of-life care case. Put together a resource pack for staff which identifies where they might seek help to manage their emotions at this time. In dealing with your own motions which ones do you find useful and why?
	3.2, 5.3 Reflect on it (p. 301)	Complete the activity. Write a short journal piece. Discuss this with your assessor and say what you have learned from this case?
	3.3 Reflect on it (p. 302)	Prepare a poster which shows how effective the different types of communication are. Or you could use the bullet points and write a short piece to say how they might be used effectively.
	3.3, 3.4 In practice (p. 302)	Put together a session for your staff which details the communication process at this time and their roles in negotiation and mediation. Alternatively if your setting does not have an end-of-life care protocol, devise one for further discussion.

LO	Assessment criteria and accompanying activities	Assessment methods *To evidence coverage of the ACs you could:*
	3.5 In practice (p. 302)	Compile a list of appropriate contacts to help resource end-of-life care in your setting and address points in the activity.
	3.6 In practice (p. 302)	Observe the work of an advocate in your setting and then ask them to discuss their role with you.
	3.6 Research it (p. 302)	Research advocate services and comment on one of the services your setting is likely to call upon.
	3.7 In practice (p. 303)	Discuss with your assessor how you manage emergency situations such as these in your care setting. Can they be improved?
	3.8, 6.2 Research it (p. 304)	Complete the activity. Discuss with your assessor how you think the use of such measures improves the care given to service users.
	3.8, 6.2, 6.3 In practice (p. 304)	Prepare a hand-out about the tool used in your setting to measure standards at end-of-life care. At a team meeting agenda an item to engage staff in discussion about the effectiveness of the tool used in your setting and how it fits with national quality indicators. What might you recommend your setting does to improve aspects of the end of life care service?
	LO3, LO6 Research it (p. 305)	Complete the activity. Make short notes on what you have found.
LO4	4.1, 4.3 In practice (p. 305)	Complete the activity. Alternatively observe the care of a patient who is nearing the end of their life and write an account of the relationships and the decisions being made.
	4.2, 4.4, 4.6 In practice (p. 306)	Prepare answers to the questions and put them into your portfolio.
	4.2, 4.6 Research it (p. 306)	Complete the activity. Discuss this with your assessor.
	4.5, 4.7 In practice (p. 306)	Complete the activity. Discuss with your assessor the process of referral to other specialists in the wider team.
LO5	5.1, 5.2, 5.6, 5.7 In practice (p. 307)	Complete a reflective account. You might also prepare a report to address the points in the activity. You could undertake a professional discussion with a member of your staff. You could give an account of the formal and informal supervision carried out within your own setting.
	5.3 In practice (p. 307)	Make a list of the resources available in your setting to support staff in managing their feelings? Write about an incident in which you as a manager ensured that staff were aware of these resources and were able to access them?
	5.8 In practice (p. 308)	Undertake a professional discussion with a member of staff in which you give feedback about their work with EOLC. Document the feedback given highlighting the areas of encouragement given. How did you show the staff member that they were valued in this instance? How might you improve this part of your role?
LO6	6.1, 6.3 In practice (p. 308)	Using your reflective journal, highlight areas of your learning which might be used to improve practice. Address points in the activity.

References

Bowlby, J. (1980) *Attachment and Loss. Loss, Sadness and Depression. Vol 3.* New York: Basic Books.

Parkes, C. M. (1972) *Bereavement. Studies of Grief in Adult Life.* London: Penguin Books.

Other sources:

Bowlby, J. (1961) 'Processes of mourning,' *The International Journal of Psycho-Analysis*, XLII (4–5).

College of Emergency Management (2012) End of life care for adults in the Emergency Department

SCIE (2013) 'Effective supervision in a variety of settings,' *SCIE Guide 50*, accessed via www.scie.org.uk

DOH (2008) *End of Life Care Strategy: Promoting high quality care for all adults at the end of life.* London: NSO.

DOH (2009) *End of Life Care Strategy: Quality markers and measures for end of life care.* London: NSO.

DOH (2009) *Implementing the New Priority Areas, Outcomes and Guiding Principles for Care at the End of Life.* London: NSO.

Gov.uk (2015) A mandate from the Government to the NHS Commissioning Board:

www.gov.uk/dh

Gov.uk More Care, Less Pathway; A Review of the Liverpool Care Pathway (accessed at www.gov.uk/government/uploads/system/uploads/attachment_data/file/212450/Liverpool_Care_Pathway.pdf)

Health Care Conference (2014) Improving end of life care – Implementing the new priority areas, outcomes and guiding principles for care at the end of life. London: Health Care Conferences UK.

National PPC Review Team (2007) The Preferred Priorities for Care, www.nhsiq.nhs.uk/resource-search/publications/eolc-ppc.aspx (accessed on 19/1/16).

Stroebe, M. and Schut, H. (1999) 'The dual process model of coping with bereavement: rationale and description,' *Death Studies*, 23(3), 197–224, http://dx.doi.org/10.1080/074811899201046

Worden, J. W. (1991) *Grief Counselling and Grief Therapy* (2e). London: Routledge.

www.nice.org.uk/guidance/NG31/chapter/Recommendations-for-research

Useful resources and further reading

Jackson, S. and Morris, K. (1994) 'Looking at partnership teaching in social work qualifying programmes', London: CCETSW.

Unit LM2a

Understanding professional supervision practice

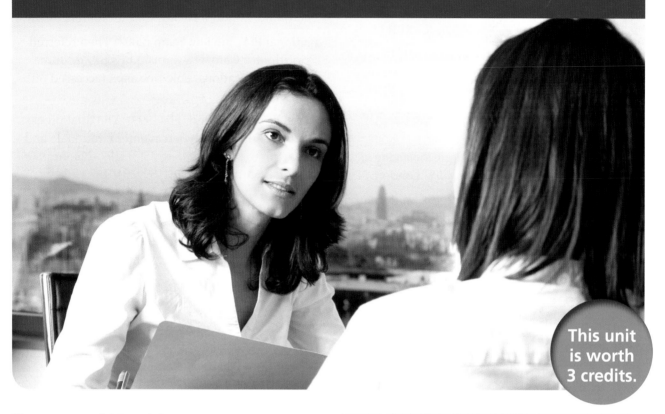

This unit is worth 3 credits.

The purpose of this unit is to assess your knowledge and understanding of professional supervision practice. The previous unit on supervision (LM2c) will have helped you to develop supervision practice in your setting and there will be some overlap with this unit. Cross references have been provided where there is overlap in some of the content. This unit aims to build that knowledge so you have a greater understanding about the role. You should certainly undertake this particular unit if you are preparing for a supervisory role as the content will help that process. Alternatively, if you already carry out a supervisory role then this will certainly enhance your practice.

Learning outcomes

By the end of this unit you will:

1 Understand the purpose of supervision.
2 Understand how the principles of supervision can be used to inform performance management.
3 Understand how to support individuals through professional supervision.
4 Understand how professional supervision supports performance.

LO1 Understand the purpose of supervision

AC 1.1 Evaluate theoretical approaches to professional supervision

Skills for Care (2007) define 'supervision' as 'an accountable process which supports, assures and develops the knowledge skills and values of an individual group or team. It is therefore a process of learning, and a number of approaches and models are available for use.

There are three primary models of supervision:

1 Developmental models.
2 Integrated models.
3 Orientation-specific models.

See Unit LM1c AC 5.4 for solution-focused models.

You will also come across:

4 Managerial supervision.
5 Clinical supervision.
6 Professional supervision.

The first models are those primarily used in a counselling or psychotherapeutic context.

Developmental models

Stoltenberg and Delworth's (1987) developmental model has three levels for supervisees – beginning, intermediate and advanced – and the focus in each level is on the development of self-awareness, motivation and autonomy.

For supervisors using this type of model it is important to accurately identify the supervisee's current stage of development and provide support which is necessary at that developmental stage (Stoltenberg and Delworth, 1987).

See LM2c AC 1.2 for more information on Stoltenberg and Delworth's model.

Integrated models

These are more eclectic in nature and integrate several models. It is not unusual for a therapist to use several models in their work and this type of supervision mirrors this. Bernard's Discrimination Model purports to be 'a-theoretical', (Bernard and Goodyear, 1992) and was originally developed as a conceptual framework to assist new supervisors providing a structure and focus for supervision. Three supervisory roles of teacher, counsellor and consultant are used with three key areas of process, conceptualisation and personalisation.

If, for example, the supervisor took on a teaching role, they may instruct and inform the supervisee. In the counselling role they might assist and facilitate rather than lecture. The area of personalisation may simply be dealing with personal issues related to the work process.

When supervisors relate as colleagues during supervision they might act in a 'consultancy' role and there may be potential here for what is referred to as a *dual relationship*. Care needs to be taken about the potential for unethical practice to occur when there are close relationships with staff. For example, the purpose of adopting a 'counsellor' role in supervision is to identify unresolved issues of a personal nature that may cloud the supervisee's judgements in their therapeutic relationship. However, if these issues require ongoing counselling, supervisees should be referred on to another therapist rather than work on those personal issues with their supervisor.

It should be noted here that this model is one used in the field of therapy and therefore tends to reflect the therapeutic relationship. It may not be useful in a health care setting.

Integrated models are also covered in unit (7) LM2c AC 1.2.

Orientation-specific models

In this type of supervision the particular model that the therapist uses will be reflected in the supervisor's model. An advantage of this approach is that the supervisee and supervisor share the same theoretical orientation, thereby allowing modelling and practice skills to be more specific to the model being used. For example, if the psychoanalytical approach to therapy is used, the assumption with supervision is that the supervisee learns the qualities of the 'analytic' attitude. The most effective way of doing this would be to experience these qualities from their supervisor in the supervisory relationship (Ekstein and Wallerstein, cited in Leddick and Bernard, 1980).

See Unit LM1c for information on solution-focused models.

As a supervisor for a care professional you are more likely to require knowledge of the following three models of supervision:

Managerial, clinical and professional supervision

- Managerial supervision is that supervision carried out by a supervisor with authority and accountability for the supervisee. This type of supervision enables staff to review their performance and to set aims and objectives in line with the organisation's objectives and service needs. They are also able to identify training and continuing development needs. This may already be a part of your appraisal process.
- In hospitals or clinical settings, the availability of clinical supervision gives staff the opportunity to review their practice on a regular basis and to reflect on the process. Cases can be discussed and practice modified in the light of what is learned. There is also an opportunity to identify further training needs.
- Similar to clinical supervision is professional supervision, where staff are able to review the professional standards by which they work and identify any training and continuing development needs they may have. It is also an opportunity to keep up to date with developments in their profession, as well as to ensure that professional codes of conduct and boundaries are being worked within.

See unit LM2c AC 1.2 for more information on all of these theories and models.

Research it

1.1 Evaluating theoretical approaches

Research and identify theoretical approaches to professional supervision which you may use, and write a short account evaluating each one and say which one you prefer and why.

AC 1.2 Analyse how the requirements of legislation, codes of practice, policies and procedures impact on professional supervision

As a healthcare support worker or care professional you are duty bound to deliver high-quality care and support to some of the most vulnerable individuals in the population. Codes of conduct not only provide guidance as to how this should happen, but you can also gain some reassurance that you are providing safe and compassionate care of a high standard.

With respect to supervision, the guidance statements within the code of conduct for Healthcare Support Workers and Adult Social Care state that you must:

1 *Ensure up-to-date compliance with all statutory and mandatory training, in agreement with your supervisor.*

2 *Participate in continuing professional development to achieve the competence required for your role.*

3 *Carry out competence-based training and education in line with your agreed ways of working.*

4 *Improve the quality and safety of the care you provide with the help of your supervisor (and a mentor if available), and in line with your agreed ways of working.*

5 *Maintain an up-to-date record of your training and development.*

6 *Contribute to the learning and development of others as appropriate.*

Source: SfC 2013 Code of Conduct for Healthcare Support Workers and Adult Social Care

In the 2014 Care Act, the issue of safeguarding individuals in various settings requires that supervision be a fundamental process, with the focus being on 'good outcomes for adults in need of care and support'. It further states that as managers are responsible for the standard of safeguarding practice, they need to ensure that supervision is used not only to challenge practice in a constructive manner, but to identify barriers to effective practice. The recommendation is that sessions may be one-to-one or in groups, but should be flexible enough to allow supervisees to raise issues they are most immediately concerned about (Adult safeguarding practice questions SCIE 2015 (www.scie.org.uk/care-act-2014/safeguarding-adults/adult-safeguarding-practice-questions/).

The focus of supervision is for the care professional to practise in such a way as to meet legal requirements and to ensure codes of practice and local policy are being followed.

The policies and procedures within your own work setting will reflect the legal position and any guidelines that need to be followed and you need to make a thorough analysis of these policies to ensure you understand how these may impact upon your work as a supervisor. Analysing your policies and codes of practice in line with legislation will ensure that staff are being given the best supervision experience in line with legal requirements.

See unit LM2c AC 1.3 for more information on how requirements of legislation, codes of practice and agreed ways of working influence professional supervision.

In practice

1.1, 1.2 Theoretical approaches and legislation

Compare two theoretical approaches to professional supervision and say how you would use them in your own work. How does the supervision practice in your setting meet the requirements of legislation, codes of practice, policies and procedures? Write a short account giving details of the process.

Reflect on it

1.2 Legislation, codes of practice, policies and procedures

Write a short reflective piece about how the requirements of legislation, codes of practice, policies and procedures impact on professional supervision.

LO2 Understand how the principles of supervision can be used to inform performance management

AC 2.1 Explain key principles of effective professional supervision

SCIE in its guidance statement 'The context for effective supervision: Developing a supervision policy' highlights the need for a supervision policy which shows commitment to supervision, and to clarify expectations regarding the standard of the process of the exercise. The policy is also required to identify how the organisation will support the process with resources, including the training and development of supervisors (www.scie.org.uk/publications/guides/guide50/contextforeffectivesupervision/supervisionpolicy.asp).

You can find more information on this in Unit LM2c AC 1.1, but the following principles of supervision are put forward by londondeaneray.ac.uk and would apply in any form of supervision:

- Ensure there is clarity about why there is a need for supervision and who has asked for it.
- Be time conscious and set parameters within a session, 'even a few minutes of focused time can be worthwhile'.
- Ensure a room is available that is private, and ensure there will be no interruptions and that nobody can overhear the conversation. Ensure confidentiality.
- Think about the seating arrangement and about how the chairs are set out.
- Be open about the extent to what the supervision is about – development or performance – and be prepared to renegotiate during the session.

Source: adapted from www.faculty.londondeanery.ac.uk/e-learning/supervision/principles-of-supervision

See unit LM2c AC 1.1 for more information on the principles, scope and purpose of professional supervision.

In practice

2.1 Key principles

Access your supervision policy and identify the principles for effective supervision within it. Do you think some changes to the policy may be needed, and what will you do about this?

Research it

2.1 Literature reviews on principles

Complete a short literature review (about five articles) about effective professional supervision and highlight the key principles for them.

AC 2.2 Analyse the importance of managing performance in relation to governance, safeguarding and key learning from critical reviews and inquiries

Scally and Donaldson (1998) defined clinical governance as:

> 'a system through which NHS organisations are accountable for continuously improving the quality of their services and safeguarding high standards of care by creating an environment in which excellence in clinical care will flourish.'

Source: Scally and Donaldson 1998, p. 61

All health care systems in this country are required to provide safe and good-quality health care, improving the patient experience, as well as continually update practice in the light of evidence from research. The scandal of the North Staffordshire Health Care Trust, for example, highlighted the treatment of patients and led to yet another inquiry into failings in the system. The Francis Inquiry and a response by the government to improve the safeguarding and the quality of care is another example of the need to monitor performance in a structured and effective manner. As Robert Francis stated in his report:

> 'The extent of the failure of the system shown in this report suggests that a fundamental culture change is needed.'

Source: Robert Francis (2014) QC

Other critical reviews you may wish to access are reviews which the government commissioned to consider some of the key issues identified by the inquiry. These are listed in the useful resources section.

A core responsibility in delivering health care is to ensure that all who receive care are safeguarded, and it is imperative that we examine and analyse how we manage such performance. As managers of health services, we are responsible for the safety and well-being of our service users, but for those individuals who are less able to protect themselves from harm, neglect or abuse, or those with impaired mental capacity, there is a greater need for diligence. Safeguarding therefore is the means by which harm and abuse to patients is prevented through the provision of high-quality care. Additionally, any allegations of harm or abuse should be responded to effectively and according to policy.

In order to maintain such high-quality care in your organisation you need to create a performance management system which:

- identifies areas of best practice and focuses on continuous improvement
- delivers better outcomes to patients
- improves health services by acting upon new initiatives and information
- ensures that organisational activities are linked to the overall goals of the organisation.

The Institute of NHS Quality states:

> 'Performance management enables organisations to articulate their business strategy, align their business to that strategy, identify their key performance indicators (KPIs) and track progress, delivering the information to decision-makers.'

It also provides a performance management tool which may be downloaded from its website to help the process. Go to: www.institute.nhs.uk/quality_and_service_improvement_tools/quality_and_service_improvement_tools/performance_management.html#sthash.efKrswZI.dpuf

You may find it useful to revisit LO2 in Unit LM2c for more information on performance management and AC 1.4 on critical reviews and inquiries.

See unit LM2c ACs 1.4 and 1.5 for more information on how findings from research, critical reviews and inquiries can be used within professional supervision and how professional supervision can protect individuals, supervisees, and supervisors.

LO3 Understand how to support individuals through professional supervision

AC 3.1 Analyse the concept of anti-oppressive practice in professional supervision

Sensitivity to and recognition of the dynamics of such power relationships must be acknowledged. As a manager and potentially the supervisor in a team you must be able to recognise the existence of power imbalances and be able to manage those imbalances. Failure to do so may result in a form of oppression, since the use of power in any relationship marginalises others and subordinates them. If a group or a person is disempowered in any way then oppression has occurred. The term oppression means we discriminate in some way, and discrimination means distinguishing differences between one or more things. This rather benign definition does not seem to confer anything negative. However, when used in the context of inequality it is associated with negative attribution (Thompson, 2011), and it is used to discriminate against someone. This implies disadvantage or oppression of an individual which impacts negatively upon their self-concept, their dignity, their opportunities or their ability to obtain social justice. Discrimination can take many forms such as stereotyping and marginalisation, and common categories of discrimination include race

and racism, gender and sexism, age and ageism, educational disadvantage, economic disadvantage and mental and disability discrimination.

Negative discrimination occurs when the identification of difference results in someone being treated unfairly on the basis of that difference. In promoting practice which is truly anti-oppressive, organisations must develop, implement and monitor policies that support this. All codes of practice for care workers must include statements about the requirement to treat others equally and fairly, and to engage in non-judgemental and anti-discriminatory practice. Such policies and guidelines help to raise awareness about unacceptable behaviours, and provide a structure for individuals to challenge such behaviours. Your supervision policy will be no exception here.

The term 'dignity' is often used in care work and it is important that all people we care for are treated with respect. In this way, good practice demands that we protect our clients and patients from discrimination and oppressive practices. Recognising the diverse nature of practice and the fact that some individuals are disadvantaged just because they are different has led to the terms anti-discriminatory or anti-oppressive practice being used.

You may wish to refer to Unit LM2c ACs 3.1 and 3.2 for more information on power imbalance.

AC 3.2, 3.3 Explain methods to assist individuals to deal with challenging situations and Explain how conflict may arise within professional supervision

Occasionally, difficult situations within supervision and team management arise. You may have to deal with cases of poor individual or team performance or complaints from members of the public about staff. It is likely that at times staff shortages become an issue and you have team members who are unhappy about the situation they are in.

Case study

3.2 Dealing with challenging situations

Nadia is a member of staff who has worked in the same role for three years. She is undertaking a foundation degree at the local university and has recently been off sick for at least one span of duty per fortnight. There seems to be a pattern developing and you are wondering what is going on. In your regular supervision session, Nadia becomes very defensive and starts to lose her temper with you. You remain calm – you are aware that this is uncharacteristic but something you need to address.

How will you deal with this situation?

Conflict within multi-agency teams is common and can disrupt performance in a major way. The fact that conflict exists, however, is not necessarily a bad thing: as long as it is resolved effectively, it can lead to personal and professional growth of the team. If managed well, conflict can be creative and productive, and creative solutions to difficult problems can often be found through positive conflict resolution. However, at all times conflict within the team or among staff should not impact upon the well-being of the service user.

Three types of differences or conflict may involve:

- **task-based conflict** – disagreements in relation to approaches to work, processes and structural issues within the teams and the organisation
- **relationship-based conflict** – conflicts between individual members of the team that generally stem from differences in personal values and beliefs
- **conflict with carers and service users over service decisions**.

Whatever the cause of the conflict, the emotions which arise can be quite damaging to the care being delivered and if badly managed ineffective care emerges. People may start to avoid each other with rifts developing as teams take sides. In the midst of this happening the service user suffers as care starts to disintegrate into ineffectiveness.

One of the crucial things to remember here is that challenging behaviour may be the only way a person can communicate at that time, and it is important for us as managers to find out what the 'function' of that particular behaviour is. For

example, in an emergency department setting, there may be a person who is shouting at staff. We may be frightened of this reaction but it may well be that the person is feeling pain, frustration, anxiety and may also be very frightened. Although the behaviour is potentially dangerous to us, by trying to understand the reason for that behaviour we can help to change the situation. It is easy to shout back or to manhandle somebody, but by standing back and trying to determine what led to the behaviour and what is actually being communicated by that behaviour we can go a long way to defuse the situation. We can use this reasoning in relation to Nadia in the case study. She may well be unable to communicate exactly what her problem is and her behaviour may simply be a reaction to this frustration.

Consider this for a moment.

If we describe behaviour in a negative manner we are likely to deal with it as such.

The term 'attention seeking' is often used in such instances and if we simply describe Nadia as such then this carries connotations of being negative, manipulative and just plain spoilt! But if we view it as a way of getting attention to a problem, we might have a different reaction to it. By working out what the 'function' of the challenging behaviour is and what it helps the person to achieve in a given situation we can then start to help the individual to deal with the situation they find difficult in more constructive ways.

For further reading see Lowe, K. and Felce, D. (1995) 'The definition of challenging behaviours in practice,' *British Journal of Learning Disabilities*, 23(3), 118–230.

We might use the following as a guide:

- Get the facts first and ask questions – we often race to find a solution but it is more useful to gather information and ask questions to really understand what is happening.
- Ask questions that get to the core problem and try to stop the person going into too much detail.
- Listen carefully.
- Reflect on the answers you are given and do not be too quick to jump in with a solution. Also do not be tempted to think you know the answer and pre-judge the person. We might well be tempted to think that Nadia is not coping with

In practice

3.1, 3.2, 3.3 Anti-oppressive practice, challenging situations and how conflict may arise

Write a short essay about anti-oppressive practice in professional supervision. Examine and analyse how you would ensure you practice in such a way.

Recall a time when you had to deal with a challenging member of staff. Say how you dealt with the situation at the time and then think about how you might do things differently now.

Prepare a short presentation to staff about how they might deal with challenging situations.

the university course and that is why she is missing shifts. You may even have heard this said by a member of staff. Avoid making such a judgement as it may be wrong.

- Act professionally.
- Aim for a balanced solution. We do not want people to feel that they have lost a battle and that management has won! Negotiate to find a solution in which both parties feel heard and have a solution both are happy with. This may not always be possible but careful negotiation can be useful.

You may also wish to refer to Unit LM2c ACs 4.6 and 5.1.

AC 3.4 Describe how conflict can be managed within professional supervision

Larson and LaFasto have developed a CONECT model for resolving conflict by conversation and this can be used whatever the cause of the conflict. See Unit LM2c ACs 5.1 and 5.2 for an explanation of the CONECT model.

Larson and LaFasto suggest that the most effective way of solving conflict in a team is for people concerned to have constructive conversation. This will allow each person to see the perspective of the other person and to gain some understanding about the way the other person feels about the situation. The conversation must result in each

In practice

3.4 Managing and resolving conflict

Write an account of a conflict you have had to deal with and how you resolved it. Reflect on how you might employ the above models.

party committing to making improvements in the relationship.

These conversations might be initiated by the people themselves or they may require the services of a neutral facilitator.

Thompson (2006) recommends the RED approach to managing conflict which is covered in Unit LM1c AC 1.7.

You may also wish to refer to Unit LM2c AC 4.6 (supporting supervisees to explore different methods of addressing challenging situations), AC 5.1 (examples from own practice of managing conflict situations) and AC 5.2 (reflect on own practice in managing conflict situations).

LO4 Understand how professional supervision supports performance

AC 4.1 Explain the responsibility of the supervisor in setting clear targets and performance indicators

One of the most important functions you have as a manager is to ensure that staff are fully aware of the organisational strategy and targets, and to link those with individual objectives. In supervising staff, performance management is an issue that needs to be part of the agenda. Staff must be clear about the aims and focus of their job role in relation to the wider aims of the organisation, and it is the supervisor's responsibility to ensure that staff are clear about how they can achieve these objectives. See Unit LM2c AC 4.5 for more information on reviewing and revising professional supervision targets. Unit LM2c LO2 and LO3 on performance management and undertaking preparation for professional supervision with supervisees would also be useful to refer to.

In practice

4.1 Targets and performance indicators

With one of your supervisees check their understanding about targets and performance indicators.

Write a short account of their answers here and say how you might improve this part of your role.

AC 4.2, 4.3 Explain the performance management cycle, and compare methods that can be used to measure performance

See Unit LM2c AC 2.1 for information on the performance management cycle and AC 2.3 on how performance indicators can be used to measure practice.

There are a number of ways in which performance management is measured, but primarily it is defined as being a cycle of continuous process which involves:

- **planning and developing** – at this stage there should be a clear indication about what needs to be done and to what standard. The employee's ability and competence to perform the task needed is looked at. If training or skills development are needed, these are also planned for here
- **progress reviewing** – at this point the employee has the chance to determine their progress so far and can gain feedback about whether any changes might be needed
- **evaluating** – this stage is all about what was done, how, what might have been done differently to engage with a better outcome and what has been learned.

Comparing methods that can be used to measure performance

The aim of any performance management system is to ensure that the organisation's goals are met and that staff are effective and productive. To achieve this there needs to be a clear strategy to support the vision and mission statement of the organisation. This has been accomplished in a number of ways in the health system. In 2001 annual performance ratings for the NHS were measured by means of the 'star rating system for English NHS trusts' with each trust being given a rating from zero to three stars. This has now gone out of use but targets for performance remain. Whilst targets have been somewhat beneficial the ways in which some targets have been met have come under criticism and scrutiny. For example, to meet A&E targets of emergency department waiting times, more staff may have been brought in at the expense of operations being cancelled elsewhere. (For more information see http://www.lse.ac.uk/newsAndMedia/news/archives/2006/GwynBevan.aspx).

For individual staff in an organisation, one method of measuring performance may be Management by Objectives (MBO) developed by Peter Drucker. The process involves the manager and employee identifying employee goals together with a list of the resources and a timeframe necessary to achieve the goals. Meetings to evaluate the outcomes and to discuss progress are held regularly and during these meetings goals may be reset. The employee's performance is measured by how many goals have been accomplished within the timeframe. (For more information see http://communicationtheory.org/management-by-objectives-drucker/).

In the NHS key performance indicators (KPIs) are a means of measuring how far progress has been made towards organisational goals and focus on a range of areas. They measure things such as length of stay in hospital, mortality rates, readmission rates and day case rates. For example, a local trust may notice that their discharge rates for certain procedures are above the national benchmark and patients are requiring more lengthy stays as a result. They may therefore wish to investigate this and make changes to bring it in line with national protocols. (For more information see http://www.institute.nhs.uk/quality_and_service_improvement_tools/quality_and_service_improvement_tools/performance_management.htm).

The aim of any performance management system is to ensure that the organisation's goals are met and that staff are effective and productive. To achieve this, there needs to be a clear strategy to support the vision and mission statement of the organisation. This then needs to be translated into specific objectives and targets for the department, and finally individual job goals and targets. In evaluating performance there

4.2, 4.3 Performance management cycle and comparing methods

Draw a diagram of the performance management cycle you use in your workplace.

What methods are you currently using to measure performance?

Which methods used to measure performance do you favour and why? Compare two of them.

needs to be a clear process through which the staff will be monitored and evaluated. Such performance objectives will be set in supervision and appraisal through open discussion between the supervisors and the supervisee, with progress towards the goals being monitored regularly.

AC 4.4 Describe the indicators of poor performance

What is likely to indicate to you that a member of staff is performing badly in their role? Perhaps they are failing to complete tasks on time or making more mistakes when doing so. Maybe they consistently break rules or do not follow procedure, and you find you need to spend more time with them because of this. Perhaps they are having excessive amounts of time off sick or their personal life is encroaching upon their time at work and causing issues with other staff members. Have you noticed that they are arriving late or leaving earlier than they should, or spending more time at break and lunch? All these are indicators that a person may not be coping in their job.

Poor performance can be a problem and it needs to be managed in a sensitive manner with the facts of the poor performance clearly recorded.

See Unit LM2c AC 2.3 for more information on analysing how performance indicators can be used to measure performance.

Reflect on it

4.4 Poor performance

Think about how you have managed poor staff performance in the past and describe your own feelings about this part of the management role.

AC 4.5, 4.6 Explain how constructive feedback can be used to improve performance, and evaluate the use of performance management towards the achievement of objectives

Constructive feedback

In being constructive about performance there must be a valid set of measures that can support our judgement. This is no place for hearsay or gut instinct. This is where a good performance management system must be in place, and if you have confidence that the performance is clearly not up to standard, then you can set up a performance review where you meet the member of staff to address the situation and help them improve their performance. Be aware that the employee is likely to feel under threat at such an interview, so you need to approach this with care.

Finding out what is causing the poor performance is a useful starting point in this meeting, and a copy of the job description is needed here. You might be able to go through what is expected of the employee and the standard of work expected, and it is likely that at this stage the reason will become clear and can be remedied.

Some reasons for poor performance are that the employee is unclear about their role, job description or what it is they are trying to achieve. They may feel they lack training or are having some personal issues that are causing them concern. It may simply be that the employee is not suited to this type of work.

By discussing the reason in a calm and clear way, the poor performance can quickly become a thing of the past.

Key term

Constructive feedback focuses on the issue in question and provides specific information. It is firmly based on observation and provides supportive evidence. There are two types of constructive feedback. One is positive or favourable and this is when we praise a performance or effort or outcome. The other is more negative and may be seen as unfavourable when we criticise a performance or outcome.

Evaluating use of performance management towards achievement of objectives

As a result of the feedback to the member of staff and the data collected from the method used to measure the performance, you are now in a position to see where you are in relation to the achievement of objectives within the workplace. For example, if you are aiming to market your service as outstanding and you have members of staff who underperform, the feedback you receive might lead you to re-evaluate the staff member's role and provide additional training. In doing so, the next review meeting may well show a marked increase in performance that clearly meets the objectives of the organisation.

You may also find it useful to refer to Unit LM2c AC 4.2 (providing positive feedback about the achievements), 4.3 (providing constructive feedback that can be used to improve performance) and 4.5 (reviewing and revising professional supervision targets to meet the identified objectives of the work setting).

Legislation
- The Human Rights Act 1998
- Equality Act 2010

In practice

4.5, 4.6 Performance management and constructive feedback

What are the indicators of poor performance? With a member of your staff, and not necessarily somebody who has exhibited poor performance, explain how you have used constructive feedback to improve performance and evaluate the use of performance management towards the achievement of objectives.

Research it

4.6 Performance management

Compare and contrast the use of performance measures in your own setting against those used elsewhere. Construct a new measurement tool for your setting as a result of the research you have carried out.

- Mental Capacity Act 2005
- Safeguarding Vulnerable Groups Act 2006
- Mental Health Act 1983
- The Care Act 2014
- NHS Act 2006

Assessment methods

LO	Assessment criteria and accompanying activities	Assessment methods *To evidence coverage of the ACs, you could:*
LO1	1.1 Research it (p. 314)	Complete the activity and write a short account evaluating theoretical approaches and say which one you prefer and why.
	1.2 Reflect on it (p. 315)	Undertake a professional discussion with your assessor about the points in the activity. Document the discussion.
	1.1, 1.2 In practice (p. 315)	Prepare a hand-out that shows a comparison of two theoretical approaches to professional supervision. Reflect on how you might use them in your own work. Discuss with your manager how the supervision practice in your setting meets the requirements of legislation, codes of practice, policies and procedures. Write a short account giving details of the process.

LO	Assessment criteria and accompanying activities	Assessment methods *To evidence coverage of the ACs, you could:*
LO2	2.1 In practice (p. 316)	Access your supervision policy for your portfolio and identify the principles for effective supervision within it. Discuss with your assessor whether you think some changes to the policy may be needed, and what you will do about this?
	2.1 Research it (p. 316)	Complete a short literature review.
	2.2 In practice (p. 317)	Write a report about what you have learned about governance, safeguarding and critical reviews and inquiries into health care, and say how you have changed your management of performance criteria in the workplace. Discuss with your manager some recommendations for change in your management of performance criteria in the workplace.
LO3	3.1 Reflect on it (p. 317)	Discuss with your assessor the sorts of power imbalance you have seen in your setting and how you might address power imbalances in your supervision practice.
	3.2 Case study (p. 318)	Read the following case study and complete the task for your portfolio. Or you might use a real life situation where you have had to deal with a challenging situation.
	3.1, 3.2, 3.3 In practice (p. 319)	Write a short essay about anti-oppressive practice in professional supervision. Address the different points in the activity. Prepare a short presentation to staff about how they might deal with challenging situations.
	3.4 In practice (p. 319)	Write an account or discuss with your assessor a conflict you have had to deal with and how you resolved it. Reflect on how you might employ the models discussed.
LO4	4.1 In practice (p. 320)	Undertake a supervision session with one of your supervisees and check their understanding about targets and performance indicators. Write a short account of their answers here and say how you might improve this part of your role.
	4.2, 4.3 In practice (p. 321)	Draw a diagram of the performance management cycle you use in your workplace and address the points in the activity.
	4.4 Reflect on it (p. 321)	Write a reflective account.
	4.5, 4.6 In practice (p. 322)	Prepare a hand-out which addresses the indicators of poor performance and discuss this at a team meeting. You might also interview a member of your staff,(and not necessarily somebody who has exhibited poor performance) and ask how they feel you have used constructive feedback to improve performance. Prepare a report to evaluate the use of performance management towards the achievement of objectives.
	4.6 Research it (p. 322)	Ask to shadow a member of another setting and make a comparison of the use of performance measures in your own setting against those used elsewhere. Construct a new measurement tool for your setting as a result of the research you have carried out.

References

CQC (2013) Registration under the Health and Social Care Act 2008; Supporting information and guidance: Supporting effective clinical supervision.

DOH (2014) *Hard Truths the Journey to Putting Patients First. Volume One of the Government Response to the Mid Staffordshire NHS Foundation Trust Public Inquiry*, 2 volumes. London: TSO.

http://webarchive.nationalarchives.gov.uk/20130401151715/https:/www.education.gov.uk/publications/eOrderingDownload/Providing_Effective_Supervision_unit.pdf.

www.scie.org.uk/publications/guides/guide50/contextforeffectivesupervision/supervisionpolicy.asp

http://blog.competencycore.com/2012/09/stage-3-evaluating-performance-part-8.html.

Larson, C. E. and LeFasto, F. M. (1989) *Teamwork: What might go right/What can go wrong*. London: Sage Publications.

Leddick, G. R. and Bernard, J. M. (1980) 'The history of supervision: A critical review,' *Counsellor Education and Supervision*, 27, 186–96. Source: www.mentalhealthacademy.com.au

Scally, G. and Donaldson, L. J. (1998) 'Clinical governance and the drive for quality improvement in the new NHS in England,' *British Medical Journal*, 317(7150), 4 July, 61–5.

SCIE (2014) Adult safeguarding practice questions. At www.scie.org.uk/care-act-2014/safeguarding-adults/adult-safeguarding-practice-questions/

SfC (2013) *Code of Conduct for Healthcare Support Workers and Adult Social Care Workers in England*. London: DOH.

Stoltenberg, C. D. and Delworth, U. (1987) *Supervising Counsellors and Therapists*. San Francisco, CA: Jossey-Bass.

Thompson, N. (2006) *People Problems*. Basingstoke: Palgrave Macmillan.

Useful resources and further reading

Innes, A., Macpherson, S. and McCabe, I. (2006) *Promoting Person-Centred Care at the Front Line*. York: Joseph Rowntree Foundation/SCIE.

Lowe, K. and Felce, D. (1995) 'The definition of challenging behaviours in practice,' *British Journal of Learning Disabilities,* 23(3), 118–23.

Thompson, N. (2005) *Understanding Social Work: Preparing for practice*. Basingstoke: Palgrave Macmillan.

Thompson, N. (2006) *People Problems*. Basingstoke: Palgrave Macmillan.

Resources related to AC 2.2:

Review by Professor Sir Bruce Keogh, the NHS Medical Director in NHS England into the Quality of Care and Treatment Provided by 14 Hospital Trusts in England.

The Cavendish Review: An Independent Review into Healthcare Assistants and Support Workers in the NHS and Social Care Settings.

Berwick, D. *A Promise to Learn – A Commitment to Act: Improving the Safety of Patients in England.*

A Review of the NHS Hospitals Complaints System: Putting Patients Back in the Picture by Rt Hon Ann Clwyd MP and Professor Tricia Hart.

Challenging Bureaucracy, led by the NHS Confederation.

Lewis, I. and Lenehan, C. The report by the Children and Young People's Health Outcomes Forum

Glossary

Abuse is defined in *No Secrets* as 'a violation of an individual's human or civil rights by any other person or persons'.

Accountability is taking responsibility and being liable or answerable for something.

Action orientation is a type of leadership in which practical action is taken to deal with a problem or situation.

Active listening is listening clearly and ensuring that you understand what the sender intends to communicate and the content of the message.

Active participation is a way of working where the individual is an active partner in their care rather than a passive one. It is the core principle of person-centred care. It refers to enabling individuals to be included in their care and being able to voice how they wish to live their life and obtain their own care.

Advocates represent individuals or speak on their behalf to ensure that their rights are supported. They support another person, enabling them to express their views and wishes to make sure they have a voice.

Agreed ways of working are your setting's policies and procedures as well as guidelines, for the care and support you provide for service users.

Aims, in the context of unit CCLD OP 5.25, are the broad statements of intent of your research project. They highlight what is to be accomplished and seek to address the expectations of the research.

Appraisal, sometimes referred to as performance appraisal, is the process by which employees and line managers discuss their performance, developmental needs and the support they need in their role. It is used to provide evidence and evaluation of recent performance and focus on future goals, opportunities and resources.

Appreciative inquiry is a management approach that engages with a positive way to embrace organisational change. It identifies the positives in an environment and highlights the things that are working well in an organisation.

Assistive technology refers to the use of aids such as picture and symbol communication boards and electronic devices, which help individuals who have difficulty with speech or language problems to express themselves.

Authoritarian/Autocratic is having total authority and control over decision making; keeping everything under close scrutiny.

Bias simply means any influence that may affect results or distort our view of the data, and can be the downfall of many experiments and research studies. If we set out to try to prove something because we have a preference for a particular outcome, then this will 'bias' our results. Alternatively, failure to acknowledge certain results which would seem not to support our preference is also a common mistake in experiments and research per se.

Care assessment simply refers to collecting data and evidence about an individual's needs with respect to care. During a care assessment, you determine what care needs the individuals have, together with the level and type of care and support required to meet those needs. This is a fundamental role of the care worker and a manager.

A **care** or **support plan** is a written document or something recorded in patient notes which is an agreement between a service user and health professional to help manage their day-to-day health and care needs.

Child protection forms a small part of safeguarding.

Coaching is a process that supports and enables an individual to unlock and maximise their potential, to develop and improve performance.

Conflict is a disagreement or argument.

Constructive feedback focuses on the issue in question and provides specific information. It is firmly based on observation and provides supportive evidence. There are two types of constructive feedback. One is positive or favourable and this is when we praise a performance or effort or outcome. The other is more negative and may be seen as unfavourable when we criticise a performance or outcome.

Contingency theories state that there is no one best style of leadership. In this case the leader's effectiveness is based on the situation.

Continuing professional development (CPD) is the planned process of improving and increasing capabilities of staff and is an on-going process. It includes training and education activity to ensure staff remain fit for practice.

Critical incident is an unintended event that occurs when an individual in health care is involved in something that results in a consequence to them – for example, a fall.

A **critical review** provides a summary of a book or text and evaluates it. In undertaking a review you need to read the text in depth and also look at other texts that are related to the same subject. You are then able to make a more reasoned judgement.

Critique is similar to evaluation and refers to an analysis. It has both positive and negative connotations as it involves recognising merit but also passing judgement or finding fault.

Culture is the customs, attitudes and beliefs that distinguish one group of people from another. It can also refer to the behaviour, values, thoughts and norms of an organisation – the unspoken rules. In a health and social care setting, this refers to the staff's beliefs about care and how these might affect the way in which they work.

Democratic/Participative is a sharing type of leadership in which employees' participation in the decision making is favoured.

Disclosure is the release of information about something.

Discrimination is the practice of unfairly treating a person or group differently from other people or groups of people, usually on the basis of an individual characteristic or difference.

Diversity in this context is equal respect for people who are from different backgrounds.

Duty of care refers to the professional's legal obligation as well as ethical responsibility to safeguard and protect the well-being of others and to perform to a standard of reasonable care when performing any acts that could harm others. Failure to do so may be termed negligence.

Emotional intelligence is the capacity some people have to recognise not only their own but others' emotions, and to be able to discriminate between different feelings and labels and deal with them properly. It is about being sufficiently self-aware about our reactions to situations and dealing with the emotions appropriately.

Empathy is being able to understand and share the feelings of another or having the ability to experience another person's condition from their perspective.

End-of-life care is for individuals who are considered to be in the last year of their life or who are receiving palliative care. It refers to enabling people to live as well as possible at this time and to die with dignity. End-of-life care continues for as long as it is needed, and may include those services provided at diagnosis, during treatment or palliative care, including the dying phase, or following death.

Equality means treating individuals or groups of individuals fairly and equally irrespective of race, gender, disability, religion or belief, sexual orientation and age.

Equal opportunity is the principle of having fair and similar opportunities in life to other people and ensuring people are not discriminated against on the basis of individual characteristics.

Ethics refers to the standards of right and wrong that describe how we ought to behave and that distinguish between acceptable and unacceptable behaviour. This, for example, includes the obligations we have as humans to refrain from murder, assault and causing harm to others, etc. Ethical standards relate to human rights, such as the right to life, or the right to privacy or to freedom. These are the ethical considerations we need to be aware of and examine to ensure that they are reasonable and morally sound.

Ethnography refers to the observation of other people's cultures and customs.

Evaluation is to judge the worth or value of something, to make an assessment of it, its importance, or effectiveness.

Evidence-based practice (EBP) refers to using information from high-quality research and applying it within practice to make informed decisions about a service user's care. It also applies when researchers encourage health and social care professionals to seek out information from high-quality research to inform their own clinical practice and decision making.

Extra care housing is a type of supported housing for older people to enable them to live independently for as long as possible with access to services that are responsive to their particular needs.

Feedback is an open two-way communication between two or more parties.

Generalisation, in the context of unit CCLD OP 5.25, is the degree to which the research findings can be applied to the whole population and not just the sample used.

Hazard is a danger or something that has potential to cause harm.

Health and safety is ensuring people are safe and come to no harm in the workplace. This will inform policies such as Control of Substances Hazardous to Health (COSHH), infection control, safe handling of medicine, moving and handling, and fire safety, for example.

The **Health and Safety Executive (HSE)** is the regulator or official supervisory body for the health, safety and welfare of people in work settings in the UK.

Hypothesis is an 'educated guess' which attempts to explain a set of facts. For example, we may guess that smoking causes lung cancer and pose such a hypothesis. We would then go on to devise an experiment to either prove or disprove our hypothesis.

Inclusion is positive behaviour to ensure all people have an opportunity to be included and not be unfairly excluded because of their individual characteristics.

Indicator, in the context of the safeguarding and protection of vulnerable adults unit, is anything that might lead us to suspect that something may be wrong with a person. Signs and symptoms (which may vary) may be the obvious indicators, although they may not always mean abuse has occurred.

Laissez-faire is the leadership style that favours leaving things to take their own course, without interference.

Lay carer is a person who is not a health professional but gives care to somebody, usually in their own home.

Mental capacity is the ability to make decisions for one's self. People who cannot do this are said to 'lack capacity'.

Mentoring is a relationship in which an individual with expertise can help another individual to progress in their career.

Methodology is an analysis of the ways in which we examine or research phenomena or hypotheses. If we apply the term to a research study, we are referring to the methods or principles we use to study the topic.

Negotiation is taking part in a discussion which aims to reach an agreement.

NLP (Neuro-Linguistic Programming) is an approach which sets out to change the mindset of the person being coached from one of problem solving to being solution-focused. It is possible to not fully understand the problem to find a solution because change happens in small steps and we all have various strengths and resources to help us. For example, we do not have to understand why the person gets anxious before a presentation, NLP techniques simply help them not to.

Nursing home is similar to residential care but with additional medical facilities on site.

Obligation is an action or restraint from action that a person is morally or legally bound to owe to (an) other(s).

Objectives, in the context of unit CCLD OP 5.25, are the steps you will be taking to answer your research questions. They show how the aims will be accomplished. Aims and objectives include the reasons, understanding and methods for conducting the research project.

Outcome-based practice, also referred to as outcomes management and outcomes-focused assessment, is one such approach to achieving desired patient care goals. It refers to activity that benefits patients and involves team work and quality assurance measures.

Outcomes management is a means to help patients, funding services and providers make care-related choices based on knowledge of the effects of these choices on the patient's life.

Palliative care is specialised medical care for people with serious illnesses, provided by multidisciplinary teams. Patients are provided with relief from the symptoms, pain and physical and mental stress of a serious illness.

The Paramountcy Principle underpins all new legislation with respect to the child. Any decision made on behalf of a child must reflect that the child's welfare is of 'paramount' concern or consideration (Children Act 2004).

Partnership working is the use of inclusive and mutually beneficial relationships in care work that improve the quality and experience of care. This refers to the relationships between individuals with long-term care conditions, their carers, and service providers and care professionals.

Personal development planning (PDP) is the process of planning for future education or career development. In order to make the most of development opportunities staff need to be guided to various opportunities for improving their knowledge and skills. This will include opportunities for improving their knowledge and skills, for example.

Person-centred care is the process of life planning for individuals based around the principles of inclusion and individualised care which respect their individuality, rights, choice, privacy, independence and dignity.

Personalisation refers to the way in which individuals are helped to become the drivers in developing systems of care and support designed to meet their unique needs.

Pilot study is a small-scale preliminary study which is conducted before the main study to check whether it is feasible, how much time it is likely to take and at what cost; and whether there might be any problems. It is designed to predict any issues that might arise before the full study is carried out and to improve on the study design; essentially it is a practice run.

Policy is a plan or principle of action proposed by an organisation, also known as guidelines or codes.

Positive risk taking means identifying the potential risks and then developing plans and actions that reflect the potential benefits and harm of exercising one course of action over another. It is a way of seeing the risk in a positive way that enhances the quality of life for an individual.

Prejudice is an unreasonable, pre-conceived judgement or conviction that is not based on knowledge, evidence or experience.

Procedures state how policies will be carried out or actioned in the setting.

Professional boundary describes the appropriate interaction between professionals and the public they serve and the policies that are in place to protect both parties.

Reflection is giving serious thought or consideration to something.

Reflective practice is the act of stopping and thinking about what we are doing in practice and analysing the decisions we make in the light of theory and the things we have learned. By doing this, we are more able to relate theory to practice to help us to generate new knowledge and ideas.

Regulation is a rule or order which is underpinned by law. In health care settings, apart from those concerned with health and safety care, regulations with respect to health protection and control of disease are also available.

Residential accommodation is usually a care home providing housing for a group of individuals who may require care on a daily basis.

Risk is the potential for something bad or unpleasant to happen and carries with it an uncertainty. We might consider the risk of investing unwisely or the risk of crossing a busy road when the traffic lights have failed.

Risk assessment refers to steps taken to protect your workers and/or service users and your business, as well as complying with the law. It looks at the likelihood of an event occurring and the impact of that occurrence should it happen. It is the way in which we evaluate the potential risks in an activity.

Risk management is the forecasting of potential risk and minimising them or avoiding them altogether. Your policies should identify how you undertake risk assessment in your area and how you intend to manage risks that arise.

Safeguarding, according to the CQC, means 'protecting people's health, well-being and human rights, and enabling them to live free from harm, abuse and neglect. It is fundamental to high-quality health and social care'. It encourages a preventative approach before problems occur.

Scaffolding is the process of moving students progressively towards better understanding and independence in their learning using various instructional techniques (adapted from http://edglossary.org/scaffolding/).

Serious case review takes place after a person is seriously injured or dies, particularly if abuse or neglect is thought to have been a causative factor. It looks at what we might learn from the occurrence in order to help prevent similar incidents from happening in the future.

Shared community is living in a shared house and sharing facilities but with one's own private room. Some support from care workers may be available.

Smart targets are those objectives that are specific, measurable, achievable, realistic/ relevant and time related.

Strategic direction is a course of action that leads to the achievement of goals in an organisation's strategy.

Talent management and development is about using all types of learning, planned and unplanned, to achieve and maintain changes in an organisation in order to gain a competitive edge.

Team culture is the behaviour, values, thoughts and norms of an organisation – the unspoken rules.

Triangulation refers to the use of several methods to test the results in a data set. In order to ensure the work being carried out is valid, the researcher is wise to use multiple methods to compare findings in the data. If the researcher relies on one method only there is no external check to test the result. By using three methods to get at the answer to one question, it is hoped that two of the methods will give similar results thereby validating the study. If the three methods all come up with conflicting results, at the very least the researcher knows that they need to refine the question and readdress the data.

Trust is having confidence in something or someone, or having the belief that something or somebody is reliable and honest.

Variable refers to an object, event, idea, feeling or another type of factor you are trying to measure.

Voluntary participation refers to the rights of participants to refuse to be part of research if they so choose. People must not be coerced into participating in research.

Well-being is a subjective state of being content and healthy.

Whistle-blowing means making a disclosure or revealing information that is in the public interest.

White Paper is a government report which highlights information or proposals on an issue and then asks for comment.

Workforce planning is the process whereby the staff with the necessary skills are allocated to the task when they are needed in order to deliver organisational objectives.

Index

Page references to Figures or Tables are in *italics* followed by the letters 'f' and 't' respectively. Entries relating to Key Terms are in **bold**